Amputations and Prosthetics

A CASE STUDY APPROACH

Second Edition

Bella J. May, PT, EdD, FAPTA

President, BJM Enterprises, PC
Dublin, California
and
Professor Emerita, Department of Physical Therapy
Medical College of Georgia, Augusta, Georgia

F. A. DAVIS COMPANY • Philadelphia

F.A. Davis Company
1915 Arch Street
Philadelphia, PA 19103
www.fadavis.com

Copyright © 2002 by F.A. Davis Company

Printed in the United States of America

Last digit indicates print number: 10 9 8 7 6 5 4 3

Acquisitions Editor: Margaret Biblis
Developmental Editor: Renee Gagliardi
Manager, Creative Development: Susan Rhyner
Production Editor: Nwakaego Fletcher-Perry
Cover Designer: Louis Forgione

As new scientific information becomes available through basic and clinical research, recommended treatments and drug therapies undergo changes. The author(s) and publisher have done everything possible to make this book accurate, up to date, and in accord with accepted standards at the time of publication. The author(s), editors, and publisher are not responsible for errors or omissions or for consequences from application of the book, and make no warranty, expressed or implied, in regard to the contents of the book. Any practice described in this book should be applied by the reader in accordance with professional standards of care used in regard to the unique circumstances that may apply in each situation. The reader is advised always to check product information (package inserts) for changes and new information regarding dose and contraindications before administering any drug. Caution is especially urged when using new or infrequently ordered drugs.

Library of Congress Cataloging-in-Publication Data

May, Bella J.

    Amputations and prosthetics: a case study approach / Bella J. May—2nd ed.
      p. cm.
    Includes bibliographical references and index.
    ISBN10: 0-8036-0839-X (pbk.)   ISBN13: 978-0-8036-0839-9
    1. Amputation—Physical therapy—Case studies. 2. Amputees—Rehabilitation—Case studies. 3. Artificial limb—Case studies. 4. Prosthesis—Case studies. 5. Extremities (Anatomy)—Amputation—Case studies.
    [DNLM: 1. Amputation—rehabilitation. 2. Prosthesis. 3. Physical Therapy—methods. 4. Amputees—psychology.] I. Title.

RD553 .M425 2002
617.5'803—dc21
    2001047436

Preface

Many changes have taken place in the field of prosthetics and in the terminology used in the practice of physical therapy (PT) since the first edition was published in 1996. I am pleased at the response to this book as a text for physical therapist (PT) and physical therapist assistant (PTA) students. I believe it is critical to maintain currency in a publication to facilitate student learning for practice today and tomorrow. The second edition incorporates the many changes in prosthetic technology as well as in the concepts related to physical therapy practice.

In the summer of 1995, the first Guide to Physical Therapist Practice was published by the American Physical Therapy Association (APTA). By then, the first edition of this text was already in production and the recommended changes in terminology could not be incorporated. Since its publication, the Guide has become an integral part of PT and PTA education and the text now reflects current terminology and practice guidelines as outlined in the second edition of the Guide to Physical Therapist Practice published by the APTA in January 2001.

New components and technological advances in fabrication continue to change prosthetic practice at a fast rate. Components that were in broad use 5 years ago have been replaced by newer, more effective, and lighter components. Research in prosthetic fabrication, fitting, and use has increased and there is more scientific data to guide practitioners. Web resources have increased and are also available to help PTs and PTAs understand changing prosthetic componentry. Each of the chapters has been thoroughly reviewed and revised to reflect these changes. Whenever possible, information on pertinent Web sites is provided.

The format of the book as a case study text remains unchanged and the student is facilitated to be an active learner in the process of gaining competence in working with individuals with amputations. The decision-making process of the PT is emphasized in the student activities; the role of the PTA is also considered in the specifically designed PTA activities. While the book contains information and concepts beyond the practice of the PTA, understanding each other's scope of practice continues to be important for effective teamwork. The accompanying faculty manual has also been revised and updated and continues to be a guide for the faculty—particularly faculty who do not have a strong background in this area.

The book continues to be a text for students in PT and PTA programs as well as a resource for practitioners seeking clinically-oriented current information on patient management.

Bella J. May, EdD, PT, FAPTA

Acknowledgments

Many of the individuals I thanked in the first edition have continued to provide help and support for this edition. Many prosthetic manufacturers and distributors willingly contributed photographs and materials and are acknowledged individually in the text. I continue to have a close working relationship with the Hanger Orthopaedics Prosthetic facility in Augusta, Georgia and prosthetists Robert Edwards, CP and Wink Anderson, CP. Their willingness to answer questions, discuss issues, share resources, and facilitate my activities has contributed greatly to my knowledge and understanding of the prosthetist's point of view. I continue to be grateful to my patients who constantly teach and guide me in my practice.

Most especially I thank my editor, Jean-Francois Vilain, who has always been supportive, facilitating, prodding, and ready to solve problems. Thank you, Jean-Francois—you made it all happen.

Bella J. May

Contributor

Joan E. Edelstein, MA, PT, FISPO
Associate Professor of Clinical Physical Therapy
Director, Program in Physical Therapy
Columbia University
College of Physicians and Surgeons
New York, New York

Contents

CHAPTER ONE

Amputations and Prosthetics: Then and Now

OBJECTIVES

At the end of this chapter, all students are expected to:

1 Discuss the key milestones in the history of amputations and prosthetics.
2 Discuss elements and events that triggered improvements in rehabilitation of individuals with amputations.
3 Discuss the composition of the prosthetic clinic team.
4 Discuss the role and function of members of the amputee clinic team.

INTRODUCTION

It is 1925 and you are studying physical therapy at Harvard University. Last June, you graduated from Radcliffe College with a degree in physical education and decided to enroll in a certificate course in physical therapeutics. You became interested in the field when your brother Brian lost his right leg below the knee in 1918 during World War I. You went to the hospital several times and watched Brian learn to use a wooden leg under the guidance of a **Reconstruction Aide.** (Reconstruction Aides were women who completed a special 6-month course in physical therapeutics after obtaining a college degree, usually in physical education.) The **prosthesis,** as the leg is called, was carved from a block of willow wood by a **prosthetist** who himself had an **amputation.** The **residual limb** (then called a stump) fit into a cylinder held on by a long leather corset with metal uprights that fit around the thigh; it had a wooden foot with rubber bumpers to simulate dorsiflexion and plantar flexion. It weighed about 9 lb (Fig. 1.1).

Now you are learning to be a physical therapist (PT). In 1925, you learn to teach patients with amputations to toughen their residual limbs by tapping on the skin with a glass bottle wrapped in a towel or with the fingertips. You also learn about wooden legs. In 1925 few people have amputations; most who do are young because most amputations are performed to correct problems resulting from some kind of trauma, either war injuries or accidents. Although individuals with amputations are able to return to a normal life, their participation in sports and similar activities is limited. There are few components and little choice in the fabrication of the prosthesis.

1

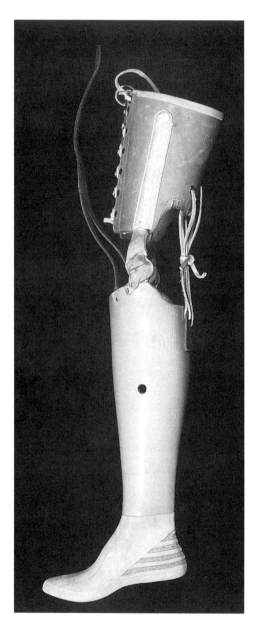

FIGURE 1.1

Conventional transtibial prosthesis similar in style to the prostheses used until the 1950s. (From Sanders, GT: Lower Limb Amputations: A Guide to Rehabilitation. FA Davis, Philadelphia, 1986, with permission.)

Jump now to today. You are a PT or physical therapist assistant (PTA) student learning about amputations and prosthetics. You may have a relative or an acquaintance who has had an amputation. It is likely that the person sustained the amputation because of peripheral vascular disease or neuropathy. He or she may have diabetes mellitus and will probably be older than age 60. The prosthesis is made of plastic; the socket was probably fabricated by a computer from an electronic image of the residual limb. The prosthesis is held on by suction or by a light elastic sleeve that rolls over the thigh or by the high plastic wings of the prosthesis. The shank is a lightweight aluminum pipe covered with a soft material shaped to resemble the other leg. The foot is designed to simulate normal motion in at least two planes, and the whole leg

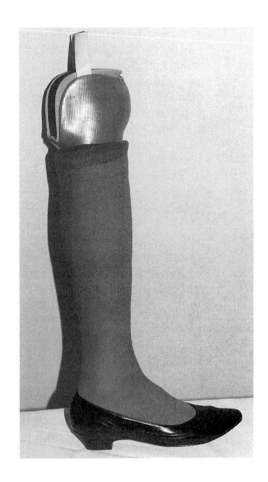

FIGURE 1.2

Modern patellar tendon bearing, suprapatellar, supracondylar endoskeleton transtibial prosthesis.

weighs less than 3 lb (Fig 1.2). The prosthetist and the client have a great variety of components to choose from, from fairly simple to highly technological.

■ Activity

1 Review the historical developments presented in this chapter. In study groups, discuss the changes that have occurred and the impetus for the changes, and become familiar with some of the terminology. Consider the future: What do you think are the important concepts to understand to be effective as a PT or PTA?

2 If available, look and feel different prostheses to gain a better understanding of the effects of technological advances.

3 Review the *Guide to Physical Therapist Practice, ed. 2,* and identify practice patterns related to peripheral vascular disease, amputations, trauma, and related surgery.[1]

HISTORY

The earliest amputations usually resulted in death from shock because of blood loss or **septicemia.** Those who survived the operation itself often died in the early postoperative period from infection and gangrene. The emphasis was on surgical speed rather than shaping the residual limb. When antisepsis and anesthesia came into use in the middle of the 19th century, specific surgical techniques, tissue conservation, and postoperative management became the focus of amputation surgery. From the first amputation, performed by Hegesistratus in 484 BC, prosthetic replacements have been designed to improve function. Hegesistratus, who escaped from the stocks by cutting off one of his feet, built himself a wooden foot to compensate. There are records of 15th century knights building and using iron artificial hands to hold their swords.[2]

Over the years, technical advances in artificial limbs have resulted from attempts to improve function, and surgical improvements have come from attempts to save lives. Changes in technology and materials led to improvements in surgery and prosthetics. Governments and legislation have also contributed, particularly after wars when government agencies provided funds for prosthetic research. A brief chronological look at the major historical developments in the field of amputation and prosthetics will help you place current concepts in perspective.

The Early Years

Surgery

In the early years, there were greater changes in surgical techniques than in prosthetics. Operative and postoperative bleeding was a major problem until 1517 when Hans von Gersdorff of Strassburg described the use of a compression tourniquet and cauterization to control bleeding.[3] He also recommended covering an amputated limb with muscle from a cow or pig bladder and dressing the wound with warm—not boiling—oil. Ambroise Paré[4] (1510–1590), a French army surgeon, reintroduced the use of **ligatures,** originally set forth by Hippocrates. This technique was more successful than crushing the amputation limb, dipping it in boiling oil, or other means of cautery that had been used during the Dark Ages to stop bleeding. Paré was the first to describe phantom sensation. Wilhelm Fabry[3] (Germany) first recommended amputation above a gangrenous part. He devised a tourniquet, a ligature tightened by a stick, to stop circulation before surgery. In 1803, Dominique-Jean Larrey,[3] Napoleon's surgeon, tried refrigeration to dull the pain of amputation surgery. He was one of the first to amputate at the hip joint. He was said to have performed as many as 200 amputations in 24 hours and is recognized as the inventor of the "flying ambulances," which he used to gather wounded soldiers during battle rather than force them to wait until the end of the conflict. In 1815 Jacques Lisfranc[4] of France devised a disarticulation amputation of the foot at the tarsometatarsal joint that became known as the Lisfranc's amputation.

James Syme[4] of Edinburgh performed the first successful amputation at the ankle joint in 1842; the procedure carries his name. He also advocated thigh amputations through the cortical bone of the condyles or the trochanters. That same year Crawford Long,[4] who practiced in Athens, Georgia, was the first physician to use ether for general anesthesia. Pierre Jean Marie Flourens,[2] a French physiologist, discovered the anesthetic properties of chloroform in 1847. The increasing availability of ether and chloroform led to improved surgical procedures and more functional amputation of limbs. In 1867

Joseph Lister[3] published his principles of antiseptic surgery that markedly reduced mortality during and after surgery. Lister also experimented with catgut as a ligature (1880) rather than silk or hemp, which body tissues could not absorb, thereby often causing inflammations and hemorrhage. In the early 1900s surgeons attempted to build bone bridges at the ends of transtibial (below knee) amputations to allow for greater end bearing. These techniques were precursors to the development of myodesis and myoplasty techniques discussed in this chapter and in Chapter 4.

In 1848 Vanghetti, an Italian surgeon, attempted to develop a technique to power upper limb prosthesis directly using muscles attached to the prosthesis.[2] The technique was further refined in Germany and Argentina as surgeons developed skin-lined muscle tunnels, an early **cineplasty,** to power upper limb prostheses.[2]

Prosthetics

Early prosthetic development is less well documented. It is likely that local artisans or individuals in need of such limbs made prostheses. An artificial leg, invented by Paré in 1561 for individuals amputated above the knee, was constructed of iron and was the first artificial leg known to employ articulated joints (Fig. 1.3). In 1696 Pieter Andriannszoon Verfuyn (Verduin), a Dutch surgeon,[3,4] introduced the first known transtibial prosthesis with an

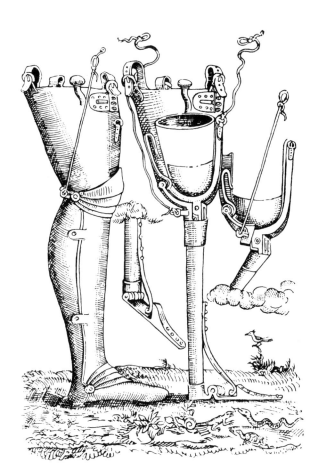

FIGURE 1.3

An above-knee artificial leg invented by Ambroise Paré (mid-16th century). (From Paré, A: Oeuvres Complètes, Paris, 1840, with permission from the National Library of Medicine.)

unlocked knee joint. In concept, it resembled the thigh-corset prosthesis used in more recent times. A thigh cuff bore part of the weight and was connected by external hinges to a leg piece with a socket made of copper and lined with leather. The leg piece terminated in a wooden foot. In 1843 James Potts[4] of London introduced a transfemoral (above-knee) prosthesis with a wooden shank and socket, a steel knee joint, and an articulated foot with leather thongs connecting the knee to the ankle. This enabled dorsiflexion (toe lift) whenever the wearer flexed the knee. The device was known as the "Anglesey (Anglesea) leg" because it was used by the Marquis of Anglesey following the loss of his leg in the Battle of Waterloo (Fig. 1.4).

During the American Civil War (1861–1865) interest in artificial limbs and amputation surgery increased because of the number of individuals surviving amputations (30,000 in the Union army) and the commitment of federal and state governments to pay for artificial limbs for veterans. J. E. Hanger,[4] who lost a leg during the Civil War, replaced the cords of his prosthesis with rubber bumpers at the ankle to control plantar flexion and dorsiflexion. The J. E. Hanger Company opened in Richmond, Virginia, in 1861, and in 1862 the U.S. Congress enacted the first law providing free prostheses to people who lost limbs in warfare.[4]

In 1863 the suction socket (Fig. 1.5), which employed the concept of using pressure to suspend an artificial limb, was patented by an American, Dubois D. Parmelee.[5] Parmelee also invented a polycentric knee unit and a multi-

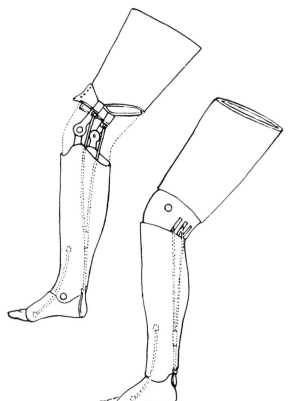

FIGURE 1.4

The Anglesey (Anglesea) leg (1816) with articulated knee, ankle, and foot. (*Left*) Below knee. (*Right*) Above knee. (From Bigg, HH: Orthopraxy: The Mechanical Treatment of Deformities, Debilities and Deficiencies of the Human Frame, ed. 3. J & A Churchill, London, 1877, with permission.)

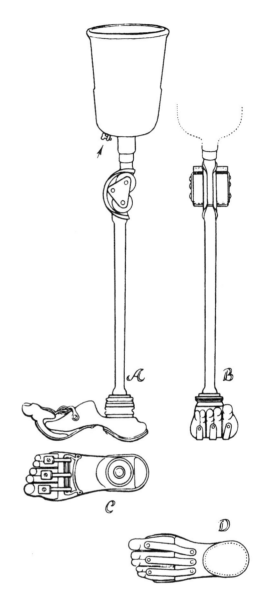

FIGURE 1.5
The D. D. Parmelee prosthesis with suction socket, patented in 1863. (From Historical development of artificial limbs. In Orthopaedic Appliances Atlas, Vol 2, Artificial Limbs. JW Edwards, Ann Arbor, Mich., 1960, p 11, with permission.)

articulated foot. In 1870 Congress passed a law that not only supplied artificial limbs to all persons honorably discharged from the military or naval service who had lost a limb while in the United States service, but also entitled them to receive one every 5 years.

The World Wars

Fewer Americans (4403) lost a limb during World War I (1914–1918) compared to the British (42,000) or to the total number of amputations (approximately 100,000) in all the armies of Europe. However, the war was an impetus for improvements in artificial limb developments.[6] Collaboration between prosthetists and surgeons in the care of veterans with amputations led to the formation of the Artificial Limb Manufacturers Association in 1917. Little progress was made in the field of prosthetics and amputation surgery in the period between the two wars, but World War II again spurred developments. The American Orthotic and Prosthetic Association was established in 1949 and developed educational criteria and examinations to certify prosthetists and orthotists.[4]

In 1945, in response to the demands of veterans for more functional prostheses, the National Academy of Sciences (NAS) initiated a study to develop design criteria that would improve the function of artificial limbs.[2] The Committee on Artificial Limbs (CAL) contracted with universities, industrial laboratories, health providers, and others to spearhead major changes in all facets of prosthetics and orthotics. From 1947 to 1976 under NAS sponsorship and Department of Veterans Affairs (VA) support, the CAL, the Committee on Prosthetic Research and Development, and the Committee on Prosthetic-Orthotic Education influenced the development of modern prosthetics and orthotics.[2] Plastics replaced wood as the material of choice, socket designs followed physiological principles of function, lighter weight components were developed, and more cosmetic alternatives were fabricated. Most of the prosthetic principles outlined in this book had their inception in the work of these committees.[2]

Surgery

Surgically, **myoplasty,** the suturing of the ends of severed muscles over the end of the bone, was first advocated[2] in 1949 but did not gain in popularity until the 1950s, when myoplasty was adopted by Dederich[7] and popularized by Burgess.[8] **Myodesis,** the suturing of severed muscles to distal bone, was advocated by Weiss[9] in the 1960s. Both myodesis and myoplasty are designed to provide muscle fixation for improved function and shape of the residual limb. In 1958 in France, Michael Berlemont demonstrated immediate postsurgical fitting of prostheses.[4] The technique, which involves placing the residual limb in a rigid postsurgical dressing fabricated using prosthetic principles, was also advocated by Weiss[9] and brought to the United States by Sarmiento[10] and Burgess.[8]

In the 1960s and 1970s, several factors combined to lead surgeons to reconsider the transfemoral amputation as the level of choice for severely ischemic limbs. Immediate postoperative fitting reduced postoperative edema, allowing healing at transtibial levels, even for individuals with severe ischemia. Improved circulatory evaluation techniques provided accurate information on the presence of collateral circulation. The use of the long posterior flap with its increased blood supply also contributed to the healing capabilities of transtibial amputations.[11] All these factors contributed to a reversal in the number of transtibial and transfemoral amputations performed for severe limb ischemia and concomitantly increased the number of individuals becoming successful prosthetic ambulators.

Prosthetics

During the same period, many changes occurred in prosthetic development. In 1954 the Canadian hip-disarticulation prosthesis, designed at Sunnybrook Hospital, Toronto, and introduced by Colin McLaurin, allowed the individual with a hip disarticulation or transpelvic (hemipelvectomy) amputation to stand and walk with moving mechanical knee and hip joints.[4] The Canadian Syme prosthesis, also designed at Sunnybrook Hospital and introduced in 1955, combined the use of plastic laminates and a solid rubber foot.[4] In 1956 the Biomechanics Laboratory at the University of California introduced the solid ankle, cushion heel foot, which became the most popular prosthetic foot.[4] In 1959 the patellar-tendon bearing prosthesis was first introduced at the University of California at Berkeley. In the same year, the Orthopedic Appliance and Limb Manufacturers Association changed its name to the American Orthotics and Prosthetics Association.[3] In the 1960s hydraulic knee mechanisms became more prevalent. In 1971 endoskeletal prostheses with an adjustable tubular structure encased by a foam-plastic material and covered by an elastic hose were introduced by Otto Bock Orthopaedic Industry.[6]

The American Board for Certification of the Prosthetic and Orthopedic Appliance Industry became the American Board for Certification in Orthotics and Prosthetics, and the first undergraduate curriculum leading to a Bachelor of Science degree in Prosthetics and Orthotics was inaugurated at New York University in 1963. Throughout the postwar period, the rehabilitation of individuals with an amputation involved the expertise of prosthetists, engineers, researchers, physicians, and PTs. Major prosthetic rehabilitation centers held workshops to share the increasing body of knowledge. Experience in and knowledge of prosthetic and orthotic rehabilitation became part of the residency requirements for orthopedic surgeons.

In 1970 the International Society for Prosthetics and Orthotics was founded to improve communication among researchers and clinicians throughout the world. To make international communications clearer and easier, a standard nomenclature was adopted to refer to level of amputation and related prostheses. The term *trans* is used when an amputation goes across the axis of a long bone such as the transtibial or transhumeral. When there are two bones together such as the tibia and fibula, the primary bone is identified. Amputations between long bones or through a joint are referred to as disarticulations and identified by the major body part, such as knee disarticulation. The term *partial* is used to refer to a part of the foot or hand distal to the ankle or wrist that may be amputated.[12] Table 1.1 shows the relationship between the old and the new terminology. The new terminology will be used throughout this book.

Modern Times

Surgery

Most amputations today are performed for vascular disease, with more than 50 percent performed on individuals with peripheral vascular disease secondary to diabetes.[13] Most amputations are performed on individuals older than age 60. The National Commission on Diabetes estimates that 5 to 15 percent of all persons with diabetes will require an amputation.[13] A recent study indicated that the number of amputations among individuals with diabetes has increased from 4.8 per 100 persons in 1991 to 6.2 per 100 in 1994. The rate of amputation among individuals with both diabetes and end-stage renal disease has increased even more—from 11.8 per 100 persons in 1991 to 13.8 per 100 in 1994.[14] Another study indicated that although the overall rate

TABLE 1.1   AMPUTATION-LEVEL NOMENCLATURE

Old Terminology	Current Terminology
Partial hand	Partial hand
Wrist disarticulation	Wrist disarticulation
Below elbow	Transradial
Elbow disarticulation	Elbow disarticulation
Above elbow	Transhumeral
Shoulder disarticulation	Shoulder disarticulation
Forequarter	Forequarter
Partial foot	Partial foot
Syme's	Ankle disarticulation
Below knee	Transtibial
Knee disarticulation	Knee disarticulation
Above knee	Transfemoral
Hip disarticulation	Hip disarticulation
Hemipelvectomy	Transpelvic

of amputation has increased somewhat with increased longevity and better care of individuals with vascular disease, a small decrease in amputation rate is found among individuals undergoing revascularization procedures.[15] Several British researchers compared the incidence of lower extremity amputation among different centers around the world.[16] Ten centers with a population greater than 200,000 in Japan, Taiwan, Spain, Italy, North America, and England were asked to collect data on all amputations performed in a 2-year period between 1995 and 1997. All centers followed a detailed protocol to ensure comparability of data. Results indicated major differences in overall incidence of amputation among centers, with the highest incidence among the Navajo population in the United States and the lowest incidence in Japan. Among European centers, the highest incidence was in England and the lowest in Spain. There were great similarities in age and gender between all centers, with the incidence of amputation being highest in individuals older than age 60 and higher in men than in women. The incidence of amputation associated with diabetes also varied greatly, with only 20 to 30 percent of amputations in Spain associated with diabetes and more than 80 percent of amputations among Navajo men associated with diabetes. The study protocol apparently did not differentiate between peripheral vascular disease associated with diabetes and that which was not associated because the researchers reported a 51 percent incidence of amputation from peripheral vascular disease among Navajo men and an 80 percent incidence among Spanish men. The incidence associated with trauma in men was generally less than 10 percent except in Taiwan, where the percentage increased to 50 percent. The data for women were reported to be similar.[17]

Trauma is the next most frequent cause of amputation, with cancer, congenital deformities, and miscellaneous causes as other reasons for amputation. In 1959 and 1960 the "thalidomide tragedy" resulted in many children born with multiple limb anomalies; this led to government-supported research, particularly in Germany, Canada, and the United States, for prostheses and aids for children with multiple amputations. Today, the major causes of juvenile amputations are trauma, congenital abnormalities, osteomyelitis, and cancer.

Limb salvage procedures, replantation, and revascularization characterize modern surgical concepts. Replantation of fingers and thumbs has been quite successful, although efforts to replant entire upper limbs have not done as well.[17] Improved techniques of fracture fixation, vessel repair, and muscle and skin flaps have enhanced limb salvage procedures. Algorithms have been developed to guide the surgeon in cases of several multiple trauma to upper or lower limbs. Infection control has improved, and chemotherapy and tumor **ablation** with reconstruction have reduced the need for amputation for metastatic disease.

Prosthetics

Modern times are characterized by the emergence of prosthetics as a science as well as an art. Research into human movement, new materials, and new technology has led to the creation of very light and functional components. The consumer is also making greater demands on the prosthesis, seeking limbs that will enable him or her to participate in all aspects of life, including sports and leisure activities. Flexible, intimate-fit sockets suspended by suction have been developed for transfemoral and transtibial amputations. Gel-filled liners provide a shock-absorbing interface between the residual limb and the hard socket. Gel liners ensure an intimate fit that suspends the prosthesis with virtually no pistoning, making the artificial limb an integral part of the lower extremity. A wide variety of prosthetic feet is designed to respond dynamically to the pressure of walking and running and to provide mediolateral motion as well as the more traditional dorsiflexion and plantar flexion. Research highlighted the importance of swing as well as stance phase in normal walking, leading to the development of hydraulic and mechanical swing-phase-control knee joints for transfemoral amputations. Multiaxis knee mechanisms allow cosmetic fitting of individuals with long transfemoral residual limbs or knee disarticulations. Research is attempting to find a method to bring sensation into the prosthetic limb. Chapter 7 describes modern componentry for lower extremity prostheses.

The upper extremity has always posed a major challenge to prosthetists. The great complexity of hand function is difficult to duplicate mechanically. The loss of sensation limits the function of the hand or hook, and researchers have yet to develop replacement for sensory function. Research in more functional prosthetic replacements as well as replantation surgery continues. Developments in external power are probably the highlight of modern upper extremity prostheses. Myoelectric controls are now used fairly routinely for transhumeral and transradial amputations. Upper extremity prosthetics is reviewed in Chapter 10.

THE TEAM APPROACH

In early times, a surgeon performed an amputation, someone made a prosthesis, and the client learned to use the appliance as best as he or she could. During and after World War I, reconstruction aides taught veterans to use their prostheses, a practice that carried into the civilian population as PTs became more prevalent. There is no formal documentation of the development of the prosthetic rehabilitation team. As surgeons and prosthetists started to share ideas regarding prosthetic developments and as the field of rehabilitation grew, the care of individuals following amputations became a part of the rehabilitation process in areas where rehabilitation centers existed. In smaller communities, the surgeon would send the client to a prosthetist who would make the limb. The client might be referred to a physical or occupational therapist for training. As prosthetic rehabilitation became more complex, teams of experts from the fields of medicine, physical therapy, occupational therapy, prosthetics and orthotics, and social services gathered in teams to evaluate client needs and make decisions.

Most amputations today are performed by vascular or general surgeons who may or may not have received special training in prosthetic rehabilitation. Orthopedic surgeons usually perform amputations necessitated by trauma, malignancy, or other nonvascular reasons, and they complete a course in prosthetics as part of their residency training. Referral to a prosthetic clinic or to physical therapy may be delayed for many weeks if the surgeon waits until the residual limb heals completely. Such delays, particularly among elderly clients, may lead to joint contractures, muscular weakness secondary to disuse, and limited mobility. Delay in starting a rehabilitation program may limit the eventual level of rehabilitation. Ideally, the PT should be involved before surgery or at least immediately after to start the process of client education, proper positioning, and residual limb care. Unfortunately, many amputations are performed in hospitals without the services of an amputee clinic or a well-trained team that can develop and supervise the program. The PT may be the only person with competence in prosthetic rehabilitation. Close contact with the vascular surgeons in your facility may serve to increase the likelihood of early referrals and improve quality care for the client.

Increased financial limitations have also interfered with effective prosthetic rehabilitation. Individuals without insurance who do not qualify for Medicaid or indigent care and who are too young for Medicare often find themselves without the resources to obtain an artificial limb. In many states, Medicaid reimbursement is often inadequate or very slow, leaving the older person with an amputation to live in a wheelchair without services for an extended period. Even individuals with insurance may find that their medical insurance plan does not provide for the components needed or that they are forced to seek prosthetic services far from their homes. It is important for the PT who comes in contact with the patient early in the episode of care to educate the patient and the family regarding appropriate continuation of care.

Members

The clinic team plans and implements comprehensive rehabilitation programs designed to meet the physical, psychological, and economic needs of the client. Most clinic teams are located in rehabilitation facilities, university health centers, or VA medical centers. The team generally includes a physician, PT, occupational therapist (OT), prosthetist, social worker, and vocational counselor. Other health professionals who contribute to the team are

TABLE 1.2   CLINIC TEAM MEMBERS AND FUNCTIONS

Physician	Clinic chief; coordinates team decision making; supervises client's general medical condition; prescribes appliances.
Physical therapist	Evaluates and treats clients through preprosthetic and prosthetic phases; makes recommendations for prosthetic components and whether or not to fit the client. May be clinic coordinator.
Prosthetist	Fabricates and modifies prosthesis; recommends prosthetic components; shares data on new prosthetic developments.
Occupational therapist	Assesses and treats individuals with upper extremity amputations; makes recommendations for components.
Social worker	Financial counselor and coordinator; provides liaison with third-party payers and community agencies; helps family cope with social and financial problems.
Dietitian	Consultant for clients with diabetes or those needing diet guidance.
Vocational counselor	Assesses client's employment potential; coordinates and may fund education, training, and placement.

Source: May, BJ: Assessment and treatment of individuals following lower extremity amputation. In O'Sullivan, SB, and Schmitz, TJ (eds): Physical Rehabilitation: Assessment and Treatment, ed 3. FA Davis, Philadelphia, 1994, with permission.

nurses, dietitians, psychologists, and, possibly, administrative coordinators. Table 1.2 outlines the major functions of team members. Clinic meeting frequency is dictated by the caseload; clients are seen regularly and decisions are made using input from all team members. A screening session held by the PTs and OTs prior to the actual clinic allows for the careful evaluation of each person and improves the effectiveness of the clinic.[18] In centers without a clinic, close communication between the client, surgeon, and PTs—with the later addition of the prosthetist—is important to ensure an optimal outcome.

Summary

Major advances have been made in the field of prosthetic rehabilitation stimulated in part by wars that increased the number of individuals who lost limbs. Dissatisfaction with heavy, uncomfortable artificial limbs, particularly following World War II, gave impetus to research in surgery and prosthetics. Today, the number of older individuals who seek a functional and productive life following amputation and the desire of all handicapped individuals for full participation in work, sports, and leisure activities, continue to stimulate advances in prosthetics and rehabilitation.

Glossary

Ablation	Removal of a part.
Amputation	The surgical removal of a limb or body part. In this text, the term will be used to refer to the removal or absence of a limb.
Cauterization	Destruction of tissue by burning or freezing; burning was used to close wounds in early days.

Cineplasty	A surgical technique that builds a tunnel through a muscle of the residual limb to power an artificial limb. Used mostly for transradial amputations. A skin-lined tunnel was made through the biceps, and a rod was inserted through the tunnel that was attached by cable to the terminal device.
Ligatures	The process of binding or tying; sutures.
Myodesis	Attaching the ends of muscles to the end of the bone in amputation surgery.
Myoplasty	Attaching the cut ends of muscles to each other, over the end of a bone in amputation surgery.
Prosthesis	Artificial replacement of a body part.
Prosthetist	An individual who makes artificial limbs for the upper or lower extremities. A prosthetist who has completed a prescribed course of study and passed a certifying examination is allowed to use the initials CP.
Reconstruction Aide	Early PTs who joined the U.S. Army during World War I. After the war, these individuals came together and formed the American Physical Therapy Association.
Residual limb	The part of the limb that remains after amputation. It is also called the stump or the residuum.
Septicemia	The presence of pathogenic organisms in the blood, which leads to infection.

References

1. APTA: Guide to Physical Therapist Practice, ed 2. Alexandria, Va., APTA, 2001.
2. Wilson, AB, Jr: History of amputation surgery and prosthetics. In Bowker, JH, and Michael, JW (eds): Atlas of Limb Prosthetics: Surgical and Prosthetic Principles. Mosby Year Book, St. Louis, 1992.
3. Garrison, FH. An Introduction to the History of Medicine. WB Saunders, Philadelphia, 1929.
4. Wilson, AB: Limb prosthetics: 1970. Artif Limbs 14:184–189, 1957.
5. Talbott, JH: A Biographical History of Medicine: Excerpts and Essays on the Men and Their Work. Grune & Stratton, New York, 1970.
6. Sanders, GT: Lower Limb Amputations: A Guide to Rehabilitation. FA Davis, Philadelphia, 1986.
7. Dederich, R: Technique of myoplastic amputations. Ann R Coll Surg Engl 40:222–227, 1967.
8. Burgess, E, et al: Immediate postsurgical prosthetics in the management of lower extremity amputees. Veterans Administration TR 10–5, Washington, DC, 1967.
9. Weiss, M: Myoplastic Amputation, Immediate Prosthesis and Early Ambulation. US Department of Health Education and Welfare, US Government Printing Office, Washington DC (no date given).
10. Sarmiento, A, et al: Lower extremity amputation: The impact of immediate post surgical prosthetic fitting. Clin Orthop 68:22–31, 1970.
11. Most, RS, and Sinnock, P: The epidemiology of lower extremity amputations in diabetic individuals. Diabetes Care 6:87–91, 1983.
12. Schuch, CM, and Pritham, CH: International standards organization terminology: Application to prosthetics and orthotics. Journal of Prosthetics and Orthotics 6(1):29–33, 1994.
13. Sanders, R, and Helfet, D: The choice between limb salvage and amputation: Trauma. In Bowker, JH, and Michael, JW (eds): Atlas of Limb Prosthetics: Surgical and Prosthetic Principles. Mosby Year Book, St. Louis, 1992.
14. Eggers, PW, et al: Nontraumatic lower extremity amputations in the Medicare end-stage renal disease population. Kidney Int 56(4):1524–33, 1999.

15. Dormandy, J, et al: The fate of patients with critical leg ischemia. [Review] Source Seminars in Vascular Surgery 12(2):142–147, 1999.
16. Unwin, N (for the Global Lower Extremity Amputation Study Group): Epidemiology of lower extremity amputation in centers in Europe, North American and East Asia. Br J Surg 87(3):328–337, 2000.
17. Ouellette, EA, et al: Partial-hand amputation: surgical principles. In Bowker, JH, and Michael, JW (eds): Atlas of Limb Prosthetics: Surgical and Prosthetic Principles. Mosby Year Book, St. Louis, 1992.
18. May, BJ: A statewide amputee rehabilitation programme. Prosthet Orthot Int 2:24–26, 1978.

CHAPTER TWO

Peripheral Vascular Diseases

OBJECTIVES

At the end of this chapter, all students are expected to:

1 Discuss the etiology and clinical features of major disorders of the peripheral vascular system that may lead to amputation.
2 Differentiate among chronic and acute arterial and venous diseases.
3 Briefly discuss medical and surgical management of peripheral vascular diseases.
4 Discuss the functional effects of peripheral vascular diseases.

In addition, physical therapy students are expected to:

5 Develop an examination plan for an individual with peripheral vascular disease.
6 Interpret the results of the tests and measures.
7 Develop a plan of care for an individual with peripheral vascular disease.

Arteriosclerosis is the major cause of lower extremity amputation today. Physical therapists (PTs) and physical therapist assistants (PTAs) may treat an individual with an ulcerated foot caused by peripheral vascular disease, and later treat the same person following lower extremity amputation. An individual with diabetes who sustains one amputation for arteriosclerosis has a 51 percent chance of sustaining a second amputation within 5 years.[1] As will be discussed in Chapter 5, care of the remaining extremity is an important part of the postamputation treatment program. The purpose of this chapter is to provide an overview of the peripheral vascular diseases that may lead to amputation or that may be present in individuals who have had an amputation. It is not meant to provide a complete study of all peripheral vascular diseases.

Case Studies

Diana Magnolia, a 54-year-old woman with a history of insulin-dependent diabetes mellitus that was diagnosed 15 years ago. She is an outpatient referred for treatment of an ulcer on the plantar surface of the left first metatarsal head.

Benny Pearl, a 67-year-old man referred 1 day after right femoral-popliteal bypass for partial occlusion of the lower femoral artery.

Charley Johnson, a 59-year-old man referred for treatment of lower extremity edema and a stasis ulcer just proximal to the right medial malleolus.

■ Case Study Activities

All Students

1 How would you diagnostically classify each of these people's conditions? Differentiate between arterial and venous disease and between acute and chronic vascular disease in terms of:

Patient complaints including type of pain.
Condition of the lower extremity seen by observation.
Initial occurrence and progression of the disease.

2 What practice pattern(s) do each of the individuals fit into?
3 Describe the pathophysiology of each diagnosis, differentiating among major signs and symptoms. What additional information do you need before you can examine or treat each client? Supplement the information in this chapter with any pathophysiology references.
4 What are the major medical and surgical strategies used in the management of these diseases?

Physical Therapy Students

5 For each person, determine your course of action at this time. What tests and measures would you use at this time and why? How would you prioritize the examination? (e.g., given a limited time, what data are critical to obtain early and what can be delayed for later?) What are the best sources of each datum (e.g., direct examination, medical chart)? Justify your selection.
6 In your laboratory sessions, practice pertinent examination activities. Role-play each of the clients as accurately as possible. Do not look ahead to the next case study information until you have completed these items.

PATHOPHYSIOLOGY AND ETIOLOGY

Clients are rarely referred to physical therapy for preventive care in the early stages of peripheral vascular disease. However, clients with peripheral vascular disease may be referred for treatment of other conditions such as following total joint replacement or cerebrovascular accident. PTs and PTAs need to be alert for the early symptoms of arterial insufficiency and teach proper foot care (see Chap. 3). Clients with severe vascular disease, such as the individuals in the case studies, may be referred for treatment, or therapists may be involved in developing an education program that can be implemented as part of routine clinic visits. Prevention of further disability is an important part of the total management of vascular disease. The reader is encouraged to review the normal physiology of the vascular system as a point of reference in learning about vascular diseases.

Acute Vascular Diseases

Venous Thrombosis

General anesthesia, immobilization, obesity, myocardial disease, venous disease, and cerebrovascular accidents are all risk factors for the formation of a **thrombus** in the superficial or deep venous system.[2] A clot or thrombus forms, often near a venous valve where venous blood may pool, and attaches to the vein wall. It grows quickly, blocking venous flow and leading to a pooling of blood behind the thrombus. The pressure stretches the venous walls causing pain and inflammation.

The term *thrombophlebitis* refers to a thrombus in the superficial venous system.[3] Thrombi in the superficial veins are easily diagnosed and rarely become emboli. There is edema around the site of the thrombus, and the involved veins are raised, red, warm, and tender to touch.

A thrombus in the deep vein system (DVT) may become an **embolus** that is then pushed through the veins to the pulmonary system, possibly causing death. Most pulmonary emboli are believed to start as a thrombus in the deep veins of the lower leg. Data on the incidence of pulmonary embolism are inconsistent because of difficulty in diagnosis; however, it is the fourth leading cause of sudden death in the United States.[4] DVT may lead to venous inflammation, valve damage, and chronic venous problems.

Pain and tenderness in the calf, swelling of the lower leg, and redness following venous distribution have all been associated with a diagnosis of DVT; however, they are not reliable signs and are associated with many other diagnoses.[5] Estimates are that there is at least a 50 percent error in diagnosing DVT from the clinical findings alone. Homans' sign, the passive dorsiflexion of the ankle that causes pain in the calf or popliteal area, is quite unreliable and nonspecific; approximately one-half of individuals with a positive Homans' sign do not have DVT.[1] *Venography,* an invasive radiographic examination of the veins, is the most reliable test for DVT; however, several other noninvasive or semi-invasive diagnostic tools have been developed. **Doppler** ultrasonography, impedence plethysmography, and duplex color flow scanning are all noninvasive tests that range in sensitivity of detection from 96 to about 73 percent. Sensitivity decreases for thrombi of the calf and for patients without specific symptoms.[6]

Cases of a suspected deep or superficial venous thrombus represent a medical emergency and should be reported to the physician for further evaluation. It is critical for the PT to be aware of the potential for DVT development. The major treatment for acute DVT is anticoagulant and thrombolytic therapy and bed rest with mild heat, gradual exercises of the lower extremities, and application of elastic stockings to control edema. If elastic wraps are used initially, care must be taken to properly distribute pressure by applying the bandage in a figure-of-eight pattern from distal to proximal. Elastic bandages require frequent rewrapping to avoid the development of a tourniquet. Thrombophlebitis is also treated with anticoagulants; however, ambulation may be resumed earlier than with a DVT. Neither DVT nor thrombophlebitis leads to amputation.

Acute Arterial Occlusion

Acute arterial occlusion may result from trauma or embolus. The client reports acute pain in an area distal to the occlusion. On examination the limb is pale and pulseless, and the client reports that it feels cold and paralyzed. Acute arterial occlusion is a medical emergency because nerve and skeletal muscles tolerate ischemia for only 4 to 6 hours, whereas skin tolerates ischemia for about 10 hours.[7] Diagnosis can be confirmed with Doppler ultrasound evaluation. Doppler ultrasound is a noninvasive measure of blood flow (Fig. 2.1). It is quite versatile and can be used to measure venous or arterial flow or to determine the status of venous valves. Briefly, the Doppler transmits a signal into the vessel and reflects back the sound waves of the movement of the blood through that vessel. It can detect pulses that otherwise may be inaudible, and it accurately measures systolic blood pressure.[8] Doppler evaluation will be discussed further in this chapter.

The treatment of an acute arterial occlusion varies with the severity of blockage and may include surgical or medical intervention. Many surgeons have favored aggressive surgical intervention in viable limbs. Balloon embolectomy is favored in patients without underlying stenosis of the vessel. If stenosis is present, the surgeon administers an intra-arterial thrombolytic agent or may perform bypass surgery. Long-term anticoagulation therapy will follow.[9] Suspected incidents of acute arterial occlusions must be referred im-

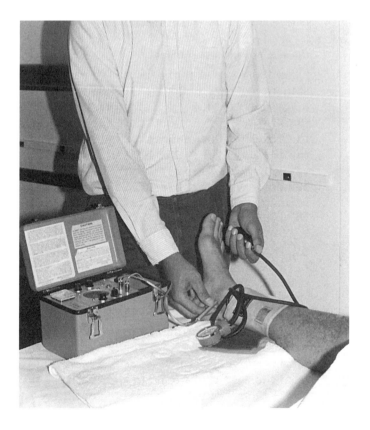

FIGURE 2.1
Doppler ultrasound may be used to measure blood flow for ABI.

mediately for medical evaluation, and treatment or irreversible tissue ischemia and amputation may result.

Chronic Vascular Diseases

Peripheral Arterial Occlusive Disease (PAOD)

Arteriosclerosis obliterans (ASO), arteriosclerosis, and arterial insufficiency
are common terms used to refer to chronic occlusive diseases of the peripheral arterial system. **Arteriosclerosis** is the term often used to refer to thickening, hardening, and narrowing of the walls of arteries. Generally, fibrous
plaques narrow the vessels, eventually leading to ischemia. The distal segment of the superficial femoral artery is a common site of involvement in
PAOD; other frequently involved sites include the common femoral artery,
the midportion of the popliteal artery, and the origins of the tibial arteries. Individuals with PAOD and diabetes also have involvement of medium and
small arteries and have worse outcomes.[10]

PAOD occurs in about 5 percent of men older than age 50 and women
older than age 60. About 25 percent of individuals with ASO eventually require reconstructive surgery, and about 5 percent eventually require major
amputation.[11] The number of cases increases if ASO is associated with diabetes. Approximately 15 percent of individuals with diabetes have ASO 15
years after onset, and 45 percent have ASO 20 years after onset of diabetes. Individuals with diabetes account for more than 50 percent of the amputations
performed in the United States today.[1,12]

Chronic Venous Insufficiency

Chronic venous insufficiency (CVI) may affect superficial or deep veins and
statistically is estimated to be underreported. Varicose veins, a chronic problem of the superficial venous system, affects 1.5 to 5.2 percent of the population.[13,14] Insufficiency of the deep vein system is likewise not well reported in
the literature, but venous ulcers are estimated to appear in about 1 percent of
the population.[15] Although many of our clients may suffer from varicose
veins, we rarely get involved unless the client has a venous ulcer or long-
standing edema from insufficiency of the deep venous system. Individuals
with arterial insufficiency, particularly with diabetes, may also have chronic
venous insufficiency.

To understand the problems encountered in the development of venous
ulcers, normal venous physiology must be understood. Deep veins and calf
muscles pump the blood toward the heart during the systolic phase of venous
contraction. Valves in the perforating veins prevent retrograde flow. During
the diastolic (relaxation) phase, the calf veins refill as blood flows from the superficial to the deep veins via the perforating veins. Venous pressure is higher
in the deep veins during the contracting (systolic) phase and higher in the superficial veins during the diastolic phase. Damage to the valves of the perforating veins affects the systolic phase. Incompetent valves allow blood to flow
from the deep to the superficial system, increasing pressure in the deep system. Venous occlusions contribute to the increased pressure as does the effect
of gravity in the upright position. The greater the hydrostatic pressure in the
superficial system during the systolic phase, the less blood will be pumped

out of the deep system toward the heart. Over time venous capillaries prolif-
erate. Increase in capillary permeability allows fluid, rich in fibrins and other
materials, to leak into the interstitial space, creating the characteristic edema
associated with chronic venous insufficiency. To manage the edematous
limb, it is important to differentiate between edema secondary to venous insufficiency and edema secondary to lymphatic disease. Table 2.1 compares arterial and venous diseases.

Thromboangiitis Obliterans (Buerger's Disease)

Thromboangiitis obliterans (TAO) is an inflammation of small- and medium-
sized arteries and veins that occurs in a very small percentage of the population. TAO, also known as Buerger's disease after the physician who first identified it, starts distally and progresses proximally, involving both upper and
lower extremities. It is initially diagnosed in young men who smoke, although the incidence of the disease in women has grown in the past decades,

TABLE 2.1 OVERVIEW OF PERIPHERAL VASCULAR DISEASES

Disease	Etiology	Pathology	Major Symptoms
Arteriosclerosis without diabetes	More men than women; older than age 50; risk factors include smoking, obesity, hypertension, hyperlipidemia, and sedentary lifestyle.	Large artery occlusive disease; affects intima of arteries with luminal narrowing. Fibrous plaques develop. Associated with hypertension and coronary artery disease (CAD).	Intermittent claudication then rest pain relieved by standing; absent or decreased pedal pulses; dry skin and hair loss on lower leg; clubbing of toenails; ischemia of toes; ulcer on weight-bearing foot surface.
Arteriosclerosis with diabetes	Older than age 40; risk factors same as ASO. Affects lower extremities more than upper extremities.	Medium and small arteries involved. Fatty streaks lead to fibrous plaques and narrowing of arteries.	Same as ASO plus decreased or absent sensation of the foot; renal complications; impaired vision; loss of muscle strength in distal segments. Multiple systems involvement.
CVI	Affects about 1% of population. Superficial and deep veins may be involved. Incidence increases with age.	Blood flows back to superficial veins secondary to damaged perforating valves; leads to increased pressure and decreased flow back to heart. New venous capillaries and increased fibrinolytic buildup prevent normal exchange and lead to cell death.	Edema, (pitting early, hard later); dilated veins; leg pain (heaviness, ache when standing relieved by elevation); cutaneous changes (brownish color, dermatitis); skin ulcers above medial malleolus.
Thromboangiitis obliterans (TAO)	Men 20–40 years; tobacco users. Incidence 12 in 100,000.	Vasospastic and arteriosclerotic components affecting small and medium arteries and veins of upper and lower extremities. Starts distally; progresses proximally.	Bilateral ischemia starting distally, leading to ulceration and amputation. Superficial phlebitis and dysesthesia; may have rubor or cyanosis; pedal claudication; rest pain.

probably related to improved diagnosis. Etiologically, TAO is directly related to smoking, is exacerbated by smoking, and improves when the client stops smoking. Symptoms include bilateral intermittent claudication starting distally, possible superficial phlebitis, and decreased cold tolerance in the hands and fingers. Clients may experience repeated episodes of pedal claudication and phlebitis. The major treatment is the cessation of all tobacco use. A small number of individuals with TAO who do not stop smoking may require amputation of one or more distal limbs. These individuals represent a very small percentage of individuals amputated for vascular disease.[16]

MEDICAL AND SURGICAL MANAGEMENT

Diagnosis

Age, gender, hypertension, diabetes, elevated serum cholesterol and low-density lipid levels in the blood, obesity, smoking, and a sedentary lifestyle are all risk factors that have been associated with PAOD. Smoking doubles the risk of PAOD in both men and women, and hypertension triples the risk.[17,18,19] The initial diagnosis is frequently made by the family practitioner, and clients are often not seen by a vascular specialist until the disease is fairly well advanced.

Intermittent claudication is often the first symptom that leads the client to seek medical attention. Intermittent claudication is a cramping calf pain that occurs when one walks, and it can increase to the point of ischemia of the muscles of the lower leg. It results from an inability of an impaired arterial system to meet the increasing demands for oxygen and glucose of exercising muscles. The pain and cramping stop as soon as the patient stops to rest, which allows the arterial circulation to catch up with the muscular demands for oxygen. As the disease progresses, the client can walk shorter and shorter distances before claudication occurs. Severe PAOD is characterized by rest pain, a cramping or aching pain in the calf or foot that occurs during sleep. Clients will get up in the night to put the limb in a dependent position and may eventually opt to sleep in a sitting position. Some edema of the lower leg may occur from maintaining the limb in a dependent position for prolonged periods. Rest pain occurs in about 24 percent of individuals experiencing intermittent claudication.[10] Severe ischemia may lead to ulcers in the ankle or foot. Two types of ulcers are related to arterial insufficiency. Individuals with large vessel disease not associated with diabetes and with severe ischemia and rest pain may develop ulcers at the ankle, the end of a toe, or between two toes. These ulcers are caused by ischemic necrosis and dry gangrene. Ulcers may also occur secondary to minor trauma or pressure on the feet. Although more common among individuals with diabetes, these ulcers may also occur in people with severe ischemia of the lower extremities. Ulcers may or may not be painful depending on the presence of diabetes, decreased sensation, and **neuropathy.** Neuropathic ulcers usually occur in areas prone to pressure such as the plantar surface of the foot or the heel. About 5 percent of individuals who have intermittent claudication sustain a lower extremity amputation secondary to gangrene of the foot.[11] Foot ulcers, a major problem among individuals with PAOD and diabetes, are discussed in more detail in Chapter 3.

Examination

Medical Examination of ASO

The physician usually diagnoses arterial insufficiency by history and physical examination. One should compare one limb with the other because one side is frequently more involved. Palpation of the femoral, popliteal, posterior tibial, and dorsalis pedis pulses helps pinpoint areas of diminished circulation. Inadequate circulation may also lead to dependent rubor; the limb is elevated at about 60 degrees for 1 minute and then placed in a dependent position. If the limb turns red, it is a rebound from the period of hypoxia and indication of dysvascularity. A walking test may also be performed, noting how far a client can walk on a treadmill before developing intermittent claudication.

Laboratory tests may include Doppler ankle/brachial index (ABI), segmental volume plethysmography, duplex ultrasonography, magnetic resonance imaging (MRI), or arteriography. The ABI test is easy to perform and quite reliable. Ankle and brachial systolic measures are obtained by inflating a blood pressure cuff above systolic pressure and determining when the resumption of flow occurs by placing the Doppler probe over the radial artery in the arm and over the tibial or dorsalis pedis arteries in the ankle. The ratio is obtained by dividing the ankle systolic pressure by the brachial systolic pressure. Normal readings range from 0.9 to 1.3, whereas a reading below 0.9 indicates arterial insufficiency to some degree. Table 2.2 indicates the implications of ranges of results.

Segmental volume plethysmography combines measures of segmental systolic pressure taken at the thigh, calf, and ankle, with assessment of pulse volume waveforms that accurately reflect vascular status.[11]

Transcutaneous oxygen measurements assess tissue metabolism as a function of perfusion by reflecting the percentage of oxygen, and thus circulation, in the tissues. These measurements may be used to predict the healing potential for an ulcer or amputation.

MRI provides the physician with an accurate estimate of blood flow velocity in a noninvasive method. The limited resolution of small peripheral arteries and its high cost limits the use of MRI in the evaluation of peripheral arterial disease.

The use of arteriography, an invasive technique where dye is injected into an artery and followed with roentgenograms, has decreased with the advent of reliable noninvasive techniques. Arteriography is usually performed prior to reconstructive surgery.

TABLE 2.2   IMPLICATIONS OF ABI READINGS

ABI Reading	Indication
0.9 to 1.3	Normal reading
0.4 to 0.9	Intermittent claudication present
0.25 to 0.4	Rest pain present
<0.25	Ulcers and gangrene

Physical Therapy Examination

Elements of Patient Management

The *Guide to Physical Therapy Practice, ed 2,* has outlined five major steps necessary for the management of any individual seeking physical therapy services. The five steps include examination, evaluation, diagnosis, prognosis, and intervention.[20]

Examination

Components of the examination include history taking, systems review, and specific data collection through the application of tests and measures. The PT must obtain a detailed history to document the extent of vascular insufficiency and other problems. Information needed includes general demographics and lifestyle information, other medical problems, medications, medical and surgical interventions, and the client's perception of the symptoms.

Arterial insufficiency rarely occurs in isolation, and it is important to know if the client has related diseases such as diabetes, hypertension, and cardiac disease. Having the client describe his or her medical problems provides some insight into the person's understanding of associated diseases. If available, the medical chart is a valuable source of information about the status of other systems.

It is very important to obtain a list of current medications, investigating their possible effects on therapeutic activities. Anticoagulants make the client more prone to bruising or bleeding. Several drugs are used to control hypertension including diuretics, beta blockers, and angiotensin-converting enzyme (ACE) inhibitors. Diuretics may lead to frequent urination. Beta blockers may limit exercise tolerance, with clients complaining of dizziness and weakness if overstressed. ACE inhibitors may also cause dizziness and a sense of weakness in some cases. Drug reactions and interactions are complex problems; clients may be taking several prescription drugs provided by different physicians and may also be taking over-the-counter medications. Some medications may interfere with rather than enhance function. Drug reactions must be suspected when client complaints or behaviors are not obviously related. Carrying a small, up-to-date pharmacology reference is recommended.

Information regarding current lifestyle is valuable in setting realistic treatment goals and encouraging compliance in home activities. What is the client's job? What are the demands at home? Recreational activities? Is the client a smoker? If yes, how much does he or she smoke? Does the client follow an appropriate diet? Although the client probably knows the negative effects of smoking and a high-cholesterol and salt diet, the PT and PTA can support and encourage necessary lifestyle changes.

Asking the client to describe current symptoms provides information on the client's perceptions. What are the current symptoms? When and how often do they occur? What is the intensity? What makes them worse? Better?

Tests and Measures

Observation of skin condition, color, presence or absence of hair, and condition of toenails are documented in some detail. Individuals with arterial insufficiency often have dry, scaly skin, no hair on the lower leg, and thick toenails (Fig. 2.2). Toes may be clubbed. Skin temperature is not a good indicator of arterial insufficiency because many conditions, many of which are benign,

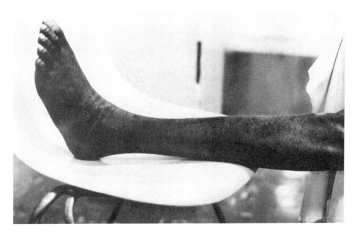

FIGURE 2.2
Leg showing arterial dysvascularity.

contribute to cold skin. The presence or absence of lower extremity pulses is noted. Collateral circulation, developed over time, may provide adequate circulation to the lower extremity even in the absence of pulses in the major vessels.

If the client has an ulcer, record the size and depth, location, amount, and color of drainage. There are many ways to document wound size; commercially available grids on acetate or sterile x-ray film can be put over the wound and traced or photographed. Depth of wound can be measured with a sterile cotton-tipped applicator.[21] Sterile techniques should be used when measuring an ulcer.

Although edema is more often associated with chronic venous insufficiency, clients with ASO may have edema related to local inflammation, associated venous disease, congestive heart disease, renal or kidney problems, or prolonged dependent position of a limb. Edema is easily documented by taking circumferential girth measurements at regular and documented intervals. Edema, particularly in the foot, can also be measured with a volumeter. The volumeter is filled with water, the foot is placed in the Plexiglas device, and the displaced water is collected in a graduated cylinder. Both limbs should be measured for comparison.

Clients with diabetes frequently exhibit decreased sensation in the foot, ankle, and possibly the lower leg. Light touch and sharp/dull differentiations are the most important sensory tests to perform. Proprioception and vibratory sense may also be impaired.

Inactivity, edema, and musculoskeletal changes may lead to decreases in range of motion (ROM) of the toes and foot that, in turn, may affect pressures generated in the shoe during ambulation. Careful goniometric measurement of all ranges of ankle motion and determination of foot and ankle strength are important parts of the examination. These parameters of both lower extremities will give an indication of the client's functional level for mobility.

Many individuals do not wear properly fitted shoes; careful examination of the client's footwear is part of the basic examination of any individual with vascular disease. Some people cannot afford proper shoes and may need to be guided in choosing special shoes to prevent ulcers. Foot problems and protective shoes are explored in greater detail in Chapter 3.

Medical Examination of Chronic Venous Insufficiency

Chronic venous disease is classified into three grades (Table 2.3). The cause of venous ulcers, a characteristic of grade III, has not been well defined. Bowse and Burnand[22] suggest that venous ulceration is related to the proliferation of venous capillaries and the increased fibrins in the fluid leaking into the interstitial space. Venous ulcers are characteristically found just proximal to the medial malleolus, where the lower three major perforating veins are located and the greatest hydrostatic pressure is concentrated when the person is in the upright position. Fluid leakage into the interstitial tissues is probably greatest in this area. Prior to the development of an ulcer, the skin usually becomes dark brown, subcutaneous fat becomes indurated, and there may be dermatitis and evidence of inflammation as well as edema. Venous ulcers are shallow and weepy with ill-defined borders.[15,22]

In contrast venography, dye is injected into the vein and radiographs are taken of the limb; it is the most accurate method of evaluating the veins. However, noninvasive tests that include the multilevel tourniquet test, plethysmography, Doppler examination, and duplex imaging are almost as accurate. The multilevel tourniquet test involves placing tourniquets in the upper and lower thigh, upper calf, and above the malleoli with the client in the supine position. The client then stands and the tourniquets are removed from the bottom up. Superficial and deep vein competence is determined by the degree of filling of the lesser and greater saphenous veins.[15]

There are two major types of plethysmography, a measure of blood flow; impedence plethysmography uses changes in voltage generated by blood flow as a reflection of volume. Air plethymosgraphy graphs the length of time it

TABLE 2.3 CVI CLASSIFICATION

Grade	Symptoms
I	Mild episodes of edema during upright activity, which resolve easily with rest and limb elevation.
	Edema, limited to the foot and possibly the ankle, is usually <1 cm.
	No changes are seen in skin condition or pigmentation.
II	Varicosities may be observable.
	Edema in foot and ankle >1 cm, which may not resolve with limb elevation.
	Client complains of heavy aching sensation with prolonged standing.
	Evidence of beginning changes in pigmentation in lower leg.
	Beginning induration of the skin.
III	Severe thick edema extending to midcalf.
	Client complains of heavy aching pain after short periods of standing.
	Dark brown pigmentation in the lower leg and ankle.
	Evidence of skin induration, dermatitis, and eczema of the lower leg.
	Weepy, shallow ulcer proximal to the medial malleolus.

takes for a vein to refill after its flow is cut off by a pneumatic cuff placed proximally on the limb.

Doppler has been previously described. The Doppler ultrasound head is placed over the vein being evaluated while the examiner squeezes the limb proximally. Changes in the flow sound reflect valve function. If the valves are functioning properly, there should be no increase in blood flow. PTs can use small portable Doppler machines for arterial or venous evaluation.[8,15,23]

Duplex ultrasound imaging provides a computer picture of the superficial and deep veins and the perforating system generated by ultrasound waves. It also images the arterial system, making it a flexible evaluation tool for the physician.[24,25]

Physical Therapy Examination of CVI

Clients with CVI may be referred to physical therapy for treatment of edema or ulcerations. The physical therapy examination includes a thorough history and patient interview to determine the current status of the symptoms and the client's ability to function in daily life. It is important to know if the edema is relieved overnight, if the client wears elastic stockings, and if the client can elevate the legs during the day. Circumferential limb measurements provide objective data for determining the effects of treatment. Measurements are taken at regular intervals (usually every 2.5 to 4 cm) for the whole limb segment (Fig. 2.3). Bony landmarks are used as reference points

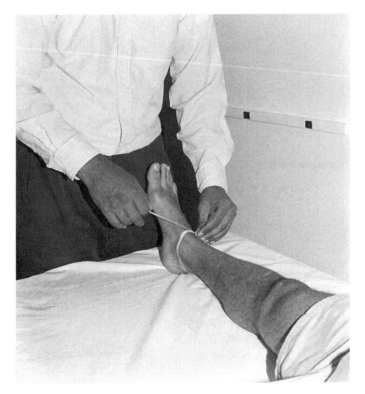

FIGURE 2.3
Taking circumferential measurements of a leg.

for each measurement (for example, 4 cm above the medial malleolus). Foot measurements need to be taken as well, usually around the head of the metatarsals, at a measured midpoint of the foot, and around the heel at the most distal point.

Although edema usually does not interfere with strength, it may limit range of ankle motion, and goniometric measurements may be necessary. The condition of the skin must be noted and the presence of ulceration documented. It is valuable to inspect the client's shoes. Foot edema leads many to wear slippers or other loose-fitting shoes that may hamper gait and may fail to protect the foot from injury. Pain is assessed in terms of its severity and when it occurs. Venous pain must be differentiated from arterial pain. Pain associated with CVI occurs after prolonged standing and is reported as a dull ache and heaviness in the lower leg. It is relieved by elevation of the legs. In contrast, arterial insufficiency leads to a sharp cramping pain of the calf. It occurs either at night or with walking. As with any other client, information on the person's understanding of the disease process, lifestyle demands, and expectations are a necessary part of the examination.

Case Studies

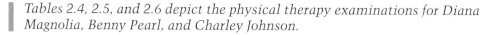

Tables 2.4, 2.5, and 2.6 depict the physical therapy examinations for Diana Magnolia, Benny Pearl, and Charley Johnson.

■ *Case Study Activities*

Determine prognosis and outcome goals for each client based on the information provided.

1 Develop a plan of intervention for each client.
2 During a laboratory session, practice any test and measurement or treatment procedure with which you are not familiar.

Management

Arterial Disease

Improvement of arterial circulation is the major goal of medical and surgical management. Surgical interventions used to improve peripheral circulation include reconstruction such as femoropopliteal bypass, balloon angioplasty, and **endarterectomy.** The greater saphenous vein, reversed to prevent interference with blood flow by the valves, is generally used for femoropopliteal bypasses, although synthetic conduits may also be used. Balloon angioplasty involves insertion of a catheter with a balloon tip inflated to the appropriate level to stretch and open the artery as it passes through. Endarectomy involves removing some of the plaque material that has accumulated inside an artery. A longitudinal study in Maryland in 1988 and 1989 revealed that, of 7210 procedures performed for peripheral arterial disease, 1185 were angioplasties, 4005 were bypasses, and 1890 were amputations. Individuals treated initially by revascularization procedures tended to be white men younger

TABLE 2.4   PHYSICAL THERAPY EXAMINATION—DIANA MAGNOLIA

HISTORY:
IDDM diagnosed 15 years ago; has always been poorly controlled; height 5′6″ weight 210 lb.
Past medical history includes hypertension and arteriosclerosis; other past medical history
noncontributory. She has not previously had an ulcer. She is followed in general medicine
clinic and goes to a podiatrist to have her toenails clipped. She is followed in the eye clinic
for early developing cataracts.

SOCIAL:
Ms. Magnolia is a waitress who lives in a small rented house in a rural town with two of her
grown children (one other child is in the Army out of the country). She spends a great deal of
time on her feet. She has no hobbies. She has medical insurance (not Major Medical,
however) through her employment. Denies the use of alcohol; smokes about 1 pack/day.

SYSTEMS REVIEW:
Noncontributory other than as noted below.

MEDICATIONS:
Insulin, 40 U daily; furosemide; and hydralazine

EXAMINATION:
Sensation:
Decreased to light touch and sharp/dull differentiation on left from below malleoli. Minimal
sensation in toes and forefoot. Decreased on right from toes to malleoli with minimal
sensation on medial border of first metatarsal. Both lower extremities are relatively hairless
from about midcalf down. The skin of the left leg is shiny particularly in the distal third of
the lower leg. The nail of the left great toe is thickened and discolored. Pedal pulses
bilaterally are absent to palpation. Both feet are cool to touch.
   Ulcer on left foot is 2.5 cm diameter; relatively shallow; no evidence of granulous tissue
and no drainage. The tissue around the ulcer is white and calloused. The tissue within the
ulcer is pinkish red. She has had the ulcer for about 6 wk.

ROM:
Left ankle: plantar flexion: active = 0°–20°; passive = 0°–25°; dorsiflexion: active = 0°
of neutral; passive = + 5°; inversion and eversion: active = 0°–5°; passive = 0°–10°.
   Left knee and hip within normal limits active and passive.
   Right ankle: plantar flexion: active and passive = 0°–25°; dorsiflexion: active and
passive = 0°– +5°; inversion and eversion active and passive = 0°–10°.
   Right hip and knee are within normal limits active and passive.

Edema:
No differences in girth noted between the lower extremities from patella tendon to 2 cm
above malleoli. Left leg is 1.5 cm larger at 2 cm above malleoli and 2 cm greater at malleoli.

Muscle Strength:
Left lower extremity dorsiflexion = Fair (3/5); plantar flexion = Fair+ (3+/5);
eversion/inversion = Poor+ (2+/5). Right lower extremity ankle musculature is Good (4/5).
   Rest of the musculature of both lower extremities is within normal limits. General body
strength appears to be within normal limits.

Pain:
Denies pain in the ulcer area. Cramping pain in the arch of her left foot interferes with
walking long distances. Occasional cramping pain at night.

FUNCTIONAL ACTIVITIES:
Patient walks without external support. Wears old loafers and socks on both feet. A gauze
pad covers the ulcer. No gait deviations. Ms. Magnolia states that she is independent in self-
care activities.

TABLE 2.5 PHYSICAL THERAPY EXAMINATION–BENNY PEARL

HISTORY:

Prior to surgery right ankle/brachial Doppler index was 0.4; segmental plethysmography indicated a significant obstruction between the upper and lower thigh. Arteriography showed a complete occlusion of the superficial femoral artery with fair collateral flow below the occlusion. History of chronic obstructive pulmonary disease (COPD), CAD. Prior to surgery, he was unable to walk more than 10 m before having pain in the right calf and foot.

SOCIAL:

Mr. Pearl and his wife live in a small frame house on the outskirts of town. They have three grown children in other parts of the country. Mr. Pearl owns and operates a service station in town. Mrs. Pearl works part-time as an LPN in a nearby hospital. In the months before surgery, he found it increasingly difficult to walk and work.

Smokes about 2 packs/day.

MEDICATION:

Nifedipine, warfarin, captopril, propoxyphene with acetaminophen, and furosemide.

EXAMINATION:

The physical examination was somewhat difficult to perform because Mr. Pearl had some difficulty following instructions and seemed a bit confused. Findings are subject to reevaluation at a later date.

Vitals:

BP, 145/95; respiration, 16; pulse, 90 at the beginning of the evaluation.

Skin:

Appears to have relatively normal sensation throughout both lower extremities. Both legs have little hair, skin is normal in appearance and warm. There is a dressing in the anterior groin area extending to the medial thigh on the right and the sutures are in place. There is no draining from the incisions.

Edema:

No evidence of edema in the lower extremities.

ROM:

On gross evaluation, the left lower extremity appears actively and passively within normal limits. Ankle ROM is grossly within normal limits. Mr. Pearl can move the right leg but full ROM testing was delayed.

Muscle Strength:

Muscle strength of the left lower extremity was grossly within normal limits. Muscle testing on the right was delayed secondary to surgery and the risk of stressing the incision. Mr. Pearl can tolerate manual resistance for ankle motions.

Pain:

Pain reported at the incision site is 4 on 0–10 scale. Mr. Pearl is afraid the bypass won't work.

FUNCTIONAL ACTIVITIES:

Mr. Pearl appears a little confused and is not a clear historian. Chart review indicates that he has not stood since surgery and cannot get from bed to chair by himself. He was able to turn from left side to back in bed. Mr. Pearl needed moderate physical help from the therapist to transfer in and out of bed into the wheelchair and step-by-step cueing. He put minimal weight on his right leg, was hesitant to try to help himself, and was slow in following directions. He made minimal attempts to wheel the chair himself despite encouragement. He appeared to tire quickly and said he wanted to go back to bed.

TABLE 2.6   PHYSICAL THERAPY EXAMINATION—CHARLEY JOHNSON

HISTORY:
Mr. Johnson reports having had varicose veins and venous problems for many years. Denies any other medical problems. Rest of system review is noncontributory.

SOCIAL:
Mr. Johnson is a textile worker who has been referred because he can no longer spend a full day standing at his machine. He is currently on sick leave from his job. He has 2 wk of sick leave credit left. He is covered by a Blue Cross/Blue Shield policy through his plant. Mr. Johnson is married with six children ranging in age from 17 to 39; two are living at home. His wife also works at the textile mill and the 17-yr-old daughter works after school and on weekends at Smith Drugs. The Johnsons live in a small wooden house which they own. Mr. Johnson used to work weekends as a security guard but had to stop about 1 mo ago because of his legs. Mr Johnson denies smoking or using alcohol.

EXAMINATION:
Height 5'7"; weight 185 lb.

Skin:
Right lower extremity: Area approximately 9.5 cm long and 6 cm wide is red, weeping and beginning to give evidence of ulceration. Dark purplish brown ring about 4 cm wide around the ulceration, which is covered with a thickened, desensitized skin. Decreased sensation all around the lower leg and proximal foot. Sensation around the toes and knee appears relatively normal. No hair on the right lower extremity below the knee.

Edema:
Edema evident in both lower extremities, greater on the right. Right ankle around malleoli = 30.5 cm, left = 28 cm; 2 in above medial malleoli = 32 cm both sides; circumference around head of metatarsals: right = 31.5 cm; left= 29 cm.

Left lower extremity: Some discoloration just above the medial malleoli with decreased sensation. Sensation is relatively normal around the toes and knee. No hair below the knee. When the patient stands for several minutes, the skin of both lower legs around the ankles and feet becomes a deeper purple.

ROM:
All ranges of motion of both lower extremities are within normal limits except as follows (active and passive ranges are the same):

	L	R
Dorsiflexion active and passive	0–9	0–3
Plantar flexion active and passive	0–15	0–10
Eversion active and passive	0–5	0–5
Inversion active and passive	0–10	0–5

Muscle Strength:
Musculature around both ankles is in the Fair+ (3+/5) range; rest of the lower extremity is in the Good to Good+ range (4+/5). Upper extremity strength appears to be within normal limits.

Pain:
Pain in the right lower extremity after standing for 15–20 min. Some pain in the left lower extremity but not as severe. Discolored areas in both legs itch frequently and severely. The itching is temporarily relieved by elevating the legs or soaking the feet in cold water.

FUNCTIONAL ACTIVITIES:
Mr. Johnson denies smoking or drinking alcoholic beverages. He states that he is independent in all self-care activities. He walked into the department using a cane in his right hand and taking a shorter step with the right leg. He is wearing black slippers and black socks.

than age 74 with Medicare or private insurance. The incidence of diabetes and hypertension, positively related to the likelihood of amputation, was significantly greater in African-Americans.[26] An Illinois study of 19,250 procedures performed during 18,603 admissions at 105 Illinois hospitals determined that severity of comorbidity such as diabetes and gangrene as well as socioeconomic status and race influenced whether revascularization or bypass procedures would be done for severe peripheral vascular problems. The average annual amputation rate was 20.77 per 100,000, femorodistal bypass rate was 24.26 per 100,000, and aortoiliac bypass was 4.70 per 100,000. A significantly greater percentage of amputations were performed on individuals in low-income areas and zip codes with large or medium African-American populations. The authors also reported that treatment at a university teaching hospital and male gender increased the odds of undergoing bypass procedures.[27] Individuals undergoing revascularization procedures are not routinely referred to physical therapy.

The major goals of physical therapy are to promote healing of any ulcer or wound, prevent further injury, and educate the client on the proper care of the extremities and on methods of enhancing the development of collateral circulation. Deficiencies in strength or ROM must be addressed. (See Chap. 3 for details of wound and ulcer care.) Education is an important part of the care of individuals with peripheral vascular disease (Table 2.7). Long-term care includes promoting the development of collateral circulation through an active

TABLE 2.7   CLIENT EDUCATION PROGRAMS

Category	Arteriosclerosis	Venous Insufficiency
Disease process	Pathophysiology in simple terms; general prognosis; how pathology can be improved; what can increase problems; answer specific questions.	
Foot and leg care	Keep feet and legs clean and dry. Apply water-absorbing lotion on dry skin, particularly after bath. Check feet daily for pressure areas. Wear supportive shoes; do not walk barefoot or with open shoes. Keep full ROM in feet and ankles. Trim toenails straight across and guard against injury; obtain professional help for problem nails.	Ankle pumps and toe motions for edema control. Elevate feet and legs regularly. Wear support stockings if prescribed. Use water-absorbing lotion on dry skin; do not use alcohol on skin. Do not scratch irritated skin. Watch for ulcer development.
Pain management	For intermittent claudication: Start a walking or bicycling program. Exercise to the point of cramping, stop and rest a moment, then resume. Exercise regularly, gradually increasing time or distance. For rest pain: Elevate head of bed; wear socks to bed; no heating pads on legs but can apply to abdomen on low heat.	Wear support stocking when standing. Stop and do ankle pumps with legs at level of heart several times a day. When sitting, keep legs elevated at level of heart. Raise foot of bed.
Lifestyle	Discuss smoking, nutrition, stress, activity level. Help client identify problem areas and find solutions.	Discuss edema control, effects of prolonged standing, effects of air temperature, use of support stockings. Help client identify problem areas and find solutions.

exercise program. Walking is excellent for individuals with arterial insufficiency. They can increase their ambulatory capabilities by walking to the point of intermittent claudication, stopping until the cramp ceases, and then walking again.[28–32] For individuals with active ulcers whose weight bearing is limited, a program of active exercises can be substituted.

Venous Diseases

The primary goal in both the medical and physical therapy management of CVI is to control venous hypertension and reduce edema. Education in proper skin care and in methods of preventing the development or recurrence of ulcers is essential. The desired outcome of treatment is not the healing of the ulcer but the prevention of further ulcers.[12] CVI cannot be cured; therefore, lifestyle changes are necessary for effective management.

The major treatment of the venous ulcer is compression using semirigid dressing, elastic stockings or wraps, or intermittent compression. Compression is believed to reduce venous hypertension by blocking transcapillary flow during contraction, thereby increasing the flow out of the deep veins. The amount of pressure needed to achieve such reduction increases with the severity of the disease. Semirigid dressings such as the Unna's boot (Miles Pharmaceutical), a zinc-impregnated semiocclusive dressing, provide wound care and compression together. The rigid dressing helps protect the limb from injury. The disadvantages are the need for frequent reapplication by a health professional, potential problems of personal hygiene, and occasional reactions to the medication. Other forms of compression bandaging may also be used. A recent study conducted in the United Kingdom, indicated that 74 percent of a sample population with venous leg ulcers treated with compression dressing healed within 26 weeks. Delayed or nonhealing was related to large ulcers, previous DVT, or previous ulceration.[33]

Standard postsurgical stockings offer uniform elastic compression from foot to knee or upper thigh; there are also individually constructed elastic stockings that provide graded compression. Knee-high custom-made elastic stockings have been shown to be effective in the treatment of CVI.[14,34] Thigh-high stockings may bind in the popliteal area and are difficult to keep in place. Most clients require compression at ankle level but rarely above the knee. Clients should be given two pairs of stockings at a time that should be replaced whenever they lose their elasticity. Clients need to be taught proper donning procedures and care of the stockings. Companies that manufacture the stockings generally provide care information to the client. If an ulcer is present, a dressing under the stocking provides extra compression to the area and keeps the stocking relatively clean. PTs and PTAs use kits available from the manufacturers to measure an individual for compression stockings. The limb needs to be measured after attempts to reduce edema through intermittent compression and elevation. It is generally advisable to measure clients for elastic stockings in the morning when edema is less.

Elastic stockings are difficult to put on; many elderly people, particularly individuals with limited hand function, find it impossible to properly don the stockings. Elastic bandages can be substituted although they are less effective. Although easier to apply, the elastic wrap loses its elasticity quickly, needs to be wrapped properly to provide appropriate pressure, must be rewrapped frequently, and occupies more space in the shoe than the stocking.

Elastic wraps need to be applied starting with the toes and follow a figure-of-eight pattern up the leg to just below the popliteal area. Overlapping the edges by at least 1 inch helps prevent skin exposure as the wrap changes position with client activity. For most clients, two 10-cm (4-inch) bandages will be needed. Compliance with the use of elastic wraps is usually poor.

Proper skin care is important for individuals with venous disease as well as for those with arterial insufficiency. Water-soluble lotion is recommended; it will not stain elastic stockings and usually feels more comfortable to the client.

Intermittent compression is an effective tool to reduce edema (Fig. 2.4). Intermittent or sequential pumps may be used. The limb is covered with stockinet prior to insertion in the inflatable sleeve. Any ulcer must be covered with a plastic bag. The client needs to be comfortably positioned in supine. Pressure is usually set to no more than 20 mm Hg less than diastolic, and it should never exceed the client's diastolic pressure; settings as low as 40 mm Hg have been found effective.[21] There are no studies outlining the effectiveness of any one on-off ratio. Generally 60 seconds on and 30 seconds off is used, although McCulloch and Hovde[23] recommend 90 seconds on and 30 seconds off. Treatments are generally 1 hour or longer. There are small home units clients can use for daily treatment. Prior to the implementation of compression therapy, the client's arterial status needs to be evaluated. Compression therapy should generally be avoided if the ABI is greater than 0.75.

Standing or sitting for prolonged periods contributes to edema. Clients need to sit or lie frequently with the legs elevated to about heart level. Al-

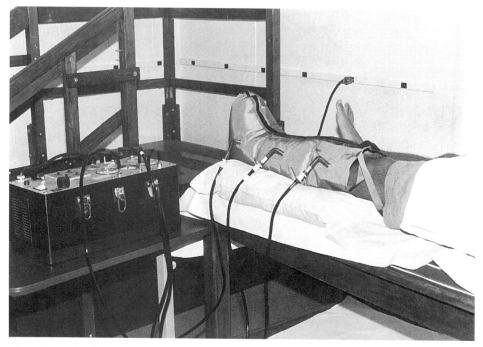

FIGURE 2.4
Applying intermittent compression to the leg.

though elevation to 45 or 50 degrees is advisable for the management of edema secondary to lymphatic disease, it is not recommended for CVI because it places too much stress on an already compromised system. Active ankle exercises are an important adjunct to the rest of the program. Muscle contraction contributes to pumping blood toward the heart in the deep venous system. The client is taught to do flexion, extension, and circumduction of the ankle slowly through the full ROM several times a day, particularly when supine. General active exercises including walking are not contraindicated and may be beneficial. Walking is a good activity for individuals with CVI, particularly if proper elastic support is worn. Walking activates the muscle pump action in the lower leg. However, individuals with both PAOD and CVI may have some difficulty with a vigorous walking program. The client should wear elastic stockings at all times when exercising and may need to spend some time lying supine following exercises to prevent or control edema.

Summary

Most clients treated for major amputations of the lower limb have some form of vascular disease. Although CVI is not a primary cause of amputation, individuals with arterial disease may also have venous insufficiency. PTs and PTAs must integrate the care of the vascular disease and the remaining extremity into the total care of the individual with a lower extremity amputation.

Glossary

Arteriosclerosis	A thickening, hardening, and narrowing of the walls of the arteries.
Atherosclerosis	A form of arteriosclerosis in which plaques composed of lipids and other materials form on the intima of the arteries.
Doppler	A noninvasive method of detecting changes in blood flow through an artery.
Embolus	A clot or mass of foreign materials that obstructs a vein or artery. An embolus may be a part of a thrombus that has broken off and traveled to a vessel too small to allow passage.
Endarterectomy	Surgical removal of the lining of an artery. May be performed on major arteries to increase blood flow.
Neuropathy	Any disease of the nervous system.
PAOD	Peripheral arterial occlusive disease.
Thrombus	A clot made of blood and other materials that forms and attaches to the walls of an artery or vein.

References

1. Most, RS, and Sinnock, P: The epidemiology of lower extremity amputations in diabetic individuals. Diabetes Care 6:87–91, 1983.
2. Graor, RA, and Bartholomew, JR: Deep vein thrombosis. In Young, JR, et al (eds): Peripheral Vascular Diseases. Mosby Year Book, St. Louis, 1991.
3. Young, JR: Clinical clues to peripheral vascular disease. In Young, JR, et al (eds): Peripheral Vascular Diseases. Mosby Year Book, St. Louis, 1991.
4. Graor, RA, and Bartholomew, JR: Pulmonary embolism. In Young, JR, et al (eds): Peripheral Vascular Diseases. Mosby Year Book, St. Louis,1991.
5. Hull, RD, et al: Clinical validity of a negative venogram in patients with clinically suspected venous thrombosis. Circulation 64:622, 1981.
6. Kafie, FE, and Williams, RA: Venous disease in the elderly. In Aronow, WS, et al (eds): Vascular Disease in the Elderly. Futura Publishing, Armonk, NY, 1997.
7. Comerota, AJ, and Leefmans, E: Acute arterial occlusions. In Young, JR, et al (eds): Peripheral Vascular Diseases. Mosby Year Book, St. Louis,1991.
8. MacKinnon, J: Doppler ultrasound examination in peripheral vascular disease. In Kloth, LC, et al (eds): Wound Healing: Alternatives in Management. FA Davis, Philadelphia, 1990.
9. Laird, JR: Pharmacologic therapies in the treatment of peripheral vascular disease: Clinical experience with reteplase, a third-generation thrombolytic. J Invas Cardiol 12(Suppl B):27B–32B, 2000.
10. Gordon, IL: Infrainguinal arterial occlusive disease in the elderly. In Aronow, WS, et al (eds): Vascular Disease in the Elderly. Futura Publishing, Armonk, NY, 1997.
11. Krajewski, LP, and Olin, JW: Atherosclerosis of the aorta and lower extremities arteries. In Young, JR, et al (eds): Peripheral Vascular Diseases. Mosby Year Book, St. Louis, 1991.
12. Reiber, GE, et al (eds): Risk factors for amputation in patients with diabetes mellitus: A case-control study. Ann Intern Med 117:97–105, 1992.
13. Browse, NL, et al (eds): Diseases of the Veins: Pathology, Diagnosis and Treatment. Edward Arnold, London, 1988.
14. Widmer, LK: Peripheral venous disorders: Prevalence and sociomedical importance—observations in 4529 apparently healthy persons, Basic III Study. Hans Huber, Bern, Switzerland, 1978.
15. O'Donnell, TF, Jr: Chronic venous insufficiency and varicose veins. In Young, JR, et al (eds): Peripheral Vascular Diseases. Mosby Year Book, St. Louis, 1991.
16. Joyce, JW: Thomboangiitis obliterans (Buerger's disease). In Young, JR, et al (eds): Peripheral Vascular Diseases. Mosby Year Book, St. Louis, 1991.
17. Kannel, WB, and McGee, DL: Update on some epidemiologic features of intermittent claudication: The Framingham study. J Am Geriatr Soc 33, 13, 1985.
18. Fowkes, FG, et al: Smoking, lipids, glucose intolerance, and blood pressure as risk factors for peripheral atherosclerosis compared with ischemic heart disease in the Edinburgh Artery Study. Am J Epidemiol 135(4):331–340, 1992.
19. Lakier, JB: Smoking and cardiovascular disease. Am J Med 93(1A):8S–12S, 1992.
20. APTA: Guide to Physical Therapist Practice. Alexandria, Va., July, 1999.
21. McCulloch, JM, and Kloth, LC: Evaluation of patients with open wounds. In Kloth, LC, et al (eds): Wound Healing: Alternatives in Management. FA Davis, Philadelphia, 1990.
22. Browse, NL, and Burnand, KG: The cause of venous ulceration. Lancet 2:243–245, 1982.
23. McCulloch, JM, and Hovde, J: Treatment of wounds due to vascular problems. In Kloth, LC, et al (eds): Wound Healing: Alternatives in Management. FA. Davis, Philadelphia, 1990.
24. Barnes, RW: Noninvasive tests for chronic venous insufficiency. In Bergan, JJ, and Yao, JST (eds): Surgery of the Veins. Grune & Stratton, Philadelphia, 1985.
25. Talbot, SR: Use of real time imaging in identifying deep venous obstruction: A preliminary report. Bruit 6:41, 1982.
26. Flanagan, LD, et al: Venous imaging of the extremities using real time B-mode ultrasound. In Bergan, JJ, and Yao, JST (eds): Surgery of the Veins. Grune & Stratton, Philadelphia, 1985.
27. Feinglass, J, et al: Peripheral bypass surgery and amputation: Northern Illinois demographics, 1993 to 1997. Arch Surg 135(1):75–80, 2000.
28. Tunis, SR, et al: Variation in utilization of procedures for treatment of peripheral arterial disease: A look at patient characteristics. Arch Intern Med 153:991–998, 1993.
29. Kloth, LC, et al: Wound Healing: Alternatives in Management. FA Davis, Philadelphia, 1990.

30. McCulloch, J: Peripheral vascular disease. In O'Sullivan, SB, and Schmitz, TJ (eds): Physical Rehabilitation: Assessment and Treatment, ed 2. FA Davis, Philadelphia, 1988.
31. Wong, RA: Chronic dermal wounds in older adults. In Guccione, AA (ed): Geriatric Physical Therapy, ed 2. Mosby, St. Louis, 2000.
32. Weiss, T, et al: Effect of intensive walking exercises on skeletal muscle blood flow in intermittent claudication. Angiology 43:63–71, 1992.
33. Guest, M, et al: Venous ulcer healing by four-layer compression bandaging is not influenced by the pattern of venous incompetence. Br J Surg 86(11):1437–40, 1999.
34. Burnand, KG, and Layer, G: Graduated elastic stockings. Br Med J 293:224–225, 1986.

CHAPTER THREE

The Diabetic Foot

Jeffrey S. Dowling, MHE, PT

Updated by Bella J. May, EdD, PT, FAPTA

OBJECTIVES

At the end of this chapter all students are expected to:

1 Identify risk factors leading to foot ulceration.
2 Describe how specific risk factors among individuals with diabetes lead to foot dysfunction.
3 Discuss the importance of education in the prevention of ulceration or reulceration.
4 Describe the key elements of the treatment program.

In addition, physical therapy students are expected to:

5 Develop an examination plan for a client at risk for ulceration or a client with an existing ulceration.
6 Establish functional outcomes for clients at various stages of ulceration.
7 Design a plan of care for clients at various stages of ulceration.
8 Select the appropriate practice patterns for patients with foot problems.

Case Study

Gladys Greene, a 63-year-old woman with a long history of diabetes, is referred to physical therapy for whirlpool and ***debridement*** of a chronic forefoot ulcer (more than 4 months in duration) on the plantar aspect of her right foot. She has been coming for outpatient treatment three times a week for the past 3 weeks. She walks into the department bearing full weight on the right lower extremity with no evidence of pain. Her foot is wrapped in a clean dressing with no signs of infection. She wears a house slipper on her right foot and a tennis shoe on her left. Her forefoot ulcer has remained essentially unchanged over the course of nine treatments.

■ *Case Study Activities*

1 What are the risk factors that may lead to foot dysfunction?
2 Determine which risk factors appear to be contributing to the persistent nature of Ms. Greene's forefoot plantar ulcer.

PATHOPHYSIOLOGY

Ms. Greene's medical record indicates the presence of peripheral vascular disease, although recent studies did not indicate the need for reconstructive surgery. The persistent nature of her forefoot ulcer is apparently related to other factors. Individuals with diabetes have a 15 percent chance of developing an ulceration of the foot or ankle during the course of the disease, either secondary to peripheral vascular disease or because peripheral **neuropathy** leads to changes in sensation and proprioception.[1,2] The foot ulcer, also called *mal perforans ulcer*, is the most common type of lesion; nearly 90 percent occur in the plantar forefoot region.[3,4] The etiology is unknown, but risk factors include mechanical stress, vascular disease, and poorly controlled diabetes. Approximately 57 to 94 percent of ulcers heal completely depending on the extent of involvement; however, ulcers place the foot at serious risk for infection and **gangrene.**[5] Early detection through thorough and frequent inspection of the feet is extremely important. However, it is predicted that most individuals with diabetes will have some sort of foot problem during their lifetimes.[2] Prompt and aggressive treatment can enhance healing and limit exacerbation.

Neuropathy

Neuropathy with some degree of sensory, autonomic, and motor involvement is a major cause of diabetic foot lesions.[2,6] The etiology may be related to the metabolic abnormalities of diabetes. The most common form is distal symmetrical sensorimotor polyneuropathy.

Sensory Neuropathy

Sensory neuropathy is the most important neuropathic risk factor, especially when it involves the small sensory fibers of pain and temperature. The individual develops an insensitive foot vulnerable to trauma. Sensory neuropathy typically has a stocking-glove type distribution involving the entire extremity distal to the knee. The severity of sensory loss is greatest distally, leaving the toes more susceptible to trauma than the ankle or leg, respectively. With a decreased ability to feel pain, the individual may repeatedly traumatize the tissue to the point of ulceration.

Autonomic Neuropathy

Neuropathic involvement of the postganglionic sympathetic fibers to the sweat glands is common. Clinical evaluation reveals dry, noncompliant skin that cracks and splits easily, leaving **fissures** that are difficult to heal and act as portals for infection. The skin is also susceptible to **callus** formation under weight-bearing areas. A thick callus over a bony prominence increases plantar pressures, resulting in a greater risk for pressure **necrosis** and ulceration.[7] Peripheral sympathetic neuropathy (Charcot foot) may result in demineralization and weakening of the bone and, with repetitive painless trauma, may lead to fracture and deformity.[8] Early signs of bony involvement or fracture are prominent dorsal veins, edema, and increased skin temperature.

Motor Neuropathy

Motor neuropathy frequently contributes to toe deformities. Dysfunction of the intrinsic muscles results in clawing of the lesser toes with hyperextension of the metatarsophalangeal joints and flexion of the proximal interphalangeal joints. Metatarsophalangeal hyperextension depresses the metatarsal heads, increasing the pressure beneath them and contributing to the forces that produce the classic mal perforans ulceration of the forefoot[9] (Fig. 3.1). The flexion contracture at the proximal interphalangeal joint can cause pressure of the toe against the toe box of the shoe leading to dorsal ulceration. Motor neuropathy can also affect a single major proximal nerve, most often the common peroneal nerve. A significant muscular deficit, such as unilateral foot drop, may occur.

Mechanical Stress

The foot is subject to friction, pressure, and shear forces during activity. Friction is the force exerted by any surface moving over another surface; the smoother the surface, the less the friction. Constant fast friction over the skin may lead to blisters; constant, slow friction over the skin may lead to callus formation. Friction forces can be created by walking with a shoe that is too loose, causing the foot to slide on each step, or by a shoe that is too tight and creates sliding pressure over certain bony prominences. Pressure is the force

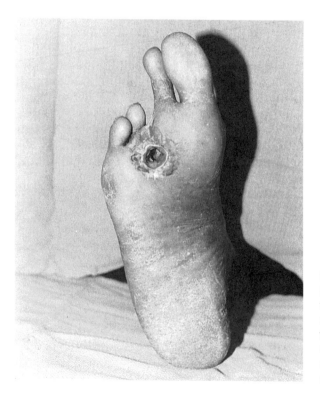

FIGURE 3.1

Mal perforans ulceration on a client with diabetes and severe peripheral neuropathy. Previous amputation of the third toe resulted in increased mechanical stress beneath the metatarsal head and the resultant ulcer formation.

created by the weight of one body on the other and is inversely proportional to the area supporting the weight; the greater the area, the less the pressure. Constant pressure over time leads to **ischemia** and tissue necrosis. An unfelt foreign object in the shoe can lead to pressure changes on the plantar surface of the foot. Walking barefoot and stepping on a sharp object will create the sudden high pressure that can lead to injury. Moderate intermittent pressure creates an inflammatory enzymatic autolysis rather than an ischemic necrosis because the blood supply is not continuously blocked.[10] The combination of friction and pressure forces created during walking are called *shear forces* and are believed to be those most responsible for tissue breakdown in the insensitive foot.[11] When ulceration occurs and subsequently heals, scarring prevents normal sliding of tissues leading to new ulcers.

Infection

Many factors may contribute to foot problems among individuals with diabetes. Prime considerations are the presence or absence of infection, neuropathy, or vascular insufficiency. Infection may precede or follow ulceration. Trauma to neuropathic or ischemic tissues can produce an ulcer that may become infected. Alternately, an individual can develop an infection that may cause an ulcer. An interdigital fissure or corn can lead to a large plantar space infection with necrotizing fasciitis. An ulcer will develop when the infection reaches the surface via a draining **sinus** or necrotic **bulla.** In either instance, infection frequently leads to microthrombi formation.[12] When the smaller, distal arteries of the foot are involved, gangrene of the toes is likely. An impaired vascular system also impairs the delivery of systemic antibiotics and oxygen to the involved tissues, making the treatment of infection more difficult. One of the major signs of early infection is an unexplained elevation of blood glucose level.

Ischemia

Chapter 2 outlines the basic concepts of peripheral vascular disease. Vascular disease with resultant circulatory insufficiency does not appear to be a primary cause of foot pathology among individuals with diabetes.[13] It does, however, contribute to tissue damage and compromised wound healing.

Other Factors

Body mass increases the pressure exerted against foot surfaces that may become critical in an insensitive foot. Limitations in joint mobility, particularly in the foot and ankle, can alter the normal biomechanical functions in gait and create excess pressure against bony prominences or soft tissue. Muscle weakness can also alter normal gait motions. The same factors could contribute to foot problems among individuals without diabetes; however, insensitivity or ischemia become critical factors that may change a minor problem into a major one.

Case Study

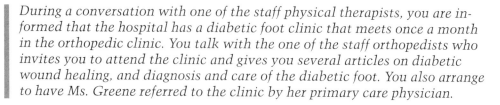

During a conversation with one of the staff physical therapists, you are informed that the hospital has a diabetic foot clinic that meets once a month in the orthopedic clinic. You talk with the one of the staff orthopedists who invites you to attend the clinic and gives you several articles on diabetic wound healing, and diagnosis and care of the diabetic foot. You also arrange to have Ms. Greene referred to the clinic by her primary care physician.

■ Case Study Activities

1   What are the dimensions of the examination process?
2   What tests and measures would you use to examine an individual with diabetes at risk for foot ulceration?
3   What practice pattern or patterns may be the most useful guide(s)?
4   Practice performing any tests and measures that may be new to you.

EXAMINATION

Several practice patterns may be useful in determining the best examination process for individuals with foot problems. Pattern 6B, multisystem impairments, 7B, and possibly 7C may be useful depending on the presence and scope of ulceration. Pattern 5F may also be useful if neuropathy is involved. The physical therapist (PT) needs to determine the applicability of multiple patterns.[14]

History

The first step in the physical therapy examination is a thorough history and systems review. The PT identifies the primary complaint, current associated symptoms, approximate date of onset, and events leading up to the foot problem. A history of similar complaints, previous ulcers, and amputations aids in determining the mechanism of injury and the effectiveness or ineffectiveness of past interventions. A long history of diabetes with previous ulcerations increases the risk of complications. The PT also determines the individual's understanding of diabetes and its impact on the lower extremities. A person who understands the risk factors related to foot dysfunction is usually more compliant with treatment. The PT and physical therapist assistant (PTA) also need to know the client's level of diabetic control. Although diabetic control is a specific concern of the physician, it is important that PTs and PTAs understand how diabetic control relates to the outcome of treatment. Inadequate control of blood glucose may interfere with normal white blood cell function, making the tissues more susceptible to infection. **Glycosylation** of structural proteins may occur in an individual with poor diabetic control.[15] Poor diabetic control may lead to renal failure, which is associated with thickening of the basement membranes and delayed healing.[16] The history and systems review must include information on other medical conditions such as hypertension or cardiac dysfunction. The history must include a review of lifestyle and habits. Work and leisure activities may contribute to foot problems, and the use of tobacco products and certain dietary practices are contributory.

Visual Inspection

The PT performs a thorough visual examination of the legs, ankles, and feet. Both shoes and socks are removed, and general overall appearance and any asymmetries are noted. Look for changes in color or texture of the skin, the presence of any deformities, and any ulcers. (See Chap. 2 for details on the vascular examination.)

Neurologic Examination

Sensory

Vibratory sense is usually the first function lost, followed by decreasing reflex activity, and finally loss of perception of pain and touch.[13] Pain sensation is one of the easiest to assess clinically by use of the Achilles squeeze test. The midpoint of the client's Achilles tendon is compressed between the examiner's index finger and thumb with moderate force. Patients without sensory neuropathy will feel pain, whereas the individual with significant sensory neuropathy will feel only pressure or nothing at all.[17]

Semmes–Weinstein monofilaments provide an easy and highly predictable method of assessment for touch sensation. The filaments are made of nylon (similar to fishing line) of various diameters set at right angles to an acrylic rod. The filaments are calibrated according to the number of grams of force required to bend them. Three filaments, 1 g, 10 g, and 75 g, are used in the assessment. The filament is applied to the plantar aspect of the foot with enough force to cause it to buckle. Perception of the 1-g monofilament is the threshold for normal sensation. The 10-g monofilament is the threshold for protective sensation, and the person with diabetes who can perceive this pressure is unlikely to sustain major foot trauma.[18] Perception of the 75-g monofilament or no perception at all indicates an increased risk for ulceration.

Motor

Standard muscle testing is used for static and dynamic strength examinations. Weakness within the foot results in deformities secondary to motor imbalance. Intrinsic weakness predisposes the foot to cavus and claw deformities. Peroneal nerve extrinsic weakness may result in an equino–adducto–varus deformity. Tibial nerve extrinsic weakness may result in a calcaneo–abducto–valgus deformity. A gross examination begins by having the client walk on the heels and then the toes; it is followed by a more detailed muscle examination as indicated by initial findings.

Vascular Examination

The femoral, popliteal, posterior tibial, and dorsalis pedis pulses are palpated; pulses are graded as 2+ = normal, 1+ = diminished, and 0 = absent. A significantly decreased or absent pulse is often associated with atherosclerotic disease.

Blanching the toe pulps with pressure by the fingertips assesses capillary refilling time from the arteriolar blood supply. The time taken for the return of normal color is counted in seconds. The normal range of refill is up to 3 seconds; longer refill time is considered delayed.

The most readily available and productive information about vascular integrity can be obtained through the use of a Doppler device. Doppler units can measure the vascular status by comparing the ratio of systolic blood pressure measurements in the foot and in the arm.[18] The units are small and portable and provide quick and objective measurements concerning the vascular supply (see Chap. 2).

Musculoskeletal Examination

A thorough and firm palpation of the foot is done. Palpation may reveal a plantar fascial inflammation in the presence of ulceration and possible infection; it is also an indicator of deep plantar space involvement. Palpation can help identify the amount of motion available in a particular joint. Limited motion may be the result of **neuroarthropathy** or soft-tissue scarring from previous inflammation and scarring.

Preulcer and Ulcer Examination

Injuries to the diabetic foot can be classified as either a potential ulceration (preulceration) or a complete ulceration. A preulceration is any undesirable change to the intact skin that left untreated would likely progress to a complete ulceration.[12] Preulcers exhibit any one or combination of the following changes: (1) an increase in temperature in a localized region in the absence of significant physical activity when compared to the contralateral foot or to that originally assessed; (2) maceration of the intra-epidermal layer, creating a boggy texture to the skin similar to that seen with an intact blister; or (3) a **hematoma** or **callus** with an underlying hematoma.

If the individual presents with a complete ulcer, the dimensions of the wound are measured, and the lesion is graded according to depth and tissue involved. Wound tracings on sterile acetate film may be more useful than diameter measurements if the borders are irregular (Fig. 3.2*A*). Serial drawings may be compared visually or digitized electronically to obtain area measurements. Photographs provide another means of documenting wound location and size. A cardinal sign of a deep ulcer that has penetrated a joint capsule is the production of a clear fluid with bubbles.

Ulcer Classification

The most widely accepted classification system for diabetic foot ulcers and lesions is based on the depth of penetration and extent of tissue necrosis. Six categories or grades range from 0 to 5. A grade of 0 is used to describe intact normal skin, grades 1 through 4 indicate progressive stages of tissue destruction, and grade 5 indicates extensive gangrene or necrosis with the need for amputation.[18]

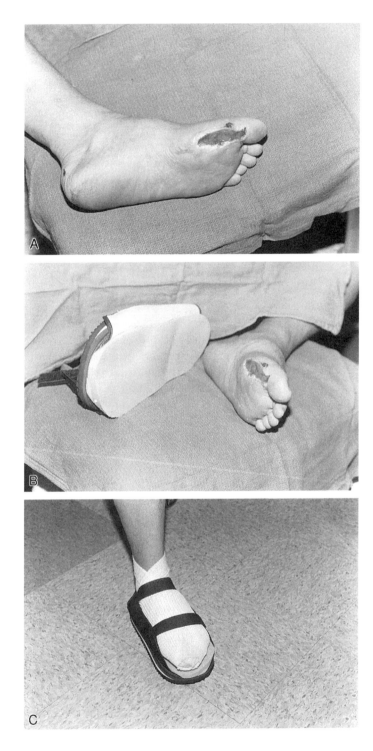

FIGURE 3.2

(*A*) Mal perforans ulceration beneath the first metatarsal head. (*B*) Plastizote liner contoured and bonded to a cast shoe to provide a pressure relief area beneath the first metatarsal head. (*C*) The client is encouraged to bear weight on the posterior aspect of the shoe to further decrease stress to the forefoot region.

TABLE 3.1 ULCER CLASSIFICATION SYSTEM

0	Absent skin lesions
1	Dense callus lesions but no preulcers or ulcers
2	Preulcerative changes
3	Partial-thickness (superficial) ulcer
4	Full-thickness (deep) ulcer but no involvement of tendon, bone, ligament, or joint
5	Full thickness (deep) ulcer with involvement of tendon, bone, ligament, or joint
6	Localized infection (abscess or osteomyelitis) in foot
7	Proximal spread of infection (ascending cellulitis or lymphadenopathy)
8	Gangrene of forefoot only
9	Gangrene of majority of foot

(Adapted from Sims, DS, et al: Risk factors in the diabetic foot: Recognition and management. Phys Ther 68(12): 1899, 1988, p 1899. Reprinted with permission of the American Physical Therapy Association.)

An alternate ulcer classification system to the Wagner system, which emphasizes surgical treatment, emphasizes the importance of early identification of foot problems in the prevention of plantar ulcers and the treatment of ulcerations nonsurgically (Table 3.1).[11]

Case Study

 The physical therapy examination for Ms. Gladys Greene is shown in Figure 3.3.

■ Case Study Activities

Physical Therapy Students:

1 Based on the findings, what are the functional outcomes for Ms. Greene?
2 Using the results of the evaluation, develop a plan of care for Ms. Greene.

Physical Therapist Assistant Students:

3 What do you think the goals of treatment will be?
4 What parts of the treatment program would you expect to have delegated to you?

MEDICAL MANAGEMENT

Revascularization

Initially, plantar ulcers may be treated with medical and nonsurgical techniques; however, if conservative approaches fail, revascularization surgery may be required.

HISTORY AND INTERVIEW:

- 63-year-old white female with adult-onset insulin-dependent diabetes diagnosed at age 36. Currently employed as a realtor. Ms. Greene lives independently in her own home with her husband. Three grown children, two grandchildren.

- Patient reports that her diabetes is reasonably well controlled with diet and daily injections of insulin.

- Previous medical history: Patient states that she has mild hypertension not requiring medication. Other medical history nonsignificant for this problem.

- Patient has had one previous ulcer about 2 years ago that resulted in the amputation of the second digit of the right foot. Patient states that she knows and understands proper foot and shoe care.

- Current medications: Rx: Insulin 40 units daily by injection; premarin 0.625 mg/day; OTC: vitamin C 500 mg and vitamin E 400 IU; calcium 1200 mg/day; aspirin 1/day.

- Chief complaint:

  - Nonhealing plantar ulcer right foot for about 2 months. No known trauma or injury.

TESTS AND MEASURES:

- BP 140/92; pulse (resting) 64; respirations normal.

- Observations: Right foot moderately edematous with slight increased temperature; flattened arch (rocker bottom appearance); hammertoe deformities of lesser toes; second digit abset with well-healed scar in web space; plantar ulceration first metatarsal head.

- Moderate amout serosanguinous drainage.

- Sensory: Lacks protective sensation plantar aspect right foot.

FIGURE 3.3
Physical Therapy Examination for Ms. Gladys Greene.

- Motor: No palpable contraction of the intrinsic muscles of right foot; weak anterior crural musculature of right leg. Weak but active contraction intrinsic muscles of the left foot. Dorsiflexion 4 on right, 4+ on left; plantar flexion 4+ on left, not tested weight-bearing on right.

  Inversion/eversion 4+ bilaterally. Rest of lower extremity musculature grossly normal bilaterally.

- Vascular: 1+ pulses posterior tibial and dorsalis pedis arteries on right; 2+ pulses on the left. Decreased but adequate blood flow bilaterally per Doppler study (approx> 1 yr ago). Left lower extremity has normal temperature to touch; no measurable edema normal coloring.

- Contracture right: lesser toes 3, 4, 5; limited dorsiflexion 1st MP joint; minimal forefoot and subtalar joint motion; ankle DF = 0; ankles PF = 35.

  Left foot: no evident contractures of toes; normal forefoot and subtalar joint motion; ankle DF = 5 degrees, PF = 35 degrees.

- Wound: Grade 5 ulceration (see Table 3.1); 2.5 cm diameter; exposed flexor tendon; no joint space involvement; no signs of infection.

- ADL: Patient ambulates with bilateral forearm crutches with minimal weight bearing on the right foot. She is independent in all ADL and functional activites including driving.

∗ For the purpose of this chapter, the examination was limited to information directly related to the ulcer.

FIGURE 3.3 (CONTINUED)
Physical Therapy Examination for Ms. Gladys Greene.

Surgical Correction of Deformity

Prophylactic surgical correction such as toenail modification and removal, hammer and claw toe repairs, bunionectomies, metatarsal head resections, metatarsal osteotomies, and resections of bony prominences are performed to reduce pressure areas. Shoe modification and orthotic devices are alternatives to surgery if the deformities are limited or surgical risks are too high. Limited range of motion in dorsiflexion places increased pressure on the plantar surface of the foot. In a study by Armstrong and colleagues, 10 individuals with diabetes and a previous history of neuropathic forefoot ulcers underwent heel cord lengthening to reduce dynamic forefoot pressure. Eight weeks postsurgery, the mean increase in postsurgical active dorsiflexion was 9 degrees, and forefoot pressure decreased by 13.2 N/cm^2. The authors suggested that heel cord lengthening could be a prophylactic measure in individuals at high risk for forefoot ulceration.[19] Details of surgical procedures are beyond the scope of this chapter; however, PTs treating individuals following such corrective surgeries are referred to the many references detailing surgical procedures.[6,20]

Infection

Infection is the most common cause of amputation and is a serious threat to the limb and the life of the individual.[2,6,16] Complications include osteomyelitis, deep tissue involvement, and gangrene. Superficial infections are usually treated with local wound care. Deep infections require surgical incision and drainage as well as the use of systemic antibiotics. An abscess is the most common type of infection in the diabetic foot.[21] The abscess must be completely opened and the infected tissue removed to increase the effectiveness of treatment. The client must also not bear weight on the affected foot during healing to prevent spread of infection to other regions of the foot.[2,22] Broad spectrum antibiotics or a combination of two or more antibiotics are used initially until the specific organism is identified and treated with the most appropriate drug. In a recent retrospective study, 14 percent of individuals treated for infected foot lesions required immediate amputation but 54 percent responded to conservative treatment. Conservative treatment consisted of long-term culture-guided antibiotics and proper wound care. The majority of lesions that responded to conservative care were classified as skin ulcers. Lesions classified as deep tissue infections or osteomyelitis did not respond as well to conservative treatment. The authors recommended the identification of specific criteria for lesions that respond or do not respond to conservative treatment.[23]

Nail and Skin Care

Toenail abnormalities, particularly thickening of the nails (*onychogryphosis*) secondary to fungal infections, are common.[24,25] The thickened nail may lead to necrosis, **subungual** hemorrhage, and ulceration at the nailbed caused by pressure from improperly fitting shoes. Nails that are allowed to grow too long may curve into a neighboring toe causing a laceration or ulceration.[26] The client also risks injury when performing "bathroom surgery" to remove an ingrown toenail or when trimming the nails with a sharp instrument such as a pointed nail file or razor blade.

Autonomic neuropathy can cause the skin of the feet to be excessively dry, leading to cracks and fissures. Parts of the foot exposed to mechanical stress may develop excessively thick calluses that also increase the risk of pressure necrosis. Any injury can lead to infection and gangrene. The client or a family member needs to learn proper nail and skin care. Intervention by a professional may be required especially with the management of hypertrophic nails and thick callosities. It must be noted, however, that individuals with diabetes have difficulty finding qualified professionals willing to cut their toenails. The risk of potential injury from even a slight nick is great, and many practitioners are not willing to risk potential lawsuits or to take the time to cut thickened and misshapened toenails. PTs should generally not become involved unless they have received special training. Family members need to be trained to provide this service.

PHYSICAL THERAPY MANAGEMENT

Wound Care

The wound should be debrided, cleaned, and covered with dressings using sterile technique and universal precautions. A heavy callus typically forms around the border of the ulcer and should be trimmed to promote epithelial growth. A topical antiseptic effective for flora found on the wound is also beneficial. No specific topical agent has been found to make any major contribution in the healing rate of neuropathic ulcers.[27] In a recent study,[28] however, human skin equivalent (HSE) was used in the treatment of 10 individuals with diabetic foot ulcers. The HSE was applied following sharp debridement of the wound. Seven of the two wounds healed completely in an average of 42 days. The authors suggested that HSE may stimulate wound contraction and epithelialization.

Decreasing Pressure during Healing

Reducing stresses on the foot by decreasing weight bearing is critical to healing an ulcer. There are many ways to reduce weight bearing including bed rest, crutch walking, specialized shoes and sandals, and total contact casts.

Bed Rest

Bed rest is the simplest method of reducing weight bearing, but it is the least practical or effective because strict compliance is rare. In the absence of normal perception to pain, the individual may still continue to walk short distances in the house, bearing weight on the unprotected and ulcerated foot. Because wound healing may take many months, prolonged periods of bed rest have adverse side effects on the person's general health, making this treatment option the least favorable.[15]

Healing Sandals and Shoes

Wearing healing sandals or shoes is another method of reducing plantar pressure (Figs. 3.2*B* & *C*). The sandals and shoes are available commercially and are lightweight and easily modified. There are a great variety of such shoes and a great variety of prices, some reasonable and some considered very expensive. Some insurance companies will pay for special shoes, while others will not. Medicaid will pay for the less expensive special shoes, and Medicare will usually reimburse for special shoes under Part B with physician certification. Most commercially available special shoes for individuals with insensitive feet are lightweight, made of soft leather, have a rocker type sole and incorporate several layers of heat moldable polyethylene foam with Plastizote (United Foam Plastics, Georgetown, Mass.) for insole construction. Plastizote is a nontoxic, closed-cell foam that does not absorb body fluids and can be washed with soap and water without damage. It has a low specific heat and can be molded directly over the foot while it is still warm. Portions of the polyethylene insole may also be cut out directly beneath the lesion to create areas of greatest pressure relief (Fig. 3.4). The foam will "bottom out" or flatten under areas of high pressure over a period of several months. The material must be replaced when it no longer provides pressure relief. The insert may be molded by a PT with special training in adaptive shoes or by a certified orthotist. Cosmesis is a problem, particularly for business individuals concerned with appearance; some companies can provide the special shoes in different colors to be more cosmetic. However, compliance may be a problem.

There are also commercially available but nonadjustable comfort shoes that may be useful for some individuals. PTs should investigate local sources of adapted shoes.

Individuals with muscular weakness secondary to neuropathy may need an orthosis in addition to a special shoe. Orthoses may be made of plastic, fiberglass, and carbon composite materials or the more traditional metal double uprights. The orthotist must consider the person's muscle status, degree and location of insensitive areas, and forces generated by normal ambulation. A number of commercially available orthoses may be adapted for use. It is important for the patient to be referred to an orthotist with experience in working with individuals with diabetes.

Gel-filled socks are available and may provide some cushioning for individuals with insensitive feet. They are more prophylactic than healing and do not eliminate the need for careful and regular observation of the feet.

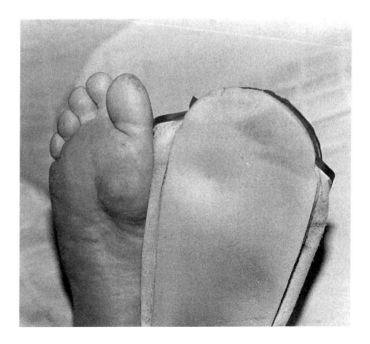

FIGURE 3.4
Plastizote liner with approximately 1 month of wear. Note areas where liner has "bottomed out" beneath the first metatarsal head and lateral border of the foot.

Total Contact Casts

The use of total contact plaster casts is well documented and remains the standard by which all other methods of ulcer treatment are measured.[29] The major difference between traditional fracture casting and total contact casting is the amount of padding applied beneath the casting material. In fracture casting, thick, bulky padding is placed between the skin and the plaster. The total contact casting uses a single layer of cotton stockinet between the skin and plaster. The wound is first assessed and then dressed with a single gauze pad. The leg and foot are covered with stockinet, and the bony prominences are padded with orthopedic felt. The innermost layers of plaster are carefully molded over the foot and leg to obtain optimal contact, whereas the outer layers are applied primarily for added stability. The distal end is closed to prevent debris from entering the cast, which could traumatize the insensitive foot. The initial cast is kept on no longer than 1 week and must be changed earlier if excessive loosening occurs secondarily. The ulcer is reevaluated, and then the cast is reapplied. Subsequent casts are replaced approximately every 2 weeks. At each cast removal or reapplication, the ulcer is reevaluated. Once the ulcer has healed, the foot should be placed in appropriate therapeutic footwear to prevent reulceration.

The effectiveness of the cast is related in part to its ability to protect the ulcer from direct trauma, reduce edema that may inhibit blood flow to the healing tissues, and immobilize the joints and soft tissue surrounding the ulceration. Compliance is not an issue because the device cannot be removed without a cast cutter. The greatest benefit comes from the cast's ability to reduce the concentration of stress at the site of the ulcer by dissipating the forces across the plantar surface of the foot while maintaining ambulation. Reductions of as much as 75 to 84 percent of peak pressure over the first and third metatarsal head have been reported in individuals walking in a total contact cast compared to normal shoes.[30] The average length of time for complete wound closure using this method of treatment occurs between 5 and 6 weeks.[31–33]

■ *Case Study Activity*

Assume your treatment was successful and wound closure was obtained. Develop a plan for Ms. Greene that will reduce her risk of future ulceration or reulceration. Be sure to address areas of specific footwear and education.

GENERAL MANAGEMENT

Prevention

Many factors may contribute to ulcer development; however, the degree to which each factor contributes to tissue destruction is unclear. Minimizing the known factors reduces the risk of ulceration or reulceration and improves the healing potential.

Risk Classification

Prevention begins with a comprehensive evaluation. The client may then be categorized according to the degree of risk for injury or reinjury. Risk classification is based on the individual's level of protective sensation, degree of vascularity, range of foot and ankle motion and muscular strength, degree of deformity that may contribute in increased plantar pressures, and history of previous injury that may increase the foot's vulnerability to future injury (Table 3.2).

Risk Management

Management is based on the level of risk. Individuals at a higher risk of ulceration need to have their feet professionally examined more frequently than those in a lower risk category. Individuals at higher risk may need specific insoles, custom-molded devices, or prescriptive footwear. Individuals at lower risk may only require education on proper footwear selection.

Education

Self-inspection

The client should be taught to perform daily foot inspection at the beginning and end of the day. More frequent inspection may be required during periods of abnormally high activity and while breaking in new shoes. The client should inspect each foot in a good light. If the individual has difficulty placing

TABLE 3.2   RISK AND MANAGEMENT CATEGORIES

Risk	Management
Category 0	
Protective sensation	Foot clinic once per year
May have a foot deformity	Patient education to include proper shoe style selection
Has a disease that could lead to insensitivity	
Category 1	
Protective sensation absent.	Foot clinic every 6 mo.
No history of plantar ulceration.	Review patient's current footwear; may need special
No foot deformity.	shoes.
Category 2	Add soft insoles (Spenco[1], nylon-covered PPT[2]).
Protective sensation absent.	Foot clinic every 3–4 mo.
No history of plantar ulcer.	Custom-molded orthotic devices are usually indicated.
Foot deformity present.	Prescription shoes are often required.
Category 3	
Protective sensation absent.	Foot clinic every 1–2 mo.
There is a history of foot ulceration or vascular laboratory	Custom orthotic devices are necessary.
findings indicate significant vascular disease.	Prescription shoes are often required.

(*Source:* Levin, ME, et al (eds): The Diabetic Foot, ed. 5. Mosby, St. Louis, 1993, p 534, with permission.)
[1]Spenco Medical Corporation, Waco, TX.
[2]Professional Protective Technology, Deer Park, NY.

the foot in a position that allows for a thorough visual inspection, a wall-mounted or handheld mirror may be helpful. If the individual has impaired vision, a friend or family member should perform inspection. Above all, whoever inspects the foot must be able to recognize the warning signs and know how to respond most appropriately.

Foot Care

In addition to self-inspection, the client should be instructed in daily foot care.[33] Individuals with diabetes should wash their feet thoroughly using warm, soapy water and a soft washcloth. The feet should be dried completely, especially between the toes to prevent maceration of the skin. Any water-based lotion may be applied to the skin to keep it soft and pliable. Lotion is not applied between the toes. Nails are trimmed straight across, not rounded at the corners, with clippers; it is safest to file the nails regularly with an emery board. Thickened calluses may be safely reduced with a foot file or pumice stone. Care of thick nails or calluses requires the assistance of a trained family member or professional.

Footwear Considerations

Proper footwear is one of the most important considerations in the prevention of ulceration or reulceration in the case of a newly healed ulcer. Shoes and orthotic devices should be selected based on the level of risk for injury.

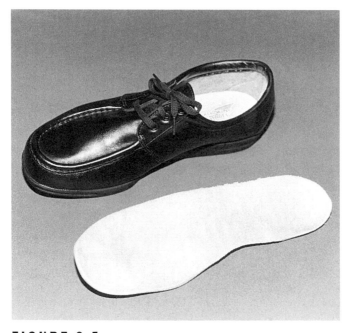

FIGURE 3.5

Extra depth shoe with removable foam liner. Note how liner has begun to contour to the shape of the foot with less than 1 week of wear.

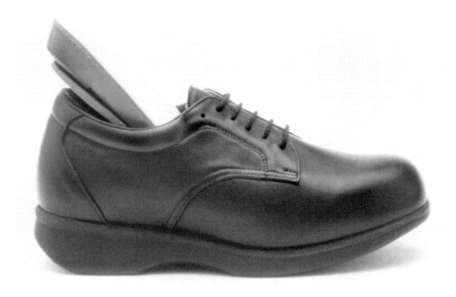

FIGURE 3.6

Commercially available shoe with adjustable inner liner(s). (Apex Foot Health Industries, *www.foot.com*, with permission.)

Those at lowest risk should select shoes made from leather because this material will adapt better than synthetic materials to the contours of the foot over time. The heel and midfoot section should fit securely on the foot to prevent slippage, and the toe box should be high and wide enough and at least 1 cm longer than the longest toe to prevent crowding and pressure on the toes. Shoes manufactured with an extra-depth toe box should be selected when deformities such as claw toes are present (Fig. 3.5). Extra depth is extremely important if additional insole material is to be added to the shoe.

Individuals with impaired sensation and deformity require custom-molded inserts made from soft thermoplastic materials or specials shoes as previously discussed (see Fig. 3.4). Individuals with severe deformity require custom-molded shoes or boots. Custom-molded footwear is relatively expensive but may be necessary to adequately accommodate the deformity. However, cost is relative when considering the cost of wound care, amputation, prosthetics, and rehabilitation following amputation (Fig. 3.6).

Cotton and wool socks provide the best padding between the foot and shoe. The socks should be clean and in good condition without holes. They should be worn without wrinkles and folds. White socks are preferred to colored socks because the dyes may cause irritation. The shoes should be inspected inside for foreign objects prior to each wearing. They should be in good repair and free from tacks or nails, which can pierce the insole and project into the foot. New shoes should be worn no more than 2 hours per day for the first week. Wear may be extended an additional 2 hours each successive week.

Summary

Ulceration of the diabetic foot is a common problem that can ultimately result in amputation; however, most ulcers heal if managed properly. Professionals who care for individuals with diabetes must be able to identify the risk factors contributing to delayed healing and know methods to reduce these factors. Above all, prevention is the ultimate goal with emphasis placed on education. Long-term security for the diabetic foot is maximized when individuals accept responsibility for the routine inspection and care of their own feet.

Glossary

Autolysis	Self-dissolution of tissue, usually by an enzyme within the body.
Bulla	A large fluid-filled blister.
Callus	A hypertrophied or thickened area of the skin.
Debridement	Removal of dead or damaged tissue from a wound.
Fissure	A cracklike opening in the skin.
Gangrene or necrosis	Death of tissue, usually from lack of circulation.
Glycosylation	Excess sugar in the cells.
Hematoma	A swelling or mass of blood.
Ischemia	Lack of blood to an area or part.
Neuroarthropathy	Joint disease combined with central nervous system disorder.
Neuropathy	A disease of the nervous system.
Sinus	A canal or passage.
Subungual	Located beneath a finger nail or toenail.

References

1. Palumbo, PJ, and Melton, LJ: Peripheral vascular disease and diabetes. In Harris, MI, and Hamman, RF (eds): Diabetes in America. NIH Pub. No. 85–1468. Bethesda, Md., 1985, National Institutes of Health, p XV 1–21.
2. Kozak, GP, et al: Diabetic foot disease: A major problem. In Kozak, GP, et al: Management of Diabetic Foot Problems, ed 2. WB Saunders, Philadelphia, 1995.
3. Birke, JA, and Sims, DS: Plantar sensory threshold in the ulcerative foot. Lepr Rev 57:261, 1986.
4. Sabato, S, et al: Plantar trophic ulcers in patients with leprosy: A correlative study of sensation, pressure and mobility. Int Orthop 6:203, 1982.
5. Reiber, G: Epidemiology of the diabetic foot. In Levin, ME, et al (eds): The Diabetic Foot, ed 5. Mosby, St. Louis, 1993.
6. Brodsky, JW: The diabetic foot. In Mann, RA, and Coughlin, MJ (eds): Surgery of the Foot and Ankle, ed 6. Mosby Year Book, St. Louis, 1993.
7. Bell, DS: Lower limb problems in diabetics: What are the causes? What are the remedies? Post Grad Med 89(8):237, 1991.
8. Levin, ME: Medical management of the diabetic foot. In Kerstein, MD (ed): Diabetes and Vascular Disease. Lippincott, Philadelphia, 1990.

9. Hamptom, G, and Birke, J: Treatment of wounds caused by pressure and insensitivity. In Kloth, LC, et al (eds): Wound Healing: Alternatives in Management. FA Davis, Philadelphia, 1990.

10. Brand, PW: The diabetic foot. In Ellenberg, M, and Rifkin, H (eds): Diabetes Mellitus: Theory and Practice, ed 3. Medical Examination Publishing, New Hyde Park, NY, 1983, pp 829–849.

11. Habershaw, D, and Chzran J: Biomechanical considerations of the diabetic foot. In Kozak, GP, et al (eds): Management of Diabetic Foot Problems, ed 2. WB Saunders, Philadelphia, 1995.

12. Levin, ME: Diabetic foot lesions. In Young, JR, et al (eds): Peripheral Vascular Disease. Mosby Year Book, St. Louis, 1991, pp 669–711.

13. Sims, DS, et al: Risk factors in the diabetic foot: Recognition and management. Phys Ther 68(12):1887, 1988.

14. APTA: Guide to Physical Therapist Practice, ed 2. Phys Ther 81: , 2001.

15. Birke, JA, and Sims, DS: Plantar sensory threshold in the ulcerative foot. Lepr Rev 57:261, 1986.

16. Campbell, DR, et al: Guidelines in the examination of the diabetic leg and foot. In Kozak, GP, et al: Management of Diabetic Foot Problems, ed 2. WB Saunders, Philadelphia, 1995.

17. Wagner, FW: The dysvascular foot: A system for diagnosis and treatment. Foot Ankle 2(2):64, 1981.

18. Schwartz, N: The diabetic foot. In Donatelli, R (ed): The Biomechanics of the Foot and Ankle. FA Davis, Philadelphia, 1990.

19. Armstrong, DG, et al: Lengthening of the Achilles tendon in diabetic patients who are at high risk for ulceration of the foot. J Bone Joint Surg Am 81(4):535–38, 1999.

20. Frykberg, RG: Podiatric problems in diabetes. In Kozak, GP, et al: Management of Diabetic Foot Problems, ed 2. WB Saunders, Philadelphia, 1995.

21. Brand, PW: Management of the insensitive limb. Phys Ther 59:8, 1979.

22. Delbridge, L, et al: Nonenzymatic glycosylation of keratin from the stratum corneum of the diabetic foot. Br J Dermatol 112:547, 1985.

23. Pittet, D, et al: Outcome of diabetic foot infections treated conservatively: A retrospective cohort study with long-term follow up. Arch Intern Med 159(8):851–56, 1999.

24. O'Neal, LW: Debridement and amputation. In Levin, ME, et al (eds): The Diabetic Foot, ed 5. Mosby, St. Louis, 1993.

25. O'Neal, LW: Surgical pathology of the foot and clinicopathology correlations. In Levin, ME, et al (eds): The Diabetic Foot, ed 5. Mosby, St. Louis, 1993.

26. Birke, JA, et al: Methods of treating plantar ulcers. Phys Ther 71(2):116, 1991.

27. Birke, JA, et al: Walking casts: Effect of plantar foot pressures. J Rehab Res Dev 22:18, 1985.

28. Brem, H, et al: Healing of diabetic foot ulcers and pressure ulcers with human skin equivalent: A new paradigm in wound healing. Arch Surg 135(6):627–34, 2000.

29. Laing, PW, et al: Neuropathic foot ulceration treated by total contact casts. J Bone Joint Surg Am 74B:133, 1992.

30. Sinacore, DR, et al: Diabetic plantar ulcers treated by total contact casting. Phys Ther 67:1543, 1987.

31. Walker, SC, et al: Total contact casting and chronic diabetic neuropathic foot ulcerations: Healing rates by wound location. Arch Phys Med Rehabil 68:217, 1987.

32. Birke, JA, et al: Healing rates in diabetic and non-diabetic plantar ulcers. Unpublished study, Gillis W. Long Hansen's Disease Center, Carville, La., 1988.

33. Eramo–Melkus, GD: Education and counseling for diabetes self-care. In Gambert, SR: Diabetes Mellitus in the Elderly. Raven Press, New York, 1990.

CHAPTER FOUR

Lower Extremity Amputation Surgery

At the end of this chapter, all students are expected to:

1 Describe the process of amputation surgery in relation to residual limb characteristics and function.
2 Describe the functional results of amputation surgery.

Case Studies

The following clients have been referred to physical therapy for postsurgical care:

Diana Magnolia had a left **transtibial** amputation yesterday secondary to diabetic gangrene and a nonhealing ulcer on the plantar surface of the right foot.

Benny Pearl had a right **transfemoral** amputation yesterday secondary to chronic arteriosclerosis obliterans (ASO).

Ha Lee Davis is an 18-year-old man who underwent traumatic transtibial amputation secondary to a motorcycle accident 2 days ago; he also sustained a severe sprain of the right wrist.

Betty Childs is a 12-year-old girl who underwent a transfemoral amputation yesterday secondary to grade IIB osteogenic sarcoma of the proximal right tibia.

■ *Case Study Activities*

All students:

1 For each client, describe what the surgeon will do with the bone, blood vessels, nerves, muscle, tissue, and skin during each amputation.

Physical Therapy Students:

2 Identify what you need to know about amputation surgery to select appropriate tests and measures and develop a plan of care.

Physical Therapist Assistant Students:

3 Identify what you need to know about amputation surgery to implement selected interventions.

INTRODUCTION

Most lower extremity amputations are performed secondary to peripheral vascular disease (more than 90 percent). Usually, amputation is preceded by attempts at limb salvage through **revascularization** procedures (see Chap. 2). The level of amputation is determined by the healing potential of the residual limb and the general health of the client. Successful healing does not require **patency** of major vessels but does necessitate patency of small vessels in the skin.[1,2,3] Surgeons use various methods to determine the lowest possible level of amputation that is likely to heal such as skin temperature, palpable pulses, and blood flow measures.[3] A recent study highlighted the use of transcutaneous oximetry, a measurement of oxygen tension through the skin, as a valid means of determining optimum level.[4] Amputations for peripheral vascular disease are usually performed through the foot (transmetatarsal), tibia (transtibial), or femur (transfemoral). **Disarticulations** are not generally performed for limb ischemia because the lower vascularization in the joints is believed to prevent successful healing. However, there is some disagreement regarding the value of performing knee disarticulations in the presence of lower limb ischemia (see discussion later in this chapter). Many studies show poor success rates for ankle disarticulation in the presence of severe limb ischemia.[1]

Level selection for traumatic amputations or for major tumors is determined by the nature of the injury and the viability of tissues. Surgeons have generally been reluctant to amputate lower extremities, even in the presence of multiple and severe traumatic injuries. However, some surgeons today advocate considering the physical, mental, and financial costs of long-term heroic limb salvage efforts. An algorithm has been developed to guide the surgeon through a decision-making process that considers a wide variety of criteria.[5] The incidence of amputation for tumors has decreased with the advent of improved detection and chemotherapy management. Whenever possible, the tumor is excised and the bone is replaced with a metal implant or an allograft, eliminating the need for amputation. Five-year survival rates have been about the same for individuals undergoing amputation and those having segmental excisions. Amputations are generally performed on individuals with large tumors who do not respond well to preoperative chemotherapy.[3]

GENERAL PRINCIPLES

Several principles of amputation surgery apply to all levels of amputation. Because most amputations are the result of vascular disease, most are performed by vascular surgeons who are not required to study prosthetic rehabilitation. Orthopedic surgeons, who perform most nonvascular amputations, must take courses in prosthetic rehabilitation.

Generally, surgeons want to save as much length as possible while providing a residual limb that can tolerate the stresses of prosthetic ambulation. Sometimes, compromises are necessary between keeping bone length and avoiding scars and other deformities that may interfere with prosthetic fitting (Fig. 4.1A and B). Newer prosthetic components, including gel liners and socks that provide a close fitting and shock-absorbing interface between the residual limb and socket, have greatly increased the comfort of a prosthesis fitted to an individual whose residual limb is bony or scarred (see Chap. 7).

Amputating a limb severs both small and large nerves; when severed, all peripheral nerves put out new tendrils that form into small neoplasms of

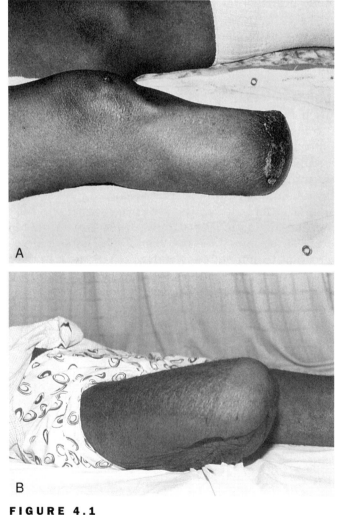

FIGURE 4.1
(A) Residual limb after transtibial amputation. (B) Residual limb after transfemoral amputation.

nerve ends (**neuromas**). If small and imbedded in soft tissue, the neuroma does not usually cause a problem. If the neuroma is large or superficial or becomes squeezed against a bone, it can cause pain that may interfere with prosthetic wear. To lessen the possibility of neuroma pain, the surgeon pulls down the major nerves firmly, resects them sharply, and allows them to retract into the soft tissue.

Muscle and soft tissue are differentially handled depending on the level of amputation. When a muscle is severed, it loses its distal attachment and, if left loose, will retract, atrophy, and scar against adjacent structures. Without attachment at both ends, a muscle cannot function. There are two ways muscle can be managed. **Myoplasty** refers to the attachment of anterior and posterior compartment muscles to each other over the end of the bone. Myoplasty is usually performed in through-the-bone amputations with myofascial closure to provide muscle stability, making sure the muscles do not slide over the end of the bone. **Myodesis** refers to the anchoring of muscles to bone. Myodesis is more rarely performed, as it requires a longer surgical procedure and causes more trauma to the bone itself. In both instances, muscles are stabilized under slight tension to provide a well-shaped residual limb.

Skin **flaps** are usually as broad as the distal end of the limb and shaped to allow the corners to retract smoothly. Anterior and posterior skin flaps place the scar in a mediolateral direction at the end of the residual limb and are generally used except for amputations of dysvascular problems (Fig. 4.2). Types of postsurgical dressings vary and are discussed in more detail in Chapter 5. A drain is often inserted just under the incision to allow for the evacuation of excess fluid. The drain is usually removed 1 or 2 days after surgery.

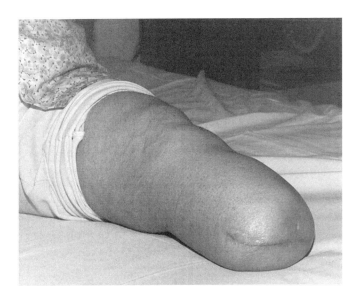

FIGURE 4.2

Residual limb from a transtibial amputation with suture of equal length flaps. (From May, BJ: Assessment and treatment of individuals following lower extremity amputation. In O'Sullivan, SB, and Schmitz, TJ (eds): Physical Rehabilitation: Assessment and Treatment, ed 3. FA Davis, Philadelphia, 1994, p 377, with permission.)

TRANSTIBIAL (BELOW KNEE)

The transtibial is the most common level of extremity amputation for periph-eral vascular disease. Prosthetic rehabilitation is more successful, and postop-erative mortality is lower with transtibial than with transfemoral amputa-tions. Several studies confirm a mortality rate of 9.5 percent following transtibial amputation in comparison to 29.5 percent following transfemoral amputation.[6,7] Traditionally, transfemoral amputations were preferred in the presence of peripheral vascular disease because it was thought that the larger vessels enhanced healing. However, studies performed in the 1960s indicated that primary healing could be obtained consistently at transtibial levels.[6,7] Bowker and associates pooled the results of several studies and reported a pri-mary healing rate of 70 percent and a secondary healing rate of 16 percent for transtibial amputations.[6] One British study of 713 clients amputated at transtibial levels because of ischemia indicated that healing was enhanced by previous attempts at revascularization that increased oxygen to the tissues.[8] A more recent study indicated that primary healing rates have remained rela-tively constant over the years ranging from 30 to 92 percent with a reamputa-tion rate of 4 to 30 percent. The authors also suggested that primary healing at transtibial levels improved to 90 percent if the popliteal pulse was present.[9] The greater prosthetic rehabilitation potential for the transtibial level of am-putation supports a greater ratio of transtibial versus transfemoral amputa-tions.

The specific level of transtibial amputation is determined by several fac-tors. In amputations following trauma, remaining viable tissue determines the level. In the presence of dysvascular disease with infection, the level is de-termined by the infection-free tissue and the vascular condition of skin flaps and soft tissue. Patency of major vessels is not necessarily a criterion for se-lecting a level. Amputations consistently heal primarily in the absence of cir-culation through the major vessels if there is bleeding through the skin flaps. The desirable length for a transtibial amputation is a matter of controversy. Some surgeons advocate leaving as much bone length as possible, believing that the longer lever arm will decrease the energy required for effective ambu-lation.[10–13] Others state that individuals with very long residual limbs develop distal skin problems because of the lack of subcutaneous padding.[14] Some sur-geons suggest that about 15 cm is optimal length.[15] The tibial tubercle is the shortest level of transtibial amputation compatible with knee function.

Many surgeons use a long posterior skin flap when performing an amputa-tion for vascular insufficiency (Fig. 4.3). The skin over the posterior leg has a better blood supply than the skin over the anterior leg. The anterior skin flap is cut at approximately the level of anticipated section of the tibia, and the posterior flap is cut 13 to 15 cm longer to ensure adequate coverage without undue tension. It is advocated that skin and subcutaneous tissue not be sepa-rated from the muscular fascia to preserve skin perfusion. The muscles are di-vided, blood vessels are ligated and divided, and the nerves are severed high with a sharp scalpel and allowed to retract into the soft tissue. The tibia and fibula are sectioned, with the fibula usually cut about 1 cm shorter than the tibia for proper shaping of the distal residual limb. Cutting the fibula much shorter than the tibia results in a sharp distal end that may be painful when fitted with a prosthesis. Leaving the fibula the same length as the tibia may

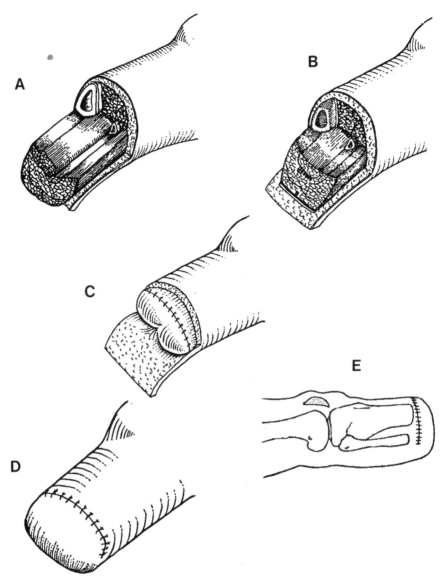

FIGURE 4.3
Transtibial amputation with long posterior skin flap. (*A*) The surgeon leaves a long posterior skin flap. (*B*) The surgeon bevels and contours the flap for a smooth distal end. (*C*) After myoplasty, the soft tissues are approximated. (*D*) The final suture is over the anterior part of the residual limb. (*E*) The relationship of the tibia and fibula.

lead to a square end that is more difficult to fit. When amputation is per-formed at the tibial tubercle level, the fibula is removed, because the biceps tendon tends to deviate the small bony remnant that is no longer anchored by soft tissue. The tibia must be beveled anteriorly at 45 to 60 degrees to allow for distribution of distal-end pressure over as wide an area as possible and to prevent osteophyte formation. Care is taken to avoid any rough bony areas. Myoplasty, rather than myodesis, is usually preferred in the presence of vas-cular disease. The posterior muscle mass is beveled to allow the flap to come forward; it is sutured anteriorly to the deep fascia of the anterolateral muscle group and to the periosteum that is reflected over the anterior aspect of the tibia. The skin is brought forward and sutured. The resulting anterior scar usually presents no problem in limb fitting (Fig. 4.4).

Recently, the advantage of the long posterior flap has come into question. In one study, the transcutaneous partial oxygen pressure (TcPo$_2$) level at the amputation site of transtibial amputations with long posterior flaps was compared to the TcPo$_2$ level of patients who underwent transtibial amputations closed with a skew (mediolateral) flap. Initially there was some reduction of TcPo$_2$ levels in all amputation flaps. However, the lower values in the long posterior flap were still evident 20 days after surgery, whereas the TcPo$_2$ levels in the skew flaps had returned to normal.[16] Some surgeons in England have advocated skew flaps—equal-length flaps cut in an anteromedial direction placing the incision in a posteroanterior direction.[17] Some studies have indicated that such flaps have better oxygen perfusion through the skin and provide a good muscle envelope for the distal tibia.[17] Another variation are sagittal flaps that are cut in an anterolateral direction and incorporate myoplasty of anterior compartment muscles to the medial gastrocnemius to cover the distal tibia.[18] There is no report of problems of prosthetic limb fitting with any of these flaps.

When amputation is performed for other than vascular reasons, anterior or posterior flaps of equal length are used, and the resultant scar is at the distal end of the limb. Equal-length flaps are often referred to as "fish-mouth" incisions because the shape of the flaps before suturing resembles a fish mouth.

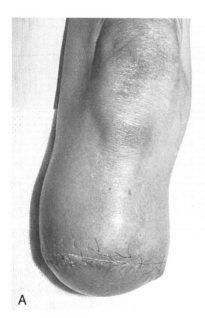
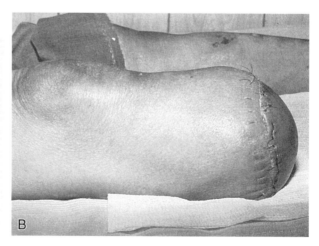

FIGURE 4.4

(*A* and *B*) Residual limb from a transtibial amputation, showing the anterior suture from a long posterior flap. (From May, BJ: Assessment and treatment of individuals following lower extremity amputation. In O'Sullivan, SB, and Schmitz, TJ (eds): Physical Rehabilitation: Assessment and Treatment, ed 3. FA Davis, Philadelphia, 1994, p. 377, with permission.)

Equal-length flaps allow for less redundant tissue at the end of the residual limb, and properly shaped flaps reduce the "dog ears," or excess tissue at the medial and lateral corners that may result from long posterior flaps.

Although the physical therapist (PT) and physical therapist assistant (PTA) have little input into the surgical technique, they need to understand what the surgeon has done to provide for effective postsurgical handling.

TRANSFEMORAL (ABOVE KNEE)

Historically, transfemoral was the most common amputation level for individuals with impaired circulation and gangrene of the foot and toes. The improved circulation above the knee increased the chances of primary healing. However, as is explained in Chapter 8, ambulation with a transfemoral prosthesis requires considerable energy, and many individuals with vascular disease never become functional walkers. In the past 30 years, the trend has changed because research indicates that amputations at the transtibial level can heal primarily, and prosthetic rehabilitation is more successful among individuals with transtibial amputations in comparison to those with transfemoral amputations. Today, more transtibial than transfemoral amputations are performed for vascular problems. The ratio has remained fairly stable over the years at 2.5 transtibial amputations for every 1 transfemoral amputation.[9] The transfemoral level is still indicated if gangrene has extended to the knee or the patient's circulatory status precludes healing at the transtibial level.

Trauma is the other major cause of transfemoral amputation; some amputations are also done for osteomyelitis or tumors. Survival and functional prosthetic rehabilitation rates are lower among individuals following transfemoral amputation. Individuals undergoing this procedure are generally sicker and have less energy reserves than individuals amputated at transtibial levels.

Equal length anterior and posterior flaps are generally used. Thigh muscles and periosteum are divided cleanly to the bone at a length just beyond the most distal part of the skin flaps. For a myoplasty, the thigh muscles are divided into four groups and elevated from the femur back to the level of proposed bone section. The blood vessels are transected just proximal to the level of bone section. The nerves are cut at a level to ensure that they will be well covered by muscle and remote from the incision. If a neuroma becomes attached to the distal scar, it may displace during walking and cause pain. The femur is divided, and the sharp peripheral edges are rounded with a rasp. Usually, the adductor magnus tendon is brought around the distal femur and sutured to the lateral distal aspect through small drill holes. The femur is held in adduction to ensure maximum tension on the muscle because it is critically important to prosthetic stability in gait to maintain the femoral shaft axis as close to normal as possible. The quadriceps and hamstrings are either anchored to each other over the end of the bone, or the quadriceps is attached directly to the femur through small drill holes with the hamstrings attached to the posterior part of the adductor magnus. Regardless of technique, the surgeon attempts to provide muscle stabilization to improve residual limb function. Some surgeons believe that myodesis is necessary to ensure adequate muscle stabilization; others suggest that myoplasty is adequate.[19-23] Some function is lost because muscles are shortened and the femur is no longer held in its normal adducted position by the tibia and fibula. (The resulting effect on gait is discussed in Chap. 8.) The muscles are trimmed before suturing, and the skin flaps are closed without undue tension with the femur in a neutral position (see Fig. 4.1B). The residual limb may be placed in a rigid dressing or in a compressive wrap.

OTHER LEVELS

Amputations through the Foot

Toe or Ray Amputation (Transphalangeal, Digital Amputation)

Toe amputations are generally indicated for localized demarcated gangrene of the distal end of the toe. A single toe can be amputated through the phalanx or disarticulated at the base of the proximal phalanx. PTs and PTAs are rarely involved with primary toe amputations, although clients with other levels of amputation may have lost one or more toes on the other side.

On occasion, an entire ray (toe plus metatarsal) may be removed. The metatarsal ray resection is indicated in some cases of congenital anomalies, gangrene secondary to frostbite, neoplasms, severe chronic infections of a single metatarsal, or a deep subaponeurotic foot abscess.

Transmetatarsal Amputation

Transmetatarsal amputation (Fig. 4.5) is removal of the toes and distal ends of the metatarsals. It is a very functional amputation for problems with toes but requires well-fitting prosthetic replacement. Foot balance is maintained because the residual limb is symmetrical in shape and major muscle attachments are preserved. Transmetatarsal amputations heal relatively slowly because of the limited blood supply in the dorsum, where the incision is located. Once healed, the foot has been shown to survive without the need for further surgery in about 71 percent of cases.[24] The incision is vulnerable to abrasion during the latter part of stance phase.

The Boyd amputation through the foot is little used today, but some surgeons advocate it for osteomyelitis of the forefoot.[25] This amputation is essentially through the calcaneus. The heel pad is left intact, and the remaining portion of the calcaneus is fused to the bottom of the tibia, thereby creating a solid and balanced foot. Problems can occur if the calcaneus does not adhere firmly to the tibia but instead migrates anteriorly, reducing the weight-bearing qualities of the foot.

Disarticulation

There are advantages and disadvantages to disarticulations over through-bone amputations. Disarticulation provides a residual limb with an intact bone, lowers chances of osteomyelitis, and, in children, maintains intact growth plates. The complete bone length of the disarticulated limb provides for a better lever arm and more prosthetic control, particularly for ankle and knee disarticulations. The disadvantages may include decreased cosmesis of the pros-

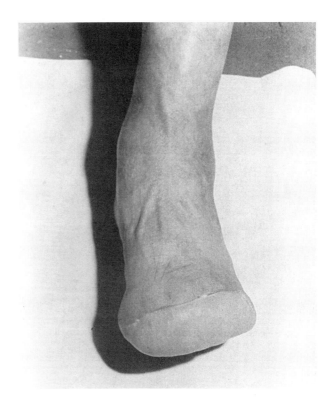

FIGURE 4.5
Residual limb after a transmetatarsal amputation.

thetic replacement and fewer available components to fit the smaller joint space. However, new technology is quickly resolving these problems.

Ankle Disarticulations

The most common ankle disarticulation procedure was developed by James Syme in 1842.[22,26] It is a weight-bearing amputation because the heel pad is swung under the tibia and fibula and attached (Fig. 4.6A). The heel flap is securely anchored to the distal end of the tibia and fibula and stabilized after skin closure, either with tape or a rigid dressing, until the heel pad has adhered securely. An unstable heel pad (Fig. 4.6B) interferes with good prosthetic fit, can be painful, and limits weight-bearing capabilities. In the Syme's procedure, muscles and tendons that cross the joint are pulled down, divided, and allowed to retract. The procedure is usually performed in a single stage except in the presence of forefoot infection. During the Korean War, many soldiers sustained severe injuries to the foot by stepping on bamboo spikes that had been smeared with human excrement. These wounds did not heal, and Syme's amputations were performed in two stages. During the first stage, the foot was removed, the heel pad brought under the tibia and sutured, and drains inserted for antibiotic irrigation. In the second stage, several weeks later when all signs of infection were gone, the malleoli were removed to the joint surface and the skin around the heel pad trimmed carefully to allow for closure without tension. The residual limb was then wrapped in plaster for healing.[25] A modified one-stage Syme amputation was reported by Sarmiento.[27,28] Prior to closing, the metaphyseal flare of the distal tibia is re-

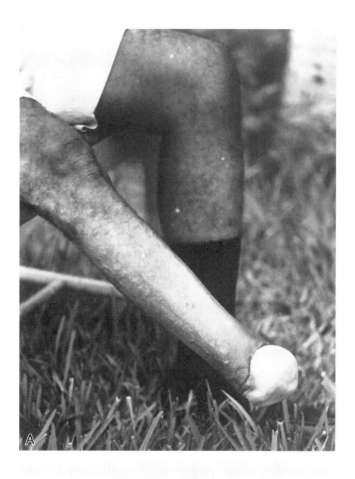

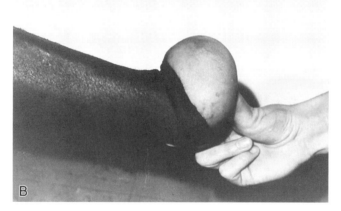

FIGURE 4.6

(*A*) Residual limb after a Syme amputation. (*B*) Unstable heel pad on a Syme residual limb.

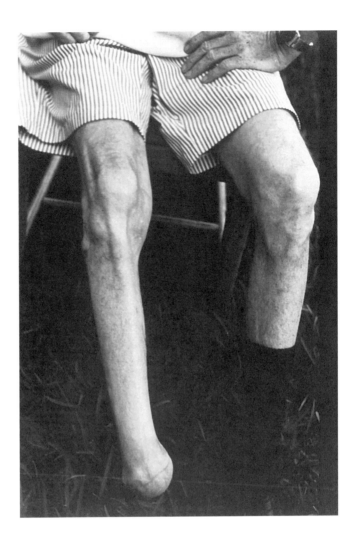

FIGURE 4.7
Residual limb after a modified
Syme amputation.

moved and the distal end of the fibula is beveled to reduce the bulbous end by
about one-third, while retaining the end-bearing feature of the limb (Fig. 4.7).
Postoperatively the limb is placed in a plaster cast until the end pad has adhered properly. In all Syme's amputations, care must be taken to maintain the
blood supply to the end pad to allow for proper healing. Generally, skin flaps
either are not trimmed or are minimally trimmed to prevent damage to the
blood supply.

Knee Disarticulations

The knee disarticulation is a relatively uncommon amputation in adults.
Knee disarticulations are generally performed for trauma and usually where
there is not enough tibia left (less than 4 cm) for a functional transtibial am-

putation. It is occasionally performed on elderly individuals with lower limb ischemia who are not considered candidates for prosthetic ambulation because adequate circulation to allow healing at the knee disarticulation level would also allow healing at the high transtibial level. With improved prosthetic replacements, some surgeons advocate using this level for more patients. The knee disarticulation is a muscle-balanced amputation level that can be used in patients with diabetes, peripheral vascular disease, as well as trauma.[29] There are a variety of surgical approaches depending on anticipated function. The most common technique uses equal length skin flaps, either sagittal or anteroposterior, to provide a soft-tissue envelope for the distal femur.[30] The envelope is created from the gastrocnemius, hamstring, and patella tendons and part of the knee joint capsule to provide an interface between residual limb and socket to absorb some of the shear forces generated in walking. The cruciate ligaments are removed; the tibial attachment of the patella ligament is also removed and attached to the remaining portions of cruciate ligaments. The patella remains in the notch between the femoral condyles out of the weight-bearing plane. A more cosmetic prosthetic socket can be used if the distal femur is modified to reduce the bulky distal end. One technique involves resecting the lateral, medial, and posterior flares.[31] Burgess advocated shortening the femur by removing the distal condyles; however, this also removes the suspension assist of the femoral condyles and may require a prosthesis with proximal suspension, particularly as the residual limb atrophies and matures.[29]

Hip Disarticulation

The hip disarticulation is a surgical procedure usually performed for malignancy of the hip or thigh that is not treatable by other means or severe trauma. On rare occasions it may be used to correct a severe congenital deformity. The Boyd technique, most commonly used, involves dissecting along fascial planes and dividing the muscles at their pelvic origins or femoral insertion. Closure without tension is permitted because all muscles have been removed except for the large gluteal flap that cushions the distal torso. The incision begins at the anterior superior iliac spine and curves distally and medially to a point about 5 cm below the adductor muscle origins. The incision continues posteriorly around the thigh to the ischial tuberosity, then to the greater trochanter and then to the anterior superior iliac spine. The muscles of the lower leg are detached at their origins, vessels and nerves are ligated, and the remaining gluteal flap is brought anteriorly with the gluteal muscles and sutured to the pectineus and origin of the adductors. The anterior position of the scar is distant from the lateral and terminal pressure areas, reducing the chance of wound contamination from fecal matter. A firm supporting compression dressing is applied to control edema and postoperative pain.[33–34]

Transpelvic (Hemipelvectomy)

This level is also usually performed for malignancy of the hip or pelvis or for severe trauma. It is similar to the hip disarticulation except that the surgery includes removal of all or part of the ilium. The patient is usually placed in a semilateral position on the side opposite to the lesion to allow the abdominal contents to move away from the surgical site. The procedure is done in three stages: anterior, perineal, and posterior. The incision is started above the inguinal ligament, extending posteriorly to the iliac crest, and then across the pubic tubercle to the crease between the thigh and perineum. The posterior incision extends from the iliac crest downward. An anterior convexity is made as the incision extends anterior to the greater trochanter and comes around the posterior aspect of the upper thigh or along the gluteal fold to meet the lower end of the anterior incision at the ischial tuberosity. The ipsilateral abdominal musculature is sectioned, and the peritoneum and attached ureter are pushed medially. The pelvis is usually separated at the pubic symphysis, and the ilium is divided between the middle and posterior thirds of the crest or at the sacroiliac joint, depending on the site of pathology. The gluteus maximus is reflected with the skin flaps and sutured to the lateral or anterior abdominal musculature. The skin is closed and the residual area wrapped with a compression dressing.[33–34]

Translumbar (Hemicorporectomy)

This rare level of amputation may be performed for malignancy of the pelvic organs, skin, or musculoskeletal structures of the lumbar area, or, occasionally, for severe sacral decubitus or similar complications of paraplegia. This complex and multistage surgical procedure involves removal of the bony pelvis, pelvic contents, lower extremities, and external genitalia following disarticulation of the lumbar spine and transection of the spinal cord. Cholestomy and other reconstructive procedures for the internal organs are necessary. Postoperative morbidity and mortality rates are high, partly because of the complexity of the procedure itself and partly because of the underlying disease.[35]

Summary

The PT and PTA must understand the basic procedures in amputation surgery to work effectively with the postsurgical client and provide guidance for proper residual limb management. When possible, clinicians are encouraged to read the operative report to note any unusual findings or surgical variations. Observing surgery is also instructive.

Glossary

Disarticulation	Amputation through a joint.
Flaps	A piece of partially detached tissue, usually including skin and underlying muscles and vessels.
Myodesis	The anchoring of muscles to bone when closing an amputation.
Myoplasty	Suturing posterior and anterior compartment muscles together over the end of the bone in an amputation.
Neuroma	Any type of tumor composed of nerve cells identified by the specific part of the nerve that is involved.

	Amputation neuroma is formed by the cut ends of peripheral nerves.
Patency	A state of being open.
Revascularization	Re-establishing patency of circulation to a part.
Transfemoral	Amputation through the femur.
Translumbar	Amputation through the lumbar area of the spinal cord and removal of all structures below the level.
Transpelvic	Amputation through the pelvis.
Transtibial	Amputation through the tibia.

References

1. McCollum, PT, and Walker, MA: Major limb amputation for end-stage peripheral vascular disease: Level selection and alternative options. In Bowker, JH, and Michael, JW (eds): Atlas of Limb Prosthetics, ed 2. Mosby Year Book, St. Louis, 1992.
2. Bowker, JH, et al: The choice between limb salvage and amputation. In Bowker, JH, and Michael, JW (eds): Atlas of Limb Prosthetics, ed 2. Mosby Year Book, St. Louis, 1992.
3. Moore, TJ: Planning for optimal function in amputation surgery. In Bowker, JH, and Michael, JW (eds): Atlas of Limb Prosthetics, ed 2. Mosby Year Book, St. Louis, 1992.
4. Misuri, A, et al: Predictive value of transcutaneous oximetry for selection of the amputation level. J Cardiovasc Surg 41(1):83–87, 2000.
5. Hiatt, MD, et al: The decision to salvage or amputate a severely injured limb. J South Orthop Assoc 9(1):72–78, 2000.
6. Bowker, JH, et al: Transtibial amputation. In Bowker, JH, and Michael, JW (eds): Atlas of Limb Prosthetics, ed 2. Mosby Year Book, St. Louis, 1992.
7. Sarmiento, A, and Warren, WD: A re-evaluation of lower extremity amputations. Surg Gynecol Obstet 129:799–802, 1969.
8. Dormandy, J, et al: Prospective study of 713 below-knee amputations for ischaemia and the effects of a prostacyclin analogue on healing. Br J Surg 81:333–37, 1994.
9. Dormandy, J, et al: Major amputations: Clinical patterns and predictors. [Review] Sem Vasc Surg 12(2):154–61, 1999.
10. McCollough, NC, III, et al: Below knee amputation. In Bowker, JH, and Michael, JW (eds): Atlas of Limb Prosthetics. Mosby Year Book, St. Louis, 1981, pp 341–68.
11. Epps, CH, Jr: Amputation of the lower limb. In Evarts, CM (ed): Surgery of the Musculoskeletal System, ed 2. Churchill Livingstone, New York, 1990.
12. Moore, TJ: Amputations of the lower extremity. In Chapman, M (ed): Operative Orthopaedics. JB Lippincott, Philadelphia, 1988.
13. Gonzalez, EG, et al: Energy expenditure in below-knee amputees: Correlation with stump length. Arch Phys Med Rehabil 55:111–19, 1974.
14. Marsden, FW: Amputation: Surgical technique and postoperative management. Aust N Z J Surg 47:384–92. 1977.
15. Burgess, EM: The below-knee amputation. Bull Prosthet Res. 10:19–25, 1988.
16. Johnson, WC, et al: Transcutaneous partial oxygen pressure changes following skew flap and Burgess-type below-knee amputation. Arch Surg 132:261–63, 1997.
17. Robinson, KP, et al: Skew flap myoplastic below-knee amputation: A preliminary report. Br J Surg 69:554–57, 1982.
18. Smith, DG, and Fergason, JR: Transtibial amputations. Clin Orthop 361:108–15, 1999.
19. Bohne, WHO: Above the knee amputation. In Atlas of Amputation Surgery. Thieme Medical Publishers, New York, 1987.
20. Burgess, E: Knee disarticulation and above-knee amputation. In Moore, W, and Malone, J (eds): Lower extremity amputation. WB Saunders, Philadelphia, 1989.
21. Harris, WR: Principles of amputation surgery. In Kostuik, JP (ed): Amputation Surgery and Rehabilitation—the Toronto Experience. Churchill Livingstone, New York, 1981.
22. Gottschalk, F: Transfemoral amputation. In Bowker, JH, and Michael, JW (eds): Atlas of Limb Prosthetics, ed 2. Mosby Year Book, St. Louis, 1992.

23. Gottschalk, F: Transfemoral amputation. Biomechanics and surgery. Clin Orthop (361):15–22, 1999.
24. Santi, MD, et al: Survivorship of healed partial foot amputations in dysvascular patients. Clin Orthop 292:245–49, 1993.
25. Grady, JF, and Winters, CL: The Boyd amputation as a treatment for osteomyelitis of the foot. J Am Podiatr Med Assoc 90(5):234–39, 2000.
26. Wagner, FW, Jr: The Syme ankle disarticulation. In Bowker, JH, and Michael, JW (eds): Atlas of Limb Prosthetics, ed 2. Mosby Year Book, St. Louis, 1992.
27. Sarmiento, A: A modified surgical-prosthetic approach to the Syme's amputation: A follow-up report. Clin Orthop 85:11–15, 1972.
28. Sarmiento, A, et al: A new surgical-prosthetic approach to the Syme's amputation: A preliminary report. Artif Limbs 10:52–55, 1966.
29. Pinzur, MS, and Bowker, JH: Knee disarticulation. Clin Orthop (361):23–28, 1999.
30. Pinzur, MS: Knee disarticulation: Surgical procedures. In Bowker, JH, and Michael, JW (eds): Atlas of Limb Prosthetics, ed 2. Mosby Year Book, St. Louis, 1992.
31. Utterback, TD, and Rohren, DW: Knee disarticulation as an amputation level. J Trauma 13:116, 1973.
32. Burgess, EM: Disarticulation of the knee: A modified technique. Arch Surg 112:1250–55, 1977.
33. Boyd, HB: Anatomic disarticulation of the hip. Surg Gynecol Obstet 84:346–49, 1947.
34. Tooms, RE: Hip disarticulation and transpelvic amputation: Surgical procedures. In Bowker, JH, and Michael, JW (eds): Atlas of Limb Prosthetics, ed 2. Mosby Year Book, St. Louis, 1992.
35. Weaver, JM, and Flynn, MB: Hemicorporectomy. J Surg Oncol 73(2):117–24, 2000.

CHAPTER FIVE

Postsurgical Management

OBJECTIVES

At the end of this chapter, all students are expected to:

1. Compare and contrast the major methods of postoperative residual limb management.
2. Implement an intervention program for a client following lower extremity amputation.
   - **2.a** Teach proper positioning.
   - **2.b** Describe and demonstrate proper residual limb bandaging and care.
   - **2.c** Implement an appropriate program of exercises.
   - **2.d** Develop an appropriate client education program.
3. Exhibit an understanding of the psychosocial and economic effects of amputation on clients of different ages.

In addition, physical therapy students are expected to:

4. Develop an examination plan for a client following lower extremity amputation.
5. Evaluate the examination data to:
   - **5.2** Establish a plan of care.
   - **5.3** Establish functional outcomes.
   - **5.4** Implement the plan with any simulated client.

Case Studies

Diana Magnolia, a 54-year-old woman who had a left transtibial amputation yesterday secondary to diabetic gangrene.

Benny Pearl, a 62-year-old man who had a revision to a right transfemoral amputation yesterday secondary to wound infection of a 4-day-old transtibial amputation. The transtibial amputation resulted from a failed femoral popliteal bypass.

Ha Lee Davis, an 18-year-old man who underwent traumatic right transtibial amputation secondary to a motorcycle accident 2 days ago. He sustained some abrasion on the upper right thigh and a sprained right wrist.

Betty Childs, a 12-year-old girl who underwent a transfemoral amputation secondary to IIB osteogenic sarcoma of the proximal right tibia yesterday.

■ *Case Study Activities*

All Students:

1 Compare and contrast the different methods of residual limb postoperative care, identifying the major advantages and disadvantages of each.

2 Discuss how you expect each person to respond to the amputation.

Physical Therapy Students:

3 Develop an examination plan for each of the clients listed above.

4 Assuming that each client has been referred the day after surgery, what tests and measurements could you implement on the first visit? Which would you have to delay? Justify your priorities in relation to the client information above and in Chapter 2.

5 Identify the appropriate practice pattern(s) for each client.

Physical Therapist Assistant Students:

6 What factors will affect taking goniometric measurements or performing a manual muscle test?

INTRODUCTION

The earlier the onset of rehabilitation, the greater the potential for success. The longer the delay, the more likely it is that complications such as joint contractures, general debilitation, and a depressed psychological state will occur. The postsurgical management[1] program can be divided into two phases: the *postsurgical phase,* which is the time between surgery and fitting with a definitive prosthesis or a decision is made not to fit the client, and the *prosthetic phase,* which starts with delivery of a temporary or permanent appliance. The major goal is to help the client regain the presurgical level of function, whether to return to gainful employment with an active recreational life, to be independent in the home and community, or even to be independent in the sheltered environment of a retirement center or nursing home. If the amputation resulted from chronic disease, the goal may be to help the person function at a higher level than that experienced immediately before surgery.

POSTOPERATIVE DRESSINGS

The postoperative dressing protects the incision and residual limb and controls postoperative edema. Edema control is critical because excessive edema in the residual limb compromises healing and causes pain. The postoperative dressing may include (1) immediate postoperative fitting or rigid dressing; (2) semirigid dressing (SRD); (3) controlled environment; or (4) soft dressing.

Rigid Dressing

In the early 1960s, orthopedic surgeons in the United States started experimenting with immediate postoperative prosthetic fitting, a technique developed in Europe that consisted of fitting the client with a plaster prosthetic socket. An attachment, at the distal end of the dressing, allowed the addition of a foot and pylon for limited weight-bearing ambulation[2-4] (Fig. 5.1). Use of immediate postoperative rigid dressings varies greatly. Generally, orthopedic surgeons use the technique more than do vascular surgeons. Immediately fitting a postoperative prosthesis:

1. Greatly limits the development of postoperative edema, thereby reducing postoperative pain and enhancing wound healing.
2. Allows earlier bipedal ambulation with the attachment of a pylon and foot.
3. Allows for earlier fitting of a definitive prosthesis by reducing the length of time needed to shrink the residual limb.[2-5]

However, it also:

1. Requires careful application by individuals knowledgeable about prosthetic principles.
2. Requires close supervision during the early healing stage.

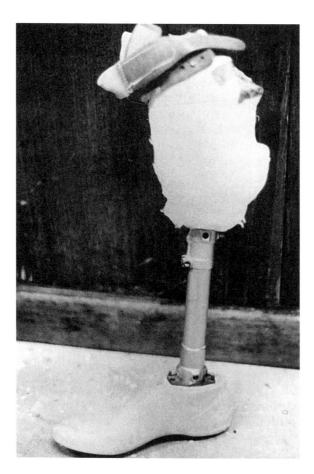

FIGURE 5.1
Rigid postoperative dressing with pylon and prosthetic foot attached.

3. Does not allow for daily wound inspection and dressing changes, unless the cast has a removable window at the distal end.

Semirigid Dressings

SRDs provide better control of edema than soft dressings, but each has some disadvantage that limits its use. SRDs are made of a paste compound of zinc oxide, gelatin, glycerin, and calamine and are applied in the operating or recovery room.[6,7] The dressing adheres to the skin, eliminating the need for a suspension belt, and allows slight joint movement. SRDs have been shown to be more effective than soft dressings in helping reduce postoperative edema.[7] The major disadvantages are that SRDs may loosen with use and are less rigid than plaster dressings.

Little first reported the use of an air splint to control postoperative edema as well as aid in early ambulation.[8,9] The air splint is a plastic double-wall bag that is pumped to the desired level of rigidity. The residual limb is covered with an appropriate postoperative dressing and inserted into the bag. The air splint allows wound inspection, but the constant pressure does not intimately conform to the shape of the residual limb, and the plastic is hot and humid requiring frequent cleaning.

Soft Dressings

The soft dressing is the oldest method of postsurgical management of the residual limb (Fig. 5.2). Two forms of soft dressings are the elastic wrap and the elastic **shrinker.** Both are:

1. Relatively inexpensive.
2. Lightweight.

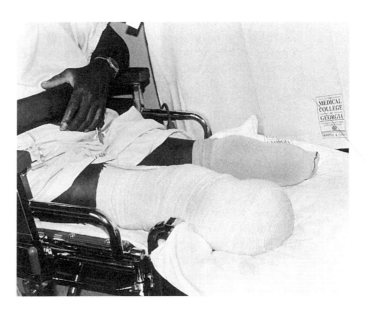

FIGURE 5.2
Postoperative soft dressing includes an elastic wrap over gauze pads.

3. Readily available.
4. Washable.

Elastic Wrap

Immediately after surgery, the elastic bandage is applied over the postsurgical dressing with moderate compression, preferably using a figure-of-eight pattern (see Fig. 5.2). The soft dressing is probably the most frequently used and is generally indicated in cases of local infection. It is easier to use than rigid dressings or SRDs, but it is not as effective as either type in controlling edema. Elastic wrap needs frequent rewrapping because movement of the residual limb against the bedclothes, bending and extending the proximal joints, and general body movements cause slippage and wrinkling. Wrinkles in the elastic bandage create uneven pressure on the residual limb that can lead to skin abrasions and breakdown. Covering the finished wrap with a stockinet helps reduce some of the wrinkling. Careful and frequent rewrapping, however, is the only effective way to prevent complications. Nursing and therapy staff need to assume responsibility for frequent inspection and rewrapping of the residual limb while the client is in hospital. After initial healing has occurred, the client or a family member should learn to apply the wrap properly. Most elderly individuals with a transfemoral amputation do not have the necessary balance and coordination to wrap effectively. Elastic wraps stretch over time and need replacement. Residual limb wrapping is described later in this chapter.

Shrinkers

Shrinkers are socklike garments knitted of rubber reinforced cotton; they are **conical** or cylindrical in shape and come in various sizes (see Fig. 5.3). Shrinkers should not be used until after the sutures have been removed and drainage has stopped. The act of donning the shrinker can put excessive distracting pressures at the distal end of the residual limb, and wound drainage will soil the shrinker. The shrinker is easy to don and is probably as effective as the elastic wrap but is less effective than rigid dressings or SRDs in controlling edema. As the residual limb becomes smaller, new shrinkers must be purchased or the existing shrinker made smaller by sewing an additional seam.

Many vascular surgeons prefer delaying elastic wrapping until the incision has healed and the sutures have been removed. Leaving the residual limb without any pressure wrap allows for development of postoperative edema that causes pain and that may interfere with circulation in the many small vessels in the skin and soft tissue. The physical therapist (PT) needs to discuss the benefits of edema control with the surgeon as early as possible and encourage the use of some form of compression dressing. Residual limb shrinkage is also necessary prior to prosthetic fitting. The residual limb must attain a stable size if the first prosthetic socket is to fit for a reasonable amount of time. Because the residual limb continues to shrink after permanent socket fitting, the more stable the residual limb is, the longer the socket will fit. However, delaying fitting for an extended period of time increases the problems associated with a lower level of mobility. Therefore, a general rule of thumb is to fit the first prosthesis when the incision is well healed and the residual limb has remained stable in size for 2 to 3 weeks. The time between

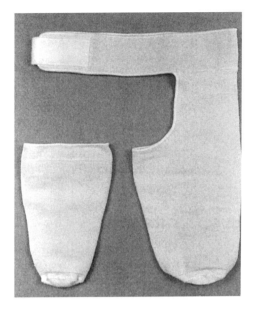

FIGURE 5.3

(*Left*) Transtibial and (*right*) transfemoral residual limb shrinkers. (From May, BJ: Assessment and treatment of individuals following lower extremity amputation. In O'Sullivan, SB, and Schmitz, TJ (eds): Physical Rehabilitation: Assessment and Treatment, ed 3. FA Davis, Philadelphia, 1994, p 381, with permission.)

amputation and initial prosthetic fitting is quite variable but is at least 6 to 8 weeks.

EXAMINATION

The *Guide to Physical Therapy Practice, ed. 2,* includes three practice patterns associated with amputations: 4J, 6A, 7A. Practice pattern 4J, impaired motor function, muscle performance, range of motion, locomotion, and balance associated with amputation is generally the most appropriate pattern, although the PT will determine the appropriate pattern or patterns through evaluation of data gathered in the examination phase.[10]

Careful examination is an integral part of the management of each client. Data are obtained continuously throughout this period as the incision heals and the person's tolerance improves. Table 5.1 outlines the typical data needed during a postsurgical examination. The availability of some data will depend in part on the treatment of the residual limb by the surgeon. The examination includes a careful history, a systems review, and the application of appropriate tests and measurements.

Range of Motion

Gross range-of-motion (ROM) estimations are usually adequate for the hip and knee of the uninvolved lower extremity and the upper extremities, but specific goniometric measurements are necessary for the uninvolved ankle (particularly for clients with vascular disease) and the amputated extremity. Many individuals with dysvascular disease have limitations of ankle motion. Such limitations can increase the stresses on the foot during walking and in-

TABLE 5.1 POSTSURGICAL EXAMINATION GUIDE

History	General demographic data
	Family and social data
	Pre-amputation status (work, activity level, degree of independence, lifestyle)
	Prosthetic goals (desire for prosthesis, anticipated activity level, and lifestyle)
	Financial (ability to pay for prosthesis)
	Prior prosthesis (if bilateral)
	Other as appropriate to specific client
General systems review	Cause of amputation (disease, tumor, trauma, congenital)
	Associated diseases/symptoms (neuropathy, visual disturbances, cardiopulmonary disease, renal failure, congenital anomalies)
	Current physiological status (postsurgical cardiopulmonary status, vital signs, out of bed [OOB], pain)
	Medications
Skin	Scar (healed, adherent, invaginated, flat)
	Other lesions (size, shape, open, scar tissue)
	Moisture (moist, dry, scaly)
	Sensation (absent, diminished, hyperesthesia)
	Grafts (location, type, healing)
	Dermatological lesions (psoriasis, eczema, cysts)
Residual limb length	Bone length (transtibial limbs measured from medial tibial plateau; transfemoral limbs measured from ischial tuberosity or greater trochanter)
	Soft tissue length (note redundant tissue)
Residual limb shape	Cylindrical, conical, bulbous end, etc.
	Abnormalities ("dog ears," adductor roll)
	Specific circumferential measurements
Vascularity (both limbs if amputation cause is vascular)	Pulses (femoral, popliteal, dorsalis pedis, posterior tibial)
	Color (red, cyanotic)
	Temperature
	Edema (circumference measurement, water displacement measurement, caliper measurements)
	Pain (type, location, duration)
	Trophic changes
ROM	Residual limb (specific for remaining joints)
	Other lower extremity (gross for major joints)
Muscle strength	Residual limb (specific for major muscle groups)
	Other extremities (gross for necessary function)
Neurological	Pain (phantom [differentiate sensation or pain], neuroma, incisional, from other causes)
	Neuropathy
	Cognitive status (alert, oriented, confused)
	Emotional status (acceptance, body image)
Functional status	Transfers (bed to chair, to toilet, to car)
	Balance (sitting, standing, reaching, moving)
	Mobility (ancillary support, supervision, closed and open environments, steps, curbs)
	Home/family situation (caregiver, architectural barriers, hazards)
	ADLs (bathing, dressing)
	Instrumental ADLs (cooking, cleaning)

crease the potential for injuries. Careful evaluation of the ROM of the remaining foot is important. Hip flexion and extension, abduction, and adduction measurements are taken early in the postoperative phase following transtibial amputation. Measurement of knee flexion and extension are taken, if the dressing allows, after some incisional healing has occurred. Hip flexion, extension, abduction, and adduction ROM measurements are taken several days after surgery following transfemoral amputation when the dressing allows. Measurements of internal and external hip rotation of the transfemoral residual limb are difficult to obtain and unnecessary if no gross abnormality or pathology is evident. Joint ROM is monitored throughout the postsurgical period.

Muscle Strength

Gross manual muscle testing of the upper extremities and uninvolved lower extremity is performed early in the postoperative period. Manual muscle testing of the amputated extremity must usually wait until some healing has occurred. Although individuals with muscle weakness of the residual limb can be satisfactorily fitted with a prosthesis, it is desirable for the client to develop at least 4 to 4+ strength in the residual limb. Particular emphasis may be placed on hip extensors and abductors, and knee flexors and extensors. The strength of these muscles should be monitored throughout the postsurgical program.

Residual Limb

Circumferential measurements of the residual limb are taken as soon as the dressing allows, then regularly throughout the postsurgical period. Measurements over the length of the residual limb are made at regular intervals. Circumferential measurements of the transtibial or Syme residual limb are started at the medial tibial plateau and are taken every 5 to 8 cm depending on the length of the limb. Length is measured from the medial tibial plateau to the end of the bone or the end of the residual limb if there is substantial soft tissue.

Circumferential measurements of the transfemoral or through-knee residual limb are started at the ischial tuberosity or the greater trochanter, whichever is more palpable, and taken every 8 to 10 cm. Length is measured from the ischial tuberosity or the greater trochanter to the end of the bone. If there is considerable excess tissue distal to the end of the bone, then length measurements are taken to both the end of the bone and the incision line. For accuracy of repeat measurements, exact landmarks are carefully noted. If the ischial tuberosity is used in transfemoral measurements, hip joint position is noted as well. Other information gathered about the residual limb includes its shape (conical, **bulbous,** redundant tissue), skin condition, sensation, and joint proprioception.

Phantom Limb/Phantom Pain

Most individuals experience **phantom sensation** following loss of a limb. In its simplest form, the phantom sensation is the feeling of the limb that is no longer there. The phantom sensation, which usually occurs initially immediately after surgery, is often described as a tingling, pressure sensation, sometimes a numbness. The distal part of the extremity is most frequently felt, although on occasion the person will feel the whole extremity. The sensation is responsive to external stimuli such as bandaging or rigid dressing; it may dissipate over time, or the person may have the sensation throughout life. Phantom sensation may be painless and usually does not interfere with prosthetic rehabilitation. It is important for the client to understand that the feeling is quite normal. In a recent study, the prevalence of phantom sensation was reported to be about 79 percent in a sample of 201 individuals more than 6 months postamputation.[11]

Phantom pain is frequently characterized as either a cramping or squeezing sensation, a shooting or a burning-like pain. Some clients report all three. Pain may be localized or diffuse; it may be continuous or intermittent and triggered by some external stimuli. It may diminish over time or may become a permanent and often disabling condition. In the first 6 months following surgery, phantom pain is related to preoperative limb pain in location and intensity. That relationship does not last, however, and preoperative pain is not believed to be related to long-term phantom pain.[12] In a recent study, about 72 percent of the respondents indicated they felt phantom limb pain at some time. Only 30 percent reported severe pain, and 32 percent indicated the pain was severely bothersome.[13]

The cause and treatment of phantom sensation or pain is controversial, and the literature is replete with studies of the phenomenon.[12–17] Melzack[18] suggests that at least 70 percent of individuals have phantom pain following amputation. He believes that clients view the phantom as an integral part of themselves regardless of where it is felt in relation to the body. Melzack believes that phantom sensation and pain originate in the cerebrum. "I postulate that the brain contains a neuromatrix, or network of neurons, that, in addition to responding to sensory stimulation, continuously generates a characteristic pattern of impulses indicating that the body is intact and unequivocally one's own."[18] He reputes the general belief that phantom sensation and pain only occur with acquired amputations after the age of 5 or 6, indicating that all individuals who are missing a limb from whatever cause, as well as individuals who lose the use of their limbs through spinal cord injury, feel the missing limbs.

The residual limb should be examined to differentiate phantom pain from any other condition such as a neuroma. Sometimes, wearing a prosthesis will ease the phantom pain. Noninvasive treatments such as ultrasound, icing, transcutaneous electrical nerve stimulation (TENS), or hand massage have been used with varying success. Mild non-narcotic analgesics are of limited value, and no particular narcotic analgesic has proven to be effective. Injection with steroids or local anesthetic has reduced the pain temporarily in the presence of trigger points. Continuous infusion of a regional analgesic postsurgically has been shown to be both effective and ineffective depending on the amount of medication and the rate of administration.[18–20] Surgical procedures such as chordotomies, rhizotomies, and peripheral neurectomies meet with limited success. Hypnosis is useful in carefully selected clients. The treatment of phantom pain can be very frustrating for the clinic team and the client.[13–21]

Other Data

The vascular status of the uninvolved lower extremity is documented. The same data as outlined in Chapter 2 are gathered.

Activities of daily living (ADLs), including transfer and ambulatory status, are evaluated; equipment and assistance needed are documented. Information on the client's home situation including any constraints or special needs are valuable in establishing the individual treatment program. Data regarding presurgical activity level and the person's own long-range goals are obtained through interview.

The person's apparent emotional status and degree of adjustment are noted. Emotional adjustment and attitude influence the eventual level of rehabilitation and are discussed in detail in Chapter 6. Exploration of the client's suitability and desire for a prosthesis is begun and continues throughout the postsurgical period. Any other problems that may affect the rehabilitation program and goals are evaluated and documented.

GOALS

Tables 5.2 to 5.5 illustrate the evaluation data for the clients.

■ *Case Study Activities*

All Students:

1   Would you expect each of the clients to achieve independent mobility with crutches or a walker prior to prosthetic fitting? Why or why not?
2   Do you expect to fit each of these individuals with an artificial limb? What might affect such a decision?

Physical Therapy Students:

3   Develop functional outcome goals for each client. What does each client have to achieve in the postsurgical period to be a prosthetic candidate?

The postsurgical period is designed to:

1. Promote a high level of independent function prior to prosthetic fitting.
2. Guide the development of the patient's necessary physical and emotional levels for eventual prosthetic fitting.

If the cause of amputation was peripheral vascular disease, a third general goal would be to teach the individual proper care of the remaining lower extremity and an understanding of the disease process.

Intervention Goals

Goals to be achieved at the end of the postsurgical period might include:

1. Reducing (preventing) postoperative edema and promoting healing of the residual limb.
2. Preventing contractures and other complications.
3. Increasing strength in the affected lower extremity.
4. Increasing strength in the remaining extremities.

TABLE 5.2   POSTSURGICAL EXAMINATION—DIANA MAGNOLIA

MEDICAL CHART REVIEW:
54-year-old female had (L) transtibial amputation yesterday secondary to gangrene from diabetic ulcers. Patient has long history of poorly controlled diabetes mellitus and a nonhealing ulcer (see Fig. 2.4). (L) transtibial with posterior flap and staples was performed. Patient tolerated procedure well. Nurse's notes indicate that the wound is clean with little drainage. The residual limb is wrapped with an elastic wrap over a soft dressing.

MEDICATIONS:
Insulin, Ampicillin, Darvocet, Xanax

INTERVIEW:
Client reports that her residual limb hurts and that she can feel her amputated toes and that they are cramped. She indicates that she sat up at the side of the bed this morning.

EXAMINATION:
Vitals:
BP 135/85; pulse 80

Residual limb measurements:
Delayed

Range of motion (ROM):
Left knee: Measurements delayed; knee fully extended on bed

Left hip: Active flexion = 100 degrees; extension (side-lying) = 5 degrees

Abduction/adduction; internal/external rotation = within normal limits

Right ankle: active dorsiflexion = 5 degrees; passive = 8 degrees; active plantar flexion = 22 degrees; passive = 25 degrees; active inversion = 15 degrees; passive 20 degrees; active eversion = 15 degrees; passive 20 degrees.

Right hip and knee active and passive ROM = within normal limits.

Muscle Strength:
Both upper extremities grossly within normal limits.
    Left hip and knee delayed but all musculature grossly active and functional.
    Right hip and knee grossly 4+/5 (Good+/Normal)
    Right ankle: dorsiflexion 3+/5 (Fair+/Normal); plantar flexion (NWB) = 4−/5 (Good−/Normal)

Pulmonary Status:
Strong dry cough; has incentive spirometer.

Vascular:
RLE shows evidence of dysvascularity; dry, hairless limb, minimal toenail clubbing, no sores or open areas. Sensation decreased to touch on plantar surface of foot and toes and dorsum of toes.

FUNCTIONAL ACTIVITIES:
Rolls supine to either side independently;
    Transfers bed to chair and back with verbal cueing and contact guard;
    Propels wheelchair independently but slowly;
    Bed to stand with walker with minimal assistance one person.
    Stood by side of bed one minute.

EMOTIONAL AND MENTAL:
Patient likes to talk and does so almost constantly. However, she does not appear to listen very well, requiring PT to repeat instructions. Verbalized concern for returning to home and work.

TABLE 5.3   POSTSURGICAL EXAMINATION—BENNY PEARL

MEDICAL CHART REVIEW:
62-year-old male had right transtibial amputation 4 days ago secondary to a failed femoral bypass; revision to transfemoral level yesterday secondary to wound infection (see Fig 2.5). Patient has history of coronary arterial disease.

Equal flap procedure closed with sutures, soft dressing. Incision clean with slight drainage. Nurse's notes indicate that Pt complains of pain in residual limb and is reluctant to move.

MEDICATIONS:
Procardia, Coumadin, Capoten, Darvocet, and Lasix

EXAMINATION:

Vitals:
BP 152/82; pulse 79.

Range of Motion:
Right hip active (PROM not tested): flexion (supine) 15–90 degrees; extension (Thomas position) lacks 15 degrees of neutral; abduction 0–20 degrees; adduction; 0–5 degrees

LLE: Hip and knee motions grossly within normal limits excepts lacks 10 degrees of neutral hip extension (tested supine). Ankle dorsiflexion to 8 degrees, plantar flexion to 20 degrees.

Muscle Strength:
Patient reluctant to hold against resistance. Both upper extremities grossly in 3+ to 4/5 (F+ to G) range. Left lower extremity grossly in 3+ to 4/5 (F+ to G) range.

Right hip not tested.

Vascular Status:
Evidence of dysvascularity in LLE. Limb is thin, little muscle bulk, no hair.

FUNCTIONAL ACTIVITIES:
Transfers chair to mat and back = minimal assistance of 1 person.

Independent in bed mobility except roll to right side or prone (not tested). Comes to sitting with minimal assistance of 1 person. Pushes own wheelchair slowly. Stood in parallel bars with minimal assistance 1 person. Ambulated 1 length parallel bars with contact guard and urging.

---

5. Assisting the patient to a) adjust to the loss of a body part, b) regain independence in mobility and self-care, and c) learn proper care of the other extremity.

Functional outcome goals for the same period must be individualized for each client and will address the client's ability to:

1. Function within the home environment.
2. Care for the residual limb and the uninvolved extremity.
3. Function in the community to some level.

The success of the rehabilitation program is partially determined by the individual's psychophysiological status and the physical characteristics of the residual limb. A well-healed, cylindrical limb with a nonadherent scar (see Fig. 4.1*A* and *B*) is easier to fit than one that is conical, short, scarred, or has redundant tissue distally or laterally (Fig 5.4*A* and *B*). Factors that might affect attainment of the goals include the client's:

1. Vascular status
2. Diabetes
3. Renal disease
4. Cardiovascular disease

TABLE 5.4   POSTSURGICAL EXAMINATION—HA LEE DAVIS

MEDICAL CHART REVIEW:
18-year-old male who underwent traumatic amputation of the right leg 19 cm below the medial tibial condyle yesterday, secondary to a motorcycle accident 2 days ago. Replantation was not an option because of the level and the traction nature of the injury. Immediate postoperative fitting cast in place with drain in place. Patient tolerated procedure well.

Patient sustained an avulsion amputation of the right lower extremity as well as a severe sprain of the right hand and wrist and multiple contusions but no fractures. Palmar splint with elastic bandage on right hand and wrist to mid forearm. Patient was alert and responsive in the emergency room.

Nurses notes indicate that the patient is alert; complains of pain in his hand and wrist. Drainage is minimal and drain is to be removed this afternoon.

Patient lives at home with parents and two siblings; is a senior in high school scheduled for graduation next month. He works part-time in a computer repair store.

MEDICATIONS:
Acetaminophen and Keflex.

EXAMINATION (at beside):
Vitals:
BP 120/65; pulse 60.

ROM and Muscle Strength:
Gross active ROM and muscle strength evaluation of both upper extremities (except right wrist and hand, and the left lower extremity) within normal limits.

Muscle test right residual limb deferred; gross active ROM of right hip within normal limits.

FUNCTIONAL ACTIVITIES:
Independent in all bed mobility and transfer activities. Patient can sit and move in bed with minimal difficulty mainly caused by inability to use right wrist and hand; transfers bed to chair independently. Can stand on left lower extremity by side of bed.

---

5. Visual impairment
6. Limitation of joint motion
7. Muscle weakness

However, care must be taken not to assume that a client with multiple physiological problems cannot achieve a high degree of independent prosthetic function. Modern technology has enabled the fitting of individuals with multiple problems and less than ideal residual limbs (see Chap. 7). In the final analysis, a client's willingness to take an active part in the rehabilitation program is necessary for achievement of rehabilitation goals. If the client does not appear to be motivated, the PT should try to understand the client's perspective and ensure that he or she understands the relationship between the postsurgical program and eventual prosthetic rehabilitation. Referral to social or psychological services may be advisable for reluctant clients.

INTERVENTIONS

■ Case Study Activities

Review the examination data in Tables 5.2 to 5.5 and your functional outcome goals, and then complete the activities below.

TABLE 5.5   POSTSURGICAL EXAMINATION—BETTY CHILDS

MEDICAL CHART REVIEW:
12-year-old obese white female who underwent a transfemoral amputation yesterday secondary to IIB osteogenic sarcoma of the proximal right tibia. Scheduled to start a special program of adjuvant chemotherapy and radiation therapy as an outpatient in about 2 weeks.

Distal third transfemoral amputation performed yesterday; tumor was encapsulated but was too large for tumor excision and limb salvage to be an option. Residual limb wrapped in a rigid dressing secured with a hip spica.

Nurse's notes indicate that Betty has been complaining of pain and has been reluctant to get out of bed. Mother has been with her most of the time.

Social Service Note:
Betty is the oldest of three siblings living with their mother in their own home. Mother, an attorney, is a single parent. Father disappeared several years ago. Grandmother is currently taking care of other children, one of whom has severe asthma requiring regular medical attention.

MEDICATIONS:
Acetaminophen and vistaril.

EXAMINATION:

Vitals:
BP 118/70; pulse 68.

ROM and Strength:
Gross active ROM and muscle strength of both upper extremities and the left lower extremity appear grossly within normal limits, although patient was reluctant to participate in therapeutic activities; ROM and strength evaluation of right residual limb deferred. Residual limb reported to be through distal third of the femur.

FUNCTIONAL ACTIVITIES:
Appears independent in bed mobility. Able to come to sitting at the side of the bed with much urging and to transfer into a wheelchair with standby assistance only. Refused to come to PT department or to stand for other than the transfer.

Patient is listless and tires easily. Patient avoided looking at the residual limb or talking about the amputation.

Physical Therapy Students:

1   Diagnostically classify each client in relation to predominant practice pattern(s). Identify and prioritize the impairments, functional limitations, and disabilities to be addressed.

2   Establish a plan of care for each client.

All Students:

3   What parts of the treatment program are appropriately performed by a physical therapist assistant?

4   Most individuals are discharged from the acute care hospital 4 to 6 days following amputation. What other data do you need to recommend a patient for further treatment to an inpatient rehabilitation center? To a home health agency? To an outpatient service?

5   In laboratory sessions, practice residual limb bandaging, postsurgical exercises, and mobility training, role-playing each client. How would you vary your approach for each client?

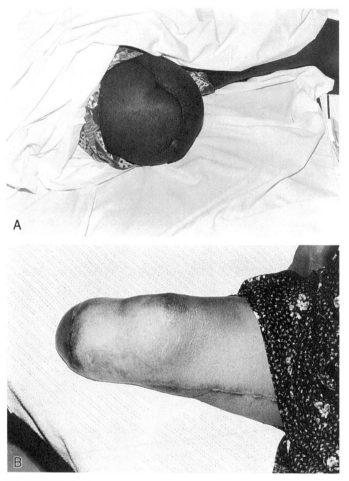

FIGURE 5.4
Short, scarred residual limbs. (*A*) Transfemoral. (*B*) Transtibial.

Residual Limb Care

Residual Limb Size

Individuals not fitted with a rigid dressing or a temporary prosthesis use elastic wrap or shrinkers to reduce the size of the residual limb. The client or a member of the family applies the bandage that is worn 24 hours a day, except when bathing.

Removable rigid dressing for transtibial residual limbs is an alternative to the elastic wrap or shrinker. The removable rigid dressing is usually a plaster cast fabricated in the shape of the prosthetic socket and applied after the incision has healed and the sutures have been removed. It is used like a temporary prosthesis with socks and is removed at night and when bathing. The semirigid dressing may also be used throughout the postsurgical period. A new dressing is applied as residual limb size decreases and the current dressing becomes loose. Regretfully, there are fewer alternatives for the transfemoral residual limb; rigid dressings and inexpensive temporary prostheses are more difficult to fabricate, and elastic wraps or shrinkers are only minimally effective. The semirigid dressing, self-suspending and not bulky, may be the most effective alternative. The semirigid dressing, however, is not in general use throughout the country. Early bipedal mobility positively affects eventual rehabilitation outcome, particularly in the elderly. It may be advisable to fit the individual with a transfemoral amputation with a definitive prosthesis early, then adjust for shrinkage by using additional socks or a liner. Adjustable sockets, discussed in Chapter 9, may also be advisable. The additional costs involved in early prosthetic fitting and socket replacement may mitigate against early fitting.

Edema in the residual limb is often difficult to control because of complications of diabetes, renal disease, cardiovascular disease, or hypertension. An intermittent compression unit can be used to reduce edema temporarily. Transfemoral and transtibial sleeves are commercially available.

The residual limb tends to become edematous after bathing as a reaction to the warm water, so nightly bathing is recommended. This is particularly important once a prosthesis has been fitted. The elastic bandage, shrinker, or removable rigid dressing is reapplied after bathing. If the person has been fitted with a temporary prosthesis, the residual limb is wrapped at night and any time the prosthesis is not worn. It is equally important that individuals fitted in surgery with a rigid dressing learn bandaging because they can encounter difficulties with edema after they remove the prosthesis at night. Learning proper bandaging is part of the therapy program for all individuals with amputations because most people need to wrap the limb at one time or another.

Skin Care

Proper hygiene and skin care are important. Once the incision is healed and the sutures are removed, the person can bathe normally. The residual limb is treated as any other part of the body; it is kept clean and dry. Individuals with dry skin should use a mild, water-based skin lotion. Care must be taken to avoid abrasions, cuts, and other skin problems. The client is taught to inspect the residual limb with a mirror each night to make sure there are no sores or impending problems, especially in areas not readily visible. If the person has diminished sensation, careful inspection is particularly important.

Clients have been known to apply a variety of "home and folk remedies" to the residual limb. Historically, it was believed that the skin had to be toughened for prosthetic wear by beating it with a towel-wrapped bottle. Various ointments and lotions have been applied; residual limbs have been immersed in substances such as vinegar, salt water, and gasoline to harden the skin. Although the skin does need to adjust to the pressures of wearing an artificial limb, there is no evidence to indicate that "toughening" techniques are beneficial. Such methods may actually be deleterious, because soft pliable skin is better able to cope with stress than tough dry skin. Client education on proper skin care can reduce the use of home remedies.

The skin of the residual limb may be affected by a variety of dermatological problems such as eczema, psoriasis, or burns from radiation therapy. Some of these conditions may mitigate against fitting or wrapping. Treatment may include ultraviolet irradiation, whirlpool, reflex heating, **hyperbaric oxygen** therapy, or medication. Care must be taken in using ultraviolet light or heat in the presence of impaired circulation. Whirlpool may also not be the treatment of choice because it increases edema. The benefits of whirlpool as a cleansing agent for skin problems, infected wounds, or incidence of delayed healing must be balanced against its disadvantages before appropriateness can be determined.

Friction massage, in which layers of skin, subcutaneous tissue, and muscle are moved over underlying tissue, can be used to mobilize adherent scar tissue. The massage is done gently after the wound is healed and no infection is present. Clients can learn to properly perform a gentle friction massage to mobilize the scar tissue and help decrease hypersensitivity of the residual limb to touch and pressure. Early handling of the residual limb by the client is an aid to acceptance and is encouraged, particularly for individuals who may be repulsed by the limb.

Residual Limb Wrapping

Most methods of residual limb wrapping incorporate figure-of-eight or angular turns, anchoring turns around the proximal joint, distributing greater pressure distally with a smooth, wrinkle-free application of the bandage. Clients tend to wrap their own residual limb in a circular manner, often creating a tourniquet that may compromise healing and will foster the development of a bulbous end. Although the client can wrap the transtibial residual limb in a sitting position, it is virtually impossible to properly wrap and anchor the transfemoral limb while sitting. Many clients cannot balance themselves in the standing position while wrapping. The ends of the bandages are better fastened with tape rather than clips or safety pins that can cut the skin and do not anchor well. Care should be taken to avoid anchoring the tape to the skin to avoid potential skin abrasions. Elastic bandages that incorporate hook and loop attachments at each end are difficult to roll properly and can cause excessive pressure because of the greater bulk of the ends.

A system of wrapping that uses mostly angular or figure-of-eight turns was developed specifically to meet the needs of the elderly and has been in use for the past 40 years.[22] Figures 5.5 and 5.6 illustrate the techniques.

The Transtibial Residual Limb

Two 4-inch elastic bandages will usually be enough to wrap most transtibial residual limbs. Very large residual limbs may require three bandages. The bandages should not be sewn together so that the weave of each bandage can be brought in contraposition to each other to provide more support. To deter the development of postsurgical edema as much as possible, a firm, even pressure against all soft tissues is desirable. If the incision is placed anteriorly, then an attempt should be made to bring the bandages from posterior to anterior over the distal end so as not to put a distracting pressure on the incision.

The first bandage is started at either the medial or lateral tibial condyle and brought diagonally over the anterior surface of the limb to the distal end. One edge of the bandage should just cover the midline of the incision in an anteroposterior plane. The bandage is continued diagonally over the posterior surface and then back over the beginning turn as an anchor. At this point, there is a choice; the bandage may be brought directly over the beginning point as indicated in step 2, or it may be brought across the front of the residual limb in an "x" design. The latter is particularly useful with long residual limbs and aids in bandage suspension. An anchoring turn over the distal thigh

BELOW—KNEE STUMP BANDAGING

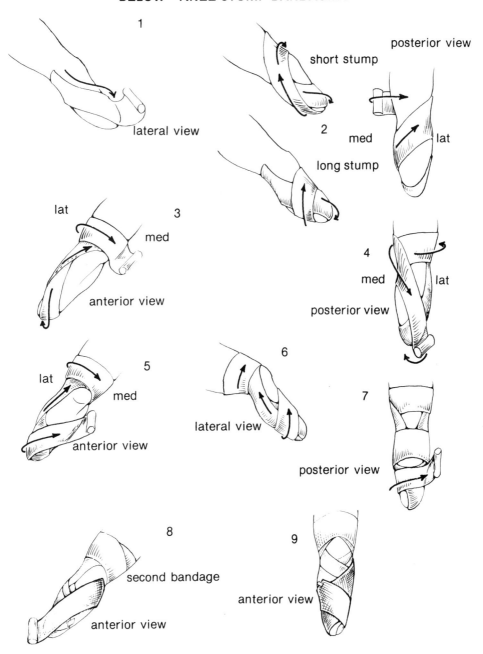

FIGURE 5.5
Wrapping the transtibial residual limb.

ABOVE-KNEE STUMP BANDAGING

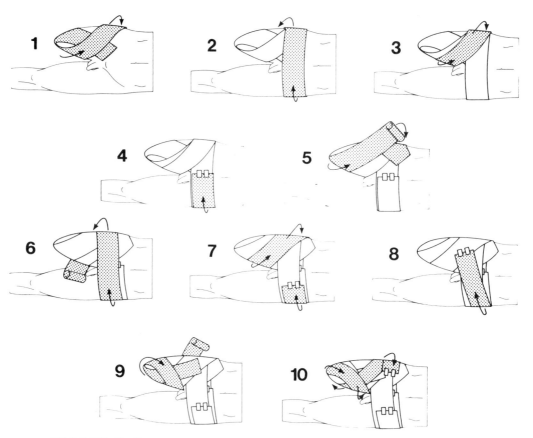

FIGURE 5.6
Wrapping the transfemoral residual limb.

is made, making sure that the wrap is clear of the patella and is not tight around the distal thigh.

After a single anchoring turn above the knee, the bandage is brought back around the opposite tibial condyle and down to the distal end of the limb. One edge of the bandage should overlap the midline of the incision and the other wrap by at least ½ inch to ensure adequate distal end support. The figure-of-eight pattern is continued as depicted in steps 4 to 7 until the bandage is completed. Care should be taken to completely cover the residual limb with a firm and even pressure. Semicircular turns are made posteriorly to bring the bandage in line to cross the anterior surface in an angular line. This maneuver provides greater pressure on the posterior soft tissue while distributing pressure anteriorly where the bone is close to the skin. Each turn should partially overlap other turns so the whole residual limb is well covered. The pattern is usually from proximal to distal and back to proximal starting at the tibial condyles and covering both condyles as well as the patellar tendon. Usually, the patella is left free to aid in knee motion, although with extremely short residual limbs, it may be necessary to cover it for better suspension.

The second bandage is wrapped like the first, except that it is started at the opposite tibial condyle from the first bandage (step 8). Bringing the weave of each bandage in contraposition exerts a more even pressure. With both bandages, an effort is made to bring the angular turns across each other rather than in the same direction.

The Transfemoral Residual Limb

For most residual limbs, two 6-inch and one 4-inch bandage will adequately cover the limb. The two 6-inch bandages can be sewn together end-to-end taking care not to create a heavy seam; the 4-inch bandage is used by itself. The client is side-lying (see Fig. 5.6), which allows a family member or therapist easy access to the residual limb.

The 6-inch bandages are used first. The first bandage is started in the groin and brought diagonally over the anterior surface to the distal lateral corner, around the end of the residual limb, and diagonally up the posterior side to the iliac crest and around the hips in a spica. The bandage is started medially so that the hip wrap will encourage extension. After the turn around the hips, the bandage is wrapped around the proximal portion of the residual limb high in the groin, and then back around the hips. Although this is a proximal circular turn, it does not create a tourniquet as long as it is continued around the hips. Going around the medial portion of the residual limb high in the groin ensures coverage of the soft tissue in the adductor area and reduces the possibility of an adductor roll, a complication that can seriously interfere with comfortable prosthetic wear. In most instances, the first bandage ends in the second spica and is anchored with tape.

If the two 6-inch bandages are not sewn together, the second 6-inch bandage is wrapped like the first but is started a bit more laterally. If they are sewn together, the pattern continues with at least two turns coming high in the groin and going around the hips. Any areas not covered with the first bandage must be covered at this time. The second bandage is also anchored in a hip spica after the first figure-of-eight and after the second turn high in the groin. Although more of the first two bandages are used to cover the proximal residual limb, care must be taken that no tourniquet is created. Bringing the bandage directly from the proximal medial area into a hip spica helps keep the adductor tissue covered and to some degree prevents rolling of the bandage.

The 4-inch bandage is used to exert the greatest amount of pressure over mid and distal areas of the residual limb. It is usually not necessary to anchor this bandage around the hips because friction with the already applied bandages and good figure-of-eight turns provide adequate suspension. The 4-inch bandage is generally started laterally to bring the weave across the weave of previous bandages. Regular figure-of-eight turns in varied patterns to cover all the residual limb are the most effective.

Bandages are applied with firm pressure from the outset. Elastic bandages can be wrapped directly over a soft postsurgical dressing so that bandaging can begin immediately after surgery. The elastic wrap controls edema more effectively if minimal gauze is used over the residual limb. Several gauze pads placed just over the incision are usually adequate protection without compromising the effect of the wrap. Care must be taken to avoid any wrinkles or folds that can cause excessive skin pressure, particularly over a soft dressing.

Shrinkers

The transtibial shrinker is rolled over the residual limb to midthigh and is designed to be self-suspending. Individuals with heavy thighs may need additional suspension with garters or a waist belt. Currently available transfemoral shrinkers incorporate a hip spica that provides good suspension except with obese individuals. Care must be taken that the client understands the importance of proper suspension because any rolling of the edges or slipping of the shrinker can create a tourniquet around the proximal part of the residual limb. Shrinkers are easier to apply than elastic bandages and may be a better alternative, particularly for the transfemoral residual limb. Shrinkers are more expensive to use than elastic wrap; the initial cost is greater, and new shrinkers of smaller sizes must be purchased as the limb volume decreases. However, shrinkers are the best option for transfemoral residual limbs and for individuals who are not able to properly wrap.

Positioning

One of the major goals of the early postoperative program is to prevent secondary complications such as contractures of adjacent joints. Contractures can develop from muscle imbalance or fascial tightness, a protective withdrawal reflex into hip and knee flexion, a loss of plantar stimulation in extension, or faulty positioning such as prolonged sitting. The client should understand the importance of proper positioning and regular exercises in preparing for eventual prosthetic fit and ambulation.

With the transtibial amputation, full ROM in the hips and knee, particularly in extension, is needed. Sitting, the client can keep the knee extended by using a posterior splint or a board attached to the wheelchair. Supine, the client should avoid placing a pillow under the knee or residual limb to avoid the development of knee or hip flexion contractures (Fig. 5.7A).

The client with a transfemoral amputation needs full ROM in the hip, particularly in extension and adduction. Prolonged sitting is to be avoided, if possible, or countered with periods of lying prone and doing active hip extensions. This is particularly important for individuals who have difficulty walking on crutches. Elevation of the residual limb on a pillow following either transfemoral or transtibial amputation can lead to the development of hip flexion contractures and should be avoided (Fig. 5.7B). Figure 5.8 depicts general rules of positioning. The early postoperative period is critical in establishing patterns of activity that will aid the client throughout the rehabilitative period.

Contractures

Some individuals will present with hip or knee flexion contractures. Mild contractures may respond to manual mobilization and active exercises, but it is almost impossible to reduce moderate to severe contractures, especially hip flexion contractures, by manual stretching. Some clinicians advocate holding the extremity in a stretched position with weights for a considerable length of time. There is little evidence that this traditional approach is successful. Active stretching techniques are more effective than passive stretching; hold-contract and resisted motion of antagonist muscles may increase ROM, par-

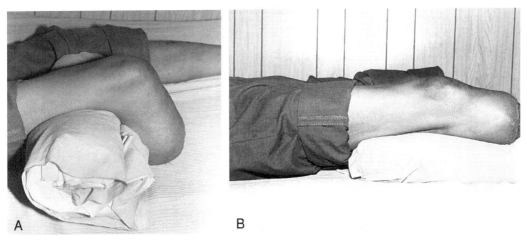

FIGURE 5.7
Improper positioning of the transtibial residual limb.

ticularly of the knee. One of the more effective ways of reducing a knee flexion contracture is to fit the client with a prosthesis aligned in a manner that
stretches the hamstrings with each step (see Chap. 8). Hip flexion contractures are more frequently found in individuals with transfemoral amputations. It is difficult to reduce a hip flexion contracture with the transfemoral
prosthesis. In some instances, depending on the severity of the contracture
and the length of the residual limb, the contracture can be accommodated in
the alignment of the prosthesis. A hip or knee flexion contracture of less than
15 degrees may not be problem caused by fit of the prosthesis. However, hip
flexion contractures of any degree are a severe impairment. Any hip flexion
contracture interferes with proper body alignment in stance and in walking
and limits the client's ability to properly bear weight on the prosthesis
through the gait cycle. Hip or hip and knee flexion contractures increase the
amount of energy required for ambulation and may deter older individuals
with multiple problems from reaching their full ambulatory potential. Prevention is the best treatment for contractures.

Exercises

The exercise program is individually designed and includes strengthening,
balance, and coordination activities. Exercises are initiated early after surgery; however, care is taken not to place stress on the incision or underlying
tissue. Gentle active movement within the pain-free range is beneficial, but
flexion should not be emphasized over extension. Gluteal sets in the first few
days after surgery can support extension, but pressure on the residual limb itself must be avoided. Bridging activities must wait until adequate healing has
occurred. The postsurgical dressing, degree of postoperative pain, and healing
of the incision determine when resistive exercises for the involved extremity
can be started. The postoperative exercise program can take many forms, and
a home program is necessary. The hip extensors, abductors, knee extensors,
and flexors are particularly important for prosthetic ambulation. Figures 5.9

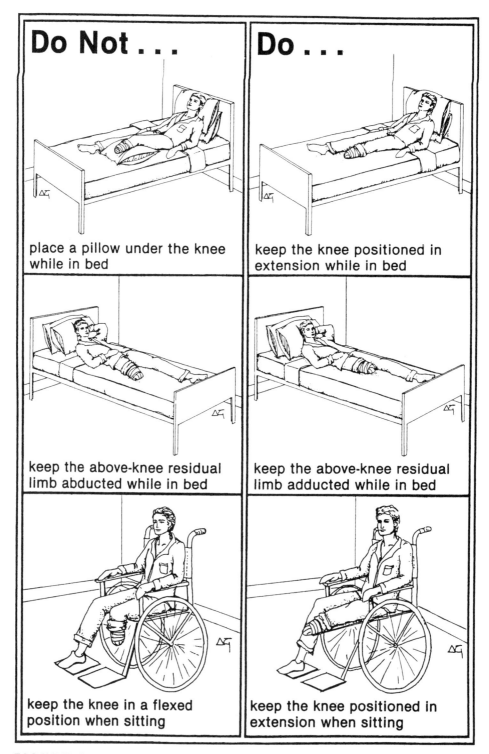

Do Not . . .

place a pillow under the knee while in bed

keep the above-knee residual limb abducted while in bed

keep the knee in a flexed position when sitting

Do . . .

keep the knee positioned in extension while in bed

keep the above-knee residual limb adducted while in bed

keep the knee positioned in extension when sitting

FIGURE 5.8

Correct and incorrect positioning following transtibial and transfemoral amputations.

and 5.10 depict a series of exercises particularly well designed to strengthen key muscles around the hip and knee. These exercises can be adapted for a home program because they are simple to perform and require no special equipment. There are a variety of methods to provide resistance in the home exercise program including the use of elastic bands (Fig. 5.11).

A general strengthening program that includes the trunk and all extremities is often indicated, particularly for the elderly person who may have been sedentary prior to surgery. Proprioceptive neuromuscular exercise routines are beneficial. The exercise program needs to be individually developed and should emphasize those muscles that are most active in prosthetic function and balance. Isometric exercises as depicted in Figures 5.9D and 5.10A may be contraindicated for individuals with cardiac disease or hypertension. Both exercises can be modified by having the client actually lift the buttocks off the treatment table in a modified bridging activity (Fig 5.12).

The younger, more active client usually does not lose a great deal of muscle strength. Many elderly individuals, however, are relatively sedentary after surgery and need encouragement to develop good strength, coordination, and cardiopulmonary endurance for later ambulation.

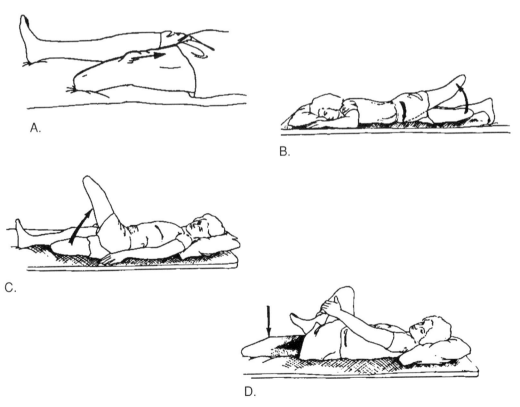

FIGURE 5.9
Exercises for the client following transtibial amputation. (*A*) Quad set. (*B*) Hip extension with knee straight. (*C*) Straight leg raise. (*D*) Extension of the residual limb with the knee of the other leg against the chest. (Adapted from Karacoloff, L [ed]: Lower Extremity Amputations. Aspen Publishers and the Rehabilitation Institute of Chicago, Rockville, MD, 1985.)

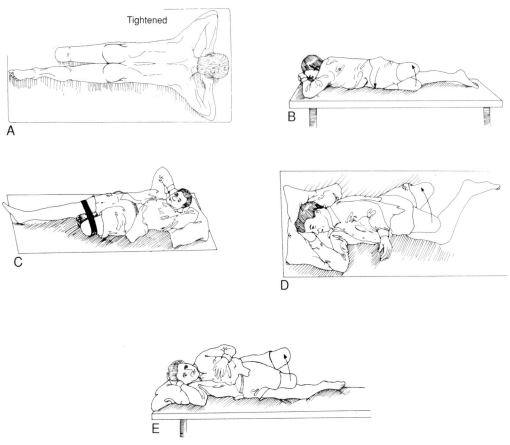

FIGURE 5.10

Exercises for the client following transfemoral amputation. (*A*) Gluteal sets. (*B*) Hip extension. (*C*) Hip abduction against elastic band. (*D*) Hip flexion and extension. (*E*) Hip abduction against gravity. (Adapted from Karacoloff, L [ed]: Lower Extremity Amputations. Aspen Publishers and the Rehabilitation Institute of Chicago, Rockville, MD, 1985.)

The exercise program is designed for progressive motor control and increasing coordination, and function. The client should progress from bed to mat activities using exercises that emphasize coordinated functional mobility. The client's postoperative status is influenced to a great extent by the preoperative activity level, length of time of disability, and other medical problems as well as the effects of the surgery itself. Because many clients are discharged from the hospital as early as a few days after surgery, referral to a rehabilitation center or home health agency is important to provide the necessary continuity of care.

Mobility

Early mobility is vital to total physiological recovery. The client needs to resume independent activities as soon as possible. Movement transitions (supine to sitting, sitting to standing) are preliminary to ambulation activities. Care must be taken during early bed and transfer movements to protect

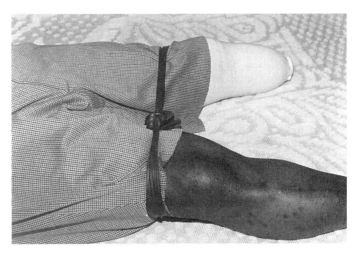

FIGURE 5.11
Elastic bands of appropriate thickness provide resistance for residual limb exercises.

the residual limb from any trauma. The client must be advised not to push on or slide the residual limb against the bed or chair. The client also needs to be cautioned against spending too much time in any one position to prevent the development of joint contractures or skin breakdowns.

Most individuals with unilateral amputations have little difficulty adjusting to the change in balance point that results from the loss of a limb. Sitting and standing balance activities are a useful part of the early postsurgical program. Upper extremity strengthening exercises with weights or elastic bands are important in preparation for crutch walking. Shoulder depression and elbow extension are particularly necessary to improve the ability to lift the body in ambulation. Individuals with bilateral amputations who have one healed residual limb will often use that limb as a prop for bed activities and

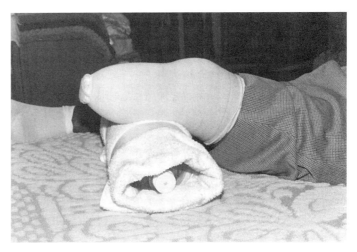

FIGURE 5.12
A bolster or a large plastic soda bottle covered with a bathtowel can be used for modified bridging exercises.

transfers. Often a debilitated person with bilateral amputations who is unable to lift the body with the arms will be able to transfer when allowed to use the old prosthesis to push on. Care must be taken not to create excess pressures and skin abrasions.

Walking is an excellent exercise and useful for independence in daily life. Gait training can start early in the postoperative phase, and the person with one intact extremity can become quite independent using a swing-through gait on crutches. Some elderly individuals have difficulty learning to walk on crutches. Some are afraid, some lack the necessary balance and coordination, whereas others lack endurance. Some studies have indicated that walking with crutches without a prosthesis requires a greater expenditure of energy than walking with a prosthesis.

Independence in crutch walking is a goal worthy of considerable therapy time. The individual who can ambulate with crutches will develop a greater degree of general fitness than the person who spends most of the time in a wheelchair. Crutch walking is good preparation for prosthetic ambulation, and the person who can learn to use crutches will not have difficulty learning to use a prosthesis. The individual who cannot learn to walk with crutches independently, however, may still become a very functional prosthetic user. If ambulation with crutches is not feasible, then the individual should be taught to use a walker.

There is a tendency among therapists to initiate mobility with a walker rather than to even try crutches, particularly with older clients and with clients who have lost a limb. There is also a time pressure with shorter hospital stays and the need to have the person as independent as possible at discharge. There are advantages and disadvantages to using a walker for support during the postsurgical period. Certainly, walking with a walker is physiologically and psychologically more beneficial than sitting in a wheelchair, but a walker should be used only if the person cannot learn to walk safely with crutches. A walker is sturdier than crutches but is awkward to use on stairs and requires a forward flexed position. It is sometimes difficult for the person who has used a walker during the postsurgical period to switch to one crutch or a cane when fitted with a prosthesis, yet the gait pattern used with a walker is not appropriate for a prosthesis. All clients need to learn some form of mobility without a prosthesis for use at night or when the prosthesis is not worn for some reason.

Temporary Prostheses

Many individuals are not fitted with any type of prosthetic appliance until the residual limb is free from edema and much of the soft tissue has atrophied, a process that can take many months of conscientious limb wrapping and exercises. During this period, the client is limited to a wheelchair or to ambulation with crutches or a walker. Most individuals cannot return to work or fully participate in ADLs while waiting for the residual limb to mature. Once fitted with a definitive prosthesis, the residual limb continues to change in size and a second prosthesis is often required within the first year. Early fitting with a temporary prosthesis can greatly enhance the postsurgical rehabilitation program (Figs. 5.13 and 5.14). A temporary prosthesis includes a socket designed and constructed according to regular prosthetic principles and attached to a pylon, a knee joint for the transfemoral level, a foot, and

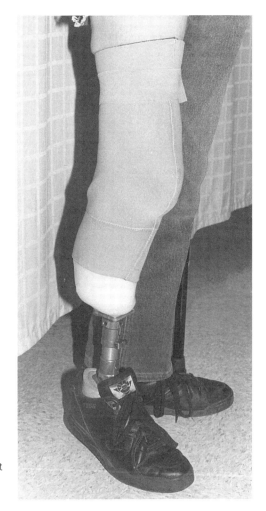

FIGURE 5.13

Temporary transtibial prosthesis. (From May, BJ:
Assessment and treatment of individuals following
lower extremity amputation. In O'Sullivan, SB, and
Schmitz, TJ [eds]: Physical Rehabilitation: Assessment
and Treatment, ed. 3. FA Davis, Philadelphia, 1994,
p 390, with permission.)

some type of suspension. Most temporary prostheses are much like the permanent prosthesis except that they do not have the cosmetic cover or finishing lamination for ease in changing sockets. In some centers, PTs have the training and equipment to fabricate temporary prostheses from plaster of Paris. These temporary limbs can be fitted earlier than the prosthetically fabricated appliances because some form of external support is generally necessary. Temporary prostheses made of plaster do not last as long, and the patient must be followed closely to make sure the limbs are in proper condition.

Generally, a temporary prosthesis can be fitted as soon as the wound has healed and the soft tissue can tolerate weight bearing, generally about 8 weeks. The advantages of a temporary prosthesis are that it:

1. Shrinks the residual limb more effectively than the elastic wrap.
2. Allows earlier bipedal ambulation, thereby reducing stress on the remaining extremity.
3. Provides safer ambulation for individuals who have difficulty walking on crutches or with a walker and one lower extremity.

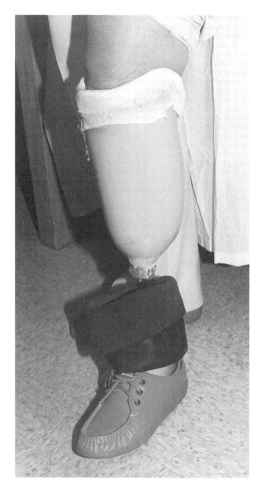

FIGURE 5.14
Temporary transtibial prosthesis with sleeve
lowered to show socket and pylon. (From May, BJ:
Assessment and treatment of individuals following
lower extremity amputation. In O'Sullivan, SB, and
Schmitz, TJ [eds]: Physical Rehabilitation:
Assessment and Treatment, ed 3. FA Davis,
Philadelphia, 1994, p 391, with permission.)

4. Is a positive motivator by providing a replacement for the missing part of
   the body.
5. Reduces the need for a complex exercise program because many people can
   return to full active daily life.

   In some centers, PTs have the training and equipment to fabricate temporary prostheses. The transtibial temporary socket may be constructed of plaster or from plastic materials. In all instances, the socket design should follow
regular prosthetic principles and should incorporate a prosthetic foot attached
to the socket with an aluminum or rigid plastic pipe for proper gait pattern
and weight distribution. A crutch tip, frequently used in earlier days, does not
adequately distribute the forces transmitted from the floor to the end of the
residual limb and is now contraindicated, particularly for the dysvascular person. The plaster prosthesis is cheaper to construct and can be changed more
frequently. It is not as sturdy as a plastic limb and usually requires the use of
crutches for safe ambulation. Depending on the attachments, proper foot
socket alignment may also be difficult to obtain if prosthetic components are
not used to attach the foot to the socket. Few therapists have been trained in
the fabrication of temporary prostheses. Some therapist-made sockets are

constructed of lightweight thermoplastic materials that can be formed over a positive cast of the residual limb; some are constructed of a fiberglass material formed directly over the residual limb. The prosthesis is usually suspended by a supracondylar cuff to which a waist belt can be added if necessary. (See Chap. 7 for a discussion of components.) The prosthesis is worn with a wool **stump sock** of appropriate thickness or ply. The light cotton sock made of stockinet material is considered to be one-ply thick. Wool socks generally come in 3- and 5-ply thicknesses (see Chap. 8) so that when the residual limb has shrunk, three 5-ply wool socks can maintain socket fit until a new socket can be constructed.

A temporary prosthesis fabricated by a prosthetist is actually a definitive prosthesis that is not finished cosmetically. These prostheses are sturdier, allowing regular prosthetic training and ambulation without external support. They are more expensive than prostheses made by a therapist, however, and cannot be changed as readily. Only therapists or other individuals who have received special training in temporary prosthetic fabrication and who have access to the appropriate equipment should attempt to construct temporary prostheses. Although it is easier to fabricate a transtibial socket, the use of a temporary prosthesis is important in the rehabilitation of the person with a transfemoral amputation.[21] The transfemoral temporary prosthesis should incorporate the regular socket, articulated knee joint, foot, and pylon. Suspension may be with Silesian bandage or pelvic band (see Chap. 7 for details of prosthetic components).

EDUCATING THE CLIENT

Case Studies

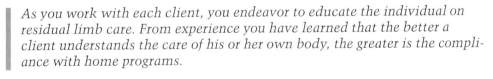

As you work with each client, you endeavor to educate the individual on residual limb care. From experience you have learned that the better a client understands the care of his or her own body, the greater is the compliance with home programs.

■ *Case Study Activities*

1   Develop a home exercise program for each of the clients. What are the critical concepts you need to include?
2   What teaching methods would work best for each client?

Educating the client and primary caregiver is an integral part of the plan of care. Information on the care of the residual limb, proper care of the uninvolved extremity, positioning, exercises, and diet if the client has diabetes, are necessary for the person to be a full participant in the rehabilitation program. Ideally, education should begin prior to the amputation, but that is rarely an option. The educational program needs to be planned for each individual and reflect the client's most effective learning style. Telling the client what to do and giving a long list of exercises is a waste of time. Using effective educational methodologies is important. Characteristics of an effective educational program include:

1. The home exercise program is limited in scope and includes only the most critical activities. Giving too much information or too many exercises is counterproductive.
2. The client and caregiver understand the rationale for the activities and how each is related to the eventual goal of prosthetic ambulation.
3. The client and caregiver are involved in determining an exercise schedule—both the length of time and the time of day.
4. There are some activities the client can do without assistance.
5. There are written and pictorial directions.
6. The client and caregiver are given a contact for questions that may be raised once the client is actually at home.

A narrated videotape of the exercises is an excellent tool. Any facility that provides care for a number of individuals with amputations can develop a videotape and then duplicate it for each client. There are also computer programs with a large library of exercises that can be downloaded to print or video media. After the client is discharged, either weekly clinic visits or home health supervision throughout the postsurgical phase provide a check on home activities and the condition of the residual limb, and is supportive to the client and family.

Many individuals with vascular disease who lose one leg are concerned about the other leg and receptive to learning proper care. (See Chap. 2 for components of an education program for individuals with peripheral vascular disease.) Ambulation on the one remaining extremity is stressful for individuals with peripheral vascular disease who need to be alert for signs of edema, pain, and changes in skin color or temperature. If the person spends considerable time sitting, it may be necessary to elevate the extremity to avoid dependent edema. Intermittent claudication (cramping of the calf) during activity is an indication of a need to stop the activity at least temporarily. The collateral circulation of the remaining extremity is developed slowly through a progressive program of exercises and ambulation. It is important to remember that too little activity may be as harmful as too much.

BILATERAL AMPUTATION

Case Studies

Mr. Canan, 79 years old, lost his right leg below the knee 4 years ago secondary to vascular insufficiency and diabetes. He was fitted with a prosthesis and became independent with a cane. He was a functional prosthetic user until about 8 months ago when he began to have problems with his left foot. He continued to wear his prosthesis but did less walking as the foot became infected. He has just had a left transtibial amputation.

Ms. Darling, 83 years old, has had both legs amputated over the last 4 months for arteriosclerotic gangrene. The right leg was amputated below the knee and the left leg above the knee. Both residual limbs are now healed, and Ms. Darling has been referred to a rehabilitation center for therapy.

■ *Case Study Activities*

1   How would the goals and treatment program for Mr. Canan and Ms. Darling differ from that of other clients?
2   From the information given, what would be the desirable functional outcomes in each instance?
3   What data would be important in determining whether either individual is a candidate for prosthetic fitting and training?

The postsurgical program for the person with bilateral lower extremity amputations is similar to the program developed for someone with a unilateral amputation except for a greater need for balanced activities and, of course, ambulation. If the individual was fitted and ambulated after unilateral amputation, the prosthesis is useful for transfer activities and limited standing in the parallel bars for balance. Occasionally, the individual may be able to use the prosthesis with external support to get around the house more easily, particularly for bathroom activities. Such ambulation generates considerable stress on the residual limb and requires considerable expenditure of energy. Care must be taken to avoid any skin breakdowns or placing too much stress on the cardiovascular system. Fitting the patient with a temporary prosthesis, as previously mentioned, is advisable, particularly if his or her amputation is at a transtibial level. The higher the initial level of amputation, the more difficult ambulation becomes.

All individuals with bilateral amputations need a wheelchair on a permanent basis. The chair should be as narrow as possible with removable desk arms and removable leg rests. Amputee wheelchairs with offset rear wheels and no leg rests are not recommended unless the therapist is sure that the person will never be fitted with a prosthesis, even cosmetically. Chair balance can be achieved by adding antitipping devices to the rear of the wheelchair or attaching small weights to the front uprights or under the seat for use when the foot rests are removed.

The postsurgical program includes mat activities for increasing body position and balance, upper extremity and residual limb strengthening exercises, wheelchair transfers, and regular ROM exercises. With bilateral amputations, individuals spend considerable time sitting and are therefore more apt to develop flexion contractures, particularly around the hip joint. The client should be encouraged to sleep prone if possible, or at least spend some time in the prone position each day. Therapy also emphasizes ROM of the residual limb. Some people move about their homes on their knees, the ends of their residual limbs, or their buttocks. Knee pads made of heavy rubber are effective protectors for the residual limbs. Protectors can also be fabricated of foam or felt. Care must be taken to avoid skin breakdowns or bursitis around the patella.[23]

Temporary prostheses are of great value in the rehabilitation of individuals with bilateral transtibial amputations. Temporary prostheses are used to evaluate ambulation potential and as aids to balance and transfer activities. If the individual was initially fitted as a unilateral amputee, the temporary prosthesis will allow some resumption of ambulation. The ambulatory potential of the person with bilateral transfemoral amputations is doubtful, particularly among the elderly.

The person with bilateral transfemoral amputations can be fitted with shortened prostheses called "stubbies" (Fig. 5.15). Stubby prostheses have reg-

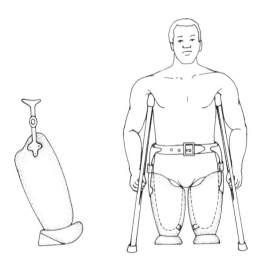

FIGURE 5.15

Stubbies. (From May, BJ: Assessment and treatment of individuals following lower extremity amputation. In O'Sullivan, SB, and Schmitz, TJ [eds]: Physical Rehabilitation: Assessment and Treatment, ed. 3. FA Davis, Philadelphia, 1994, p 392, with permission.)

ular sockets, no articulated knee joints or shank, and modified rocker bottoms turned backward to prevent the person from falling backward. Because the client's center of gravity is much lower to the ground and the prostheses are nonarticulated, stubbies are relatively easy to use. Stubbies allow the individual with bilateral transfemoral amputations to acquire erect balance and participate in ambulatory activities quickly and with only moderate expenditures of energy. Acceptance of stubbies by clients is quite low, however; some like to use them for ADLs in the home but rely on a wheelchair outside the home. Although prescribed rather rarely, stubbies are most effective for individuals with short residual limbs or those who will not be able to ambulate with regular prostheses.

NONPROSTHETIC MANAGEMENT

The postsurgical period is designed to determine the individual's suitability for prosthetic replacement. Not all people with amputations are candidates for prostheses regardless of personal desire. The cost of the prosthesis and the energy demands of prosthetic training require the use of some judgment in selecting individuals for fitting. Criteria for prosthetic fitting will be explored in more detail in Chapter 8.

Individuals who are not fitted with a prosthesis can become independent in a wheelchair.[24] The therapy program includes all transfer and ADLs and education in the proper care of the residual limb. Wrapping the residual limb is no longer necessary unless the person is more comfortable with the limb covered. The program emphasizes sitting balance, moving safely in and out of the wheelchair, and other activities to support as independent a lifestyle as the person's physical and psychological condition allows.

Summary

The postsurgical program is very important in the rehabilitation of individuals following amputation. The program emphasizes recovery from surgery, rehabilitation to a functional lifestyle, preparation for prosthetic fitting, or evaluation to determine if prosthetic fitting is feasible. The postsurgical program needs to be coordinated among the hospital and posthospital team members to ensure continuity of care in the most efficient manner.

Glossary

Bulbous	A residual limb with a large round distal end and smaller proximal end.
Conical	A residual limb that is smaller circumferentially at the distal end than at the proximal end.
Hyperbaric oxygen	Increasing the oxygen content of the blood by placing a part of or the total body in a chamber and increasing the oxygen pressure to a level greater than that of the atmosphere.
Phantom sensation	The feeling that the part of the body that has been removed or is desensitized is still there.
Phantom pain	A noxious sensation coming from the absent or desensitized body part. Phantom pain can take many forms.
Shrinker	A socklike garment made of elasticized material used to reduce edema in a residual limb.
Stump sock	A cotton or wool sock designed to fit over the residual limb and worn with the prosthesis.

References

1. May, BJ: Postsurgical management for lower extremity amputation. In O'Sullivan, SB, and Schmitz, TJ (eds): Physical Rehabilitation: Assessment and Treatment, ed 3. FA Davis, Philadelphia, 1993.
2. Burgess, EM: Amputations of the lower extremities. In Nickel, VL: Orthopedic Rehabilitation. Churchill-Livingstone, New York, 1982.
3. Sarmiento, A, et al: Lower-extremity amputation: The impact of immediate post surgical prosthetic fitting. Clin Orth 68:22, 1967.
4. Harrington, IJ, et al: A plaster-pylon technique for below-knee amputation. J Bone Joint Surg Br 73:76, 1991.
5. Cutson, TM, et al: Early management of elderly dysvascular below-knee amputees. J Prosthetics Orthotics 6: 62–66, 1994.
6. Sterescu, LE: Semi-rigid (Unna) dressing for amputation. Arch Phys Med Rehabil 55:433–34, 1974.
7. MacLean, N, and Fick, GH: The effect of semirigid dressings on below-knee amputations. Phys Ther 74:668–73, 1994.
8. Little, JM: A pneumatic weight bearing prosthesis for below-knee amputees. Lancet 1(7693):271, 1971.
9. Little, JM: The use of air splints as immediate prosthesis after below-knee amputation for vascular insufficiency. Med J Aust 2:870, 1970.
10. APTA: Guide to Physical Therapist Practice, ed 2. APTA, Alexandria, Va., 2001.
11. Ehde, DM, et al: Chronic phantom sensations, phantom pain, residual limb pain and other regional pain after lower limb amputation. Arch Phys Med Rehabil 81:1039–44, 2000.
12. Jensen, TS, et al: Immediate and long-term phantom limb pain in amputees: Incidence, clinical characteristics and relationship to pre-amputation limb pain. Pain 21:267, 1985.
13. Iacono, RP, et al: Pain management after lower extremity amputation. Neurosurgery 20:496, 1987.

14. Fisher, A, and Meller, Y: Continuous postoperative regional analgesia by nerve sheath block for amputation surgery—A pilot study. Anesth Analg 72:300, 1991.
15. Malawer, MM, et al: Postoperative infusional continuous regional analgesia. Clin Orthop 266:227, 1991.
16. Mouratoglou, VM: Amputees and phantom limb pain: A literature review. Physiother Pract 2:177, 1986.
17. Sherman, RA, et al: Phantom pain: A lesson in the necessity for careful clinical research on chronic pain problems. J Rehab R D 25:vii, 1988.
18. Melzack, R: Phantom limbs. Sci Am 266(4):123, 1992.
19. Malawer, MM, et al: Postoperative infusional continuous regional analgesia: A technique for relief of postoperative pain following major extremity surgery. Clin Orthop 266:227–37, 1991.
20. Fisher, A, and Meller, Y: Continuous postoperative regional analgesia by nerve sheath block for amputation surgery—A pilot study. Anesth Analg 72: 300–03, 1991.
21. Elizaga, AM, et al: Continuous regional analgesia by intraneural block: Effect on postoperative opioid requirements and phantom limb pain following amputation. J Rehab R D 31:179–87, 1994.
22. May, BJ: Stump bandaging of the lower extremity amputee. Phys Ther 44:808, 1964.
23. Parry, M, and Morrison, JD: Use of the Femurett adjustable prosthesis in the assessment and walking training of new above-knee amputees. Prosthet Orthot Int 13:36, 1989.
24. Edelstein, J: Special considerations—rehabilitation with prostheses: Functional skills training. In Bowker, JH, and Michael, JW (eds): Atlas of Limb Prosthetics, ed 2. Mosby Year Book, St. Louis, 1992.

CHAPTER SIX

Psychosocial Issues

OBJECTIVES

At the end of this chapter all students are expected to:

1 Recognize, discuss, and respond appropriately to the anxieties, frustrations, and coping mechanisms used by individuals following amputation.
2 Compare and contrast the psychosocial responses between individuals with traumatic and acquired amputations and between older and younger clients.
3 Exhibit an understanding of the psychosocial and economical effects of amputation on clients of different ages.
4 Describe effective communication mechanisms that enhance the therapeutic relationship with clients, families, and significant others.

Case Studies

Review the information presented in Chapter 5 on Diana Magnolia, Benny Pearl, Ha Lee Davis, and Betty Childs.

■ *Case Study Activities*

1 Compare and contrast the possible emotional responses of Diana Magnolia and Bennie Pearl as compared to Ha Lee Davis and Betty Childs. What similarities and differences would you expect and why?
2 What would you expect the major psychosocial and economical concerns to be for each of the clients?
3 In laboratory or group sessions, role-play the initial and ongoing contact between the physical therapist (PT) and physical therapist assistant (PTA) and the client.

GENERAL CONCEPTS

There are many factors that determine an individual's psychological response to amputation. The person's basic personality is a prime consideration. Individuals who are self-confident and secure generally adjust to the loss, whereas timid or self-conscious individuals may exhibit greater psychological trauma. Individuals with a strong support system are also less likely to suffer long-term psychological distress. Some people are cheerful and easygoing by nature and will make an easy adjustment to the loss. For others, joking and laughing may be a mechanism for self-deception, and for hiding fears about the possible incapacitating effects of the amputation. Some clients may choose jobs or try to perform activities they are not physically able to do. Prosthetic, social, occupational, and financial factors can either soften or intensify the degree of reaction. Individuals whose jobs or major recreational pursuits will be affected by the loss of the limb may have more difficulty than people whose lifestyle is more adaptable to the functional changes imposed by amputation.[1] The level of amputation is not thought to be related to the severity of the reaction.

Many clients are not fully aware of the consequences of amputation and may fear other physical limitations as a result of the surgery. Fear of impotence or sterility may lead some men to make grandiose statements or display reckless behavior to mask the fear.[2] Thorough explanations of the amputation process and implications by the surgeon or other health worker may alleviate many of these fears.

Individuals with a history of depression, who have a high degree of investment in their appearance, or who value dependency may exhibit more disabling psychological stress. Rybarczyk and associates [3] found a strong correlation between clinical depression as measured by standardized scales and social discomfort (described as social contacts making references to the amputation). Twenty-five percent of individuals surveyed were found to be clinically depressed. Clinically depressed individuals tend to perceive themselves in poor health and without a strong support system. Individuals who avoid references to their amputations or prostheses and who avoid social contacts in the early rehabilitative period may be more likely to develop clinical depression. Nicholas and associates[4] surveyed 94 individuals fitted with a prosthesis and reported that the major social concerns were a sense of defenselessness and unease about appearance.

Clients generally dream of themselves as not being amputated. This image may be so vivid that they fall as they get up at night and attempt to walk to the bathroom without a prosthesis or crutches. Individuals who have lost their leg through injury may dream about the accident in which they were injured. Such reenactments may lead to insomnia, trembling fits, speech impediments, and difficulty with concentration. Realistic adjustment often comes as the person learns to use the artificial substitute. Good predictors for adjustment to the prosthesis are motivation to master the prosthesis and desire to return to an active lifestyle.

Psychiatric, psychological, and counseling services are available to help clients cope with the emotional aspects of limb loss (see Chap. 1 for the role of these individuals). However, most individuals do not require such assistance. Understanding and support from family and health-care workers is usually adequate.

STAGES OF ADJUSTMENT

Individuals who lose a limb, either from disease or trauma, may go through several stages in the process of acceptance and adjustment. Bradway and associates suggested four stages of emotional adjustment to amputation.[5] The first occurs before surgery when the individual begins to be aware than an amputation may happen. It is not unusual to have a client who is being treated for a vascular ulcer say to a PT or PTA, "I'm afraid I may lose my foot." A PT's first instinct is to say, "Oh no, no, don't even think that!" Although this response is temporarily reassuring, it is not particularly helpful. A reflecting response such as "I can understand your concerns about your foot" may encourage the client to explore feelings about a possible amputation and raise questions or concern about prosthetic replacement, pain, financial limitations, and dependency. PTs and PTAs need to create an open and receptive environment and be willing to listen. Grief is the first reaction to the official initial announcement that an amputation is necessary.[2,5,6]

The second stage of reaction, immediately after surgery, is usually of short duration. Individuals who have undergone emergency or traumatic amputation may appear euphoric and overly cheerful. Individuals who anticipated the amputation may express relief at having an outcome and being able to start on the rehabilitative process. There may be some expression of grief as well. The experience may be similar to the death of a loved one. A part of the body has been irrevocably lost, and the person may feel incomplete and mourn the lost extremity. The person may experience insomnia, restlessness, and have difficulty concentrating. There is little evidence, however, that attitude toward the amputation at this stage has any relationship to eventual level of emotional or functional adjustment.[5]

The third stage occurs as the person becomes involved in the postoperative program and really faces the permanence of the loss. Some individuals exhibit denial with either euphoria or withdrawal from social contacts.[7] Younger individuals may deny the amputation by trying to exhibit physical capabilities in the use of wheelchair or crutches.[8,9] Many individuals do not mourn the actual loss of the limb, but the anticipated loss of a previous life style. Individuals may mourn or fear the possible loss of a job or the ability to participate in a favorite sport or other activity. Men who lose a limb often fear the loss of sexual capability and potency; some may equate the loss of the limb with castration.[10] In the early stages, the client's grief may alternate with feelings of hopelessness, despondency, bitterness, and anger. The person may experience feelings of internal loss and mutilation. Some people state they would prefer to be dead and wonder why this has happened to them. Clients may be jealous of others who have not suffered as they have; they may blame themselves or their surgeon for the loss. Socially they may feel lonely, isolated, and the object of pity or horror.[1,2,5]

Throughout this stage the client may have many questions, and it is important that he or she knows what to expect during the entire process. The steps of rehabilitation and the expectations should be carefully explained but only when the person asks questions or appears ready for the information. Overloading the individual with a plethora of information too early will ensure only that the information will not be heard. It is a common mistake among less experienced PTs and PTAs to try to educate the patient in all aspects of prosthetic rehabilitation immediately after surgery. Shorter hospital stays create extra pressure to prepare the individual as completely as possible for a future as an "amputee." Although it is important for the individual to know and understand as much as possible about the future, overwhelming a person with too much information at one time may only increase the feeling of helplessness. Families need to be educated as much as the patient. It is helpful to have written materials for the patient and family to take home and study at their leisure. Written materials should include information on residual limb care, postsurgical exercises, and prostheses and mobility training.

Individuals with amputations who have made satisfactory adjustments in their lives and successfully completed rehabilitation can support and encourage the new client in private or group sessions. Treating the individual in an area where clients in later stages of rehabilitation can be seen engaging in therapy is often helpful. Showing the client a prosthesis and using films or slides may also help.

Professionals skilled in group dynamics run support groups in rehabilitation centers as well as provide medical or technical advice regarding such issues as diabetes, medications, or peripheral vascular disease. Family and friends are often invited to attend. The atmosphere is nonthreatening so clients can express their feelings and frustrations. Although support groups are common in rehabilitation settings, they are less common in the community at large. Not all individuals go to rehabilitation centers following amputation surgery; therefore, the PT and PTA in the hospital, home health, or outpatient settings need to provide the support.

The final stage of adjustment is related to reintegration into a functional lifestyle. Clients have various attitudes toward the prosthesis. Some are particularly concerned about its appearance, hoping that it will conceal their disability and give the illusion of an intact body. Others are concerned primarily with the restoration of function. When the artificial limb is fitted, the client must face the fact that the natural limb has been lost irrevocably. If individuals with amputations have been told that the prosthesis will replace their own limb, they may have unrealistic expectations that appearance and function will be as good as in the nonamputated extremity. Those who are not candidates for a prosthesis need guidance on community reintegration appropriate to their functional levels.

Many clients make a satisfactory adjustment to the loss of a limb and are reintegrated into a full and active life. Some clients may try to avoid distressing thoughts of the lost limb through conscious self-control or by avoiding situations or people that remind them of the lost limb. Some may display temper tantrums or irrational resentment. Some may revert to childlike states of helplessness and dependence.

A client may not follow any of the stages or sequences described above. It is important to remember that the individual's preamputation personality and ability to adjust to the demands of everyday life are the greatest determinant of that person's ability to adjust to amputation. The description of the stages is a guide to help the PT and PTA understand some of the reactions to amputation.

Complete rehabilitation includes not only preparation of the individual physically and psychologically for the community, but also preparation of the community for the individual with an amputation. Public education media can be used to inform people of the potential abilities of persons with amputations in society and employment. As with other physically challenged individuals, those with amputations need to be accepted and integrated into the community because of their abilities and not their disabilities.

AGE CONSIDERATIONS

Psychological distress following any disability increases with age, all other factors being equal. However, the elderly do not show any greater difficulty in psychological adjustment than the adult population as a whole.[1]

Infants and Young Children

Shock is the usual parental reaction to the birth of a child with a congenital anomaly or to an amputation resulting from injury or tumor. Parents may go through periods of denial and anger and experience feelings of guilt and shame before accepting their child's amputation. Some parents may be overwhelmed and inconsolable; others may not fully appreciate the implications of disability. Parents of children with acquired amputations may accept the deficit more easily than parents of children with congenital amputations because of the genetic implication. Rehabilitation team members should be concerned with parental adjustment because parental acceptance of the amputation and the prosthesis will likely correlate with the child's adjustment.

Children are fitted early, as soon as they are developmentally ready for the prosthesis. A child with an upper extremity loss can be fitted as soon as he or she starts bilateral hand activities, whereas a child with a lower limb loss can be fitted as he starts to pull to stand. Children usually incorporate the prosthesis into their body image, some refusing to remove the prosthesis for sleep. It is important for the parents and PTs to touch the residual limb normally to indicate acceptance.

Older Children and Adolescents

Regardless of their client's age, the rehabilitation team must consider the emotional reactions of older children and adolescents. Too often, detailed discussions about the amputation and postoperative care are conducted with the parents, and the child is overlooked. The child should be aware of what to expect during anesthesia, surgery, and the recovery period. Misinformation or distortions should be detected and corrected.

Mourning is a normal process for the child as well as the adult. Children, when depressed, are likely to regress to a more infantile level of behavior and must be given the opportunity to express their feelings through play or talk. The early adolescent may grieve over the loss of self-image, whereas the adolescent may be afraid of rejection and social ostracism. Adolescence is a dynamic phase during which profound changes lead people to feel sexually attractive and capable of reproduction. Self-esteem is very vulnerable at this time. The adolescent may feel inadequate after amputation and may need reassurance from significant others. Contact with other young clients may be quite constructive. Involvement in sports programs is especially helpful. Reaction to the loss of a limb is affected by the child's previous experiences and the reaction of family members. Parental reaction profoundly influences the way the child copes.

The Elderly Client

The elderly individual with a lower extremity amputation is motivated to seek effective rehabilitation services and a meaningful lifestyle. The immediate reaction to amputation is no different than that of any other individual except that the amputation usually is anticipated. The reaction depends in part on the severity of preoperative pain and the extent of attempts to save the limb. Individuals who have suffered considerable pain may be grateful that the pain has ended. Clients who have undergone extensive medical and surgical procedures may experience a sense of failure that the efforts were not successful. If preoperative attitudes are unrealistically hopeful, then postoperative disturbances may be more severe. The elderly person should not be led to expect a total cure. Learning to use an artificial limb may be a slow and discouraging ordeal, and the client may not express distress or depression in front of the optimism of others. However, the PT and PTA must keep in mind that the majority of older individuals, particularly those whose limb was amputated at the transtibial level, make excellent adjustments to prosthetic function.[11] Sharing and support from other elderly clients can be helpful.

Stress in the Elderly

Elderly individuals are subject to considerable stress from concerns about financial limitations, loss of control over their lives, and fear of becoming dependent. An elderly individual who requires an amputation must often cope with multiple physical problems. Loss is a part of normal aging; loss of physiological capabilities, loss of a spouse or friends, loss of the self-esteem related to one's career or job, and now, loss of a limb. It is helpful to give the client as much control over decision making as possible, to provide opportunities to be involved in goals setting, and to sequence activities.[12] As with any client, PTs and PTAs need to be aware of the stressors affecting the clients and assist with coping by being reflective listeners and enablers.

Cognition and Motivation

It is a myth that elderly individuals cannot learn a new skill, have difficulty remembering, and cannot achieve at the same level as younger individuals. Some elderly individuals may have difficulty learning new skills, but most are fully able to adapt successfully to amputation and lead a full and normal life. Although some do suffer from dementia, others who are labeled as having dementia because of confusion in the acute care setting may actually only be responding to medications, metabolic imbalances, infection toxicity, insecurity in a strange environment, or the sequellae of anesthesia. The Mini Mental Status Examination and the Blessed Orientation Memory Test are both reliable and simple evaluations that can be administered by a PT to determine a client's level of orientation and mental function.[13-15] It is important to remember that cognitive dysfunction does not, in itself, preclude satisfactory rehabilitation. Understanding the client's cognitive capabilities helps the PT and PTA structure learning experiences appropriately. An individual with cognitive impairment may have difficulty following two- and three-stage commands but can to follow single-phase instructions. For example, saying to a client, "Now you need to reach down and take your foot off the foot plate, then lift the foot plate and use this little lever to push the foot rest out of the way" may be overwhelming, both because of the number of instructions and the terminology. On the other hand, the PT or PTA might suggest, "To be able to get up safely from your chair you need to have these foot rests out of the way" (pointing to the foot rests). The client might respond by initiating some movements to get the foot off the foot pedal. The PT or PTA can then respond to the client's movements by making additional suggestions as indicated. Using one-stage instructions means that only one movement suggestion is made at one time. "Now that your foot is on the floor, you need to pull the plate up out of your way" (pointing to the plate). Using familiar terms and activities helps the cognitively impaired client make connections and respond appropriately. Goal-oriented statements may also be clearer to a client. We do many activities almost automatically: getting up from a chair, turning in bed, and walking. Most of us have developed particular patterns of movements over the years. The PT and PTA can draw on such patterns by suggesting the movement goal, "How about sitting on the side of the bed?"

MOTIVATION AND COMPLIANCE

Motivation and compliance are closely interrelated, but compliance is not obedience. Everyone is motivated toward some goal. To the extent that the client's and the health professional's goals are congruent and the client performs as the health professional expects, the client is said to be motivated and compliant. However, if the client has different goals and does not follow the program the health professional has outlined, the client is considered to be noncompliant. This is one reason why it is important to clarify the client's goals and organize the rehabilitation program to help the client meet those goals. Kemp has developed a formula of motivation that considers the client's wants, beliefs, rewards, and the cost of the performance.[16]

$$\text{Motivation} = \frac{\text{Wants} \times \text{Beliefs} \times \text{Rewards}}{\text{Costs}}$$

The client's wants are essentially the client's goals, what the client wants to accomplish. Beliefs relate to what the client thinks of the activity, future, and disability. Rewards are the outcomes, pleasure, accomplishments, and positive feelings the client obtains from the activity or program. Finally, the cost stands for the consequences of participation in an activity. Is the activity painful? Is it very energy demanding? Does it interfere with other more pleasurable activities?[16] The PT or PTA must consider all the elements of the equation in establishing a rehabilitation program and in planning simple activities such as home exercises.

CAREGIVERS

In most instances the PT and PTA will be working with a caregiver as well as with the client. The caregiver is an integral part of the team and must be involved in the rehabilitation program. Caregivers can be members of the family, close friends, neighbors, or paid helpers. Caregivers have their own emotional reactions to the amputation and the client's illness. Caregiving is a demanding and often tiring activity that can upset family balance and create considerable stress. The PT and PTA need to be open to the needs of the caregiver and work closely with her or him. It is important to determine the caregiver's goals, fears, and concerns. Is the caregiver afraid of handling the client or the residual limb? Is the caregiver resentful of the time demands that caregiving imposes? What was the premorbid relationship between the client and the caregiver?

The PT and PTA can provide useful information to the caregiver regarding the disability and prognosis, as well as helpful techniques for coping with daily life. Providing time for the caregiver to ask questions and voice concerns can be an integral part of the therapeutic intervention. Many caregivers are afraid of "doing something wrong" and need to develop confidence in their caregiving skills. Effective teaching strategies need to be used with caregivers as well as clients to ensure a smooth transition into the home program.[17]

Summary

Most people who undergo an amputation eventually adjust to the disability without professional psychiatric intervention. Many PTs and PTAs are not comfortable with emotional or psychological issues related to limb loss. Each health-care provider needs to face his or her own feelings about any specific disability, and his or her own fears and concerns related to the loss of a limb, and its effects on lifestyle and sexual function. The PT and PTA need to employ effective communication techniques in helping each individual reach his or her highest functional potential. Active listening, acceptance, understanding, and openness are key elements to effective communication.

References

1. Racy, JC: Psychological adaptation to amputation. In Bowker, JH, and Michael, JW (eds): Atlas of Limb Prosthetics: Surgical, Prosthetic and Rehabilitation Principles, ed 2. Mosby Year Book, St. Louis, 1992.
2. Friedman, LW: The Psychological Rehabilitation of the Amputee. Charles C. Thomas, Springfield, Ill. 1978.
3. Rybarczyk, BD, et al: Social discomfort and depression in a sample of adults with leg amputations. Arch Phys Med Rehabil 73:1169–73, 1992.
4. Nicholas, JJ, et al: Problems experienced and perceived by prosthetic patients. J Prosthet Orthot 5 (1):36–39, 1993.
5. Bradway, JK, et al: Psychological adaptation to amputation: An overview. Orthot Prosthet 38(3):46–50, 1984
6. Parkes, CM, and Napier, MM: Psychiatric sequelae of amputation. Br J Hosp Med 4:610–14, 1970.
7. Parkes, CM: Psychosocial transitions: Comparison between reactions to loss of a limb and loss of a spouse. Br J Psychiat 127:204–10, 1975.
8. Brown, PW: Bilateral lower extremity amputation. J Bone Joint Surg Am 52A (4):687–700, 1970.
9. Noble, D, et al: Psychiatric disturbances following amputation. Am J Psych 110:609–13, 1954.
10. Mourad, M, and Chiu, WS: Marital-sexual adjustment of amputees. Med Aspects Hum Sex 47–52, February 1974.
11. Gauthier-Gagnon, C, et al: Enabling factors related to prosthetic use by people with transtibial and transfemoral amputation. Arch Phys Med Rehabil 80(6):706–713, 1999.

12. Jackson-Wyatt, O: Age-related changes in amputee rehabilitation. Top Geriatr Rehabil 8:1–12, 1992.
13. Schunk, C: Psychological and cognitive considerations. In May, BJ (ed): Home Health Care and Rehabilitation: Concepts of Care. FA Davis, Philadelphia, 1993.
14. Blessed, G, et al: The association between quantitative measures of dementia and of senile change in the cerebral grey matter of elderly patients. Br J Psychiatr 114:797–811, 1968.
15. Folstein, MF, et al: Minimental state: A practical method for grading the cognitive state of patients for the clinician. J Psychiatr Res 12:189–98, 1975.
16. Kemp, BJ: Motivation, rehabilitation, and aging: A conceptual model. Top Geriatr Rehabil 3 (3):41–51, 1988.
17. May, BJ: Caregivers. In May, BJ (ed): Home Health Care and Rehabilitation: Concepts of Care, ed 2. FA Davis, Philadelphia, 1999.

CHAPTER SEVEN

Prosthetic Components

At the end of this chapter, all students are expected to:

1   Differentiate between endoskeletal and exoskeletal prostheses.
2   Compare and contrast the major types of feet, knee joints, **socket** designs, and methods of suspension for transfemoral and transtibial prosthetic replacements.
3   Describe major components used in lower extremity disarticulation prostheses.

In addition, physical therapy students are expected to:

4   Make recommendations for prosthetic components for a simulated client.

Case Studies

Our four clients are:

Diana Magnolia, a 58-year-old woman with a transtibial amputation secondary to diabetic gangrene.

Ha Lee Davis, an 18-year-old man with a transtibial amputation secondary to a motorcycle accident.

Benny Pearl, a 72-year-old man with a transfemoral amputation secondary to arteriosclerotic gangrene.

Betty Childs, a 12-year-old girl with a transfemoral amputation secondary to bone cancer.

■ *Case Study Activities*

1   Discuss the functions of the major components in the transtibial, transfemoral, and disarticulation prostheses.
2   Reflect on the extent to which a person's lifestyle affects prosthetic replacement and selection of components.
3   What components would you select for each of the clients?

GENERAL CONCEPTS

The prosthetic prescription may be written by the surgeon who performed the amputation or the chief of an amputee clinic. Clients may also obtain a prosthesis or **component** directly from the prosthetist, although reimbursement may necessitate a prescription. Some surgeons may refer a client directly to the prosthetist, leaving the actual selection of components to the prosthetist; others may refer clients to an amputee clinic if one is locally available. In other instances, the physical therapist (PT) working with the client in the postoperative phase, a home health situation, an outpatient clinic, or a rehabilitation facility may determine when the client is ready for a temporary or definitive appliance and request a prosthetic prescription. Unlike certain devices, prostheses and orthoses are not legally controlled and may be purchased by any individual without the intervention of a health-care provider. However, recommendation by a prosthetic rehabilitation team following thorough examination provides the patient with the optimum selection of componentry. The extent to which any PT may be involved in making recommendations for prosthetic replacement depends on the work setting; however, in the current health-care market, it is important for every PT to understand the function of major prosthetic components to assist with selection as well as to develop and implement an appropriate plan of care.

PROSTHETIC PRESCRIPTION

The prosthesis needs to be comfortable, functional, and cosmetic, usually in that order. If the prosthesis is not comfortable, the client will not wear it; pain or discomfort can be the greatest impediment to successful prosthetic rehabilitation. The prosthesis must also be functional. It must allow the individual to perform desired activities that he or she would not be able to do without a prosthesis and do them with the lowest possible expenditure of energy. For most individuals, a well-fitting prosthesis will allow them to perform a greater range of mobility activities than they could on crutches or with a wheelchair. This may not be true for elderly individuals with transfemoral amputations or those with bilateral amputations. When the energy demands for prosthetic mobility are greater than for mobility without a prosthesis, the prosthesis is rarely worn. Finally, the prosthesis must be as cosmetic as possible. The importance of cosmesis varies with each person and each situation. It is not uncommon for individuals to wear a prosthesis without cosmetic cover, preferring the better foot response to the improved cosmesis. Many individuals have no difficulty wearing shorts with a prosthesis, while for others, appearance is of greater importance. The client's needs and desires must be explored in some detail prior to selecting individual components. It is also very important to educate the client about the many options. A trip to the prosthetic shop can be a valuable part of the postsurgical program.

Many factors must be considered in selecting the optimum prosthesis for each client. In an older time, choices were limited. Newer technology and materials have resulted in a plethora of prosthetic components, some very sophisticated and very expensive. An active individual can have a different prosthesis for sports and for everyday use. Some prosthetic feet adjust to changes in heel height, allowing an individual to switch from sports to dress shoes. Prostheses can be made very lightweight, improving function and reducing energy expenditure. A discussion of each available component and material is well beyond the scope of this book and would probably be outdated by the time the book is published. Therefore, the major types of prosthetic components will be discussed and the most commonly used items described. Each PT and physical therapist assistant (PTA) needs to work closely with the regional prosthetists to learn the names and configurations of components in use locally.

Client Factors

Many factors influence the selection of components. The client's general health, weight, activity level, motivation, and ability to set realistic goals must be considered. The therapist, prosthetist, and client must know and understand the demands that will be placed on the prosthesis. Concomitantly, the client needs to understand the limitations of the prosthesis. Unfortunately, many people have unrealistic expectations, believing they will be able to walk as they did before the amputation. Although such expectations may be true for healthy active individuals with unilateral transtibial amputations, they are often not true for elderly individuals with multiple health problems. Unrealistic expectations are a particular problem for individuals amputated at the transfemoral level. Prior prosthetic use may also influence the type of prosthesis prescribed. Some clients do not want to change from a known component to something new. An individual with a second amputation already fitted on one side may need to have the existing prosthesis matched.

Residual Limb Factors

The length, shape, skin condition, circulation, range of motion, and maturation of the residual limb influence the type of prosthesis. Invaginated scars and poorly placed thick or adherent incisions can affect the choice of suspension and socket. Sometimes different materials can be used to achieve a comfortable fit in the presence of residual limb problems. The PT can provide information to the prosthetist regarding sensitive areas on the residual limb or other special fitting considerations.

Cost

Regretfully, the cost of components is often a determining factor. Third-party payers frequently support only a limited range of components, and many clients cannot personally afford the higher-priced items. Efforts at cost containment often limit selection of technologically advanced components that may contribute to a higher level of function. Medicare has established some guidelines for classification of potential functional capabilities; these guidelines determine Medicare reimbursement for components (Table 7.1). Medicaid will often only fund the most basic prosthesis regardless of the person's individual needs or prognosis. The PT needs to take every opportunity to be involved in

TABLE 7.1   MEDICARE FUNCTIONAL OUTCOME GUIDELINES

Code	Description
K0	No ambulatory potential with or without a prosthesis.
K1	Prosthesis would allow limited household ambulation on level surface, with little cadence change.
K2	Prosthesis would allow limited community ambulation; can perform steps and curbs; some cadence change.
K3	Prosthesis would allow independence in community; ambulation with varying cadence and activity levels. Needed for full participation in vocational or leisure activities.
K4	Prosthesis would allow full independence and participation in high-level activity, athletics, vocational or leisure.

component selection and use his or her knowledge of the client's functional abilities to justify the use of such components. Some prosthetic components require a higher level of maintenance, thus the proximity to the prosthetic and treatment facilities may be a factor in the prosthetic prescription.

Prostheses

The lower extremity prosthesis includes a foot, knee joint for transfemoral and higher levels, a socket with or without liner, and a method of suspension. The prosthesis may be **endoskeletal** or **exoskeletal** in structure (Fig. 7.1). The endoskeletal prosthesis uses a lightweight metal pylon to connect the foot to the socket (transtibial) or knee unit (transfemoral). The **shank** may be covered by a foam cover that matches the color and configuration of the other leg. Endoskeletal prostheses use a modular concept in that components of standard design and dimensions are readily interchangeable and adjustable. Through this system, various combinations of components can be tried to find the optimum combination for a given patient. The endoskeletal modular system offers simpler and faster maintenance. It also permits more frequent and easier adjustments of alignment. It permits socket interchange without destroying the prosthesis. The flexible foam cover provides an improved appearance and can be removed for adjustments when necessary. Adjustable devices are particularly beneficial to children because the growth process necessitates frequent changes. Endoskeletal prostheses are more cosmetic, but the cover is not as durable as the exoskeletal devices.

Exoskeletal prostheses are constructed of wood or rigid polyurethane covered with a rigid plastic lamination. The rigidity of the shank makes them more durable and more resistant to external wear than the endoskeletal prostheses. Exoskeletal prostheses may be initially less expensive than endoskeletal devices. Lower extremity prosthetic components, particularly pylons and knee mechanisms, are usually rated for maximum size and weight. Most components are rated up to 250 to 300 lb with only a few rated for higher weights. The PT must work with the prosthetist to make sure that the selected components are appropriate both for the weight of the individual as well as for the anticipated activity level.

Sockets

The prosthetic socket is the foundation of the prosthesis. It is the interface between the patient and the prosthesis. The skill of the prosthetist in making

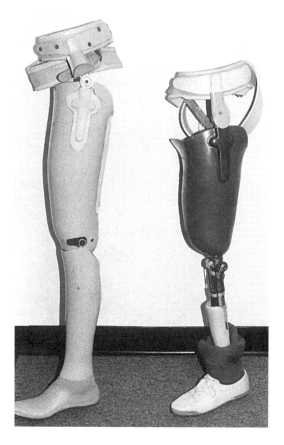

FIGURE 7.1

(*Left*) Exoskeletal transfemoral prosthesis with stance-control mechanical knee mechanism. (*Right*) Endoskeletal transfemoral prosthesis with cosmetic cover rolled down.

the small adjustments necessary to individualize the socket can be critical to the success of prosthetic rehabilitation. Socket design varies with the level of amputation and the configurations of the individual residual limb. Specific design considerations are discussed in the following sections devoted to each major prosthesis. Some general principles of socket design apply to all prostheses. PTs and PTAs should understand basic design principles to properly evaluate the fit of a prosthesis and to do initial troubleshooting when clients have pain or exhibit gait deviations.

The prosthetic socket must support body weight and hold the residual limb firmly and comfortably during all activities (Fig. 7.2*A* and *B*). Each area of the residual limb tolerates pressure differently; therefore, the tissues are selectively loaded so that the most weight is borne by pressure-tolerant tissue, such as wide and flat bony areas or tendons, and least by pressure-sensitive tissue such as nerves that are close to the skin and sharp bony prominence. This is accomplished by relief (socket concavity) over pressure-sensitive areas and socket convexity over the pressure tolerant areas. Additionally, the socket needs to grip the residual limb firmly to reduce or eliminate movement between the socket and the skin. Increased movement between the residual limb and socket creates increased instability for the client during activities and greater risk for skin abrasions. Total contact between the residual limb and the socket is required to aid in proprioceptive feedback and to prevent dependent edema and skin problems.

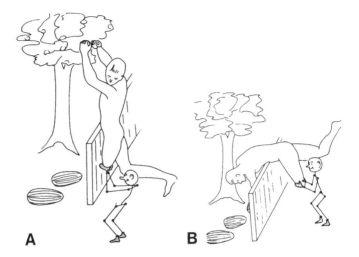

A   **B**

FIGURE 7.2

The prosthesis must (*A*) support the body weight and (*B*) hold the residual limb firmly during all activities. (From Hall CB: Prosthetic socket shape as related to anatomy in lower extremity amputees. Clin Orthop 37, 1964, with permission.)

There are many ways the prosthetist may fabricate the individual prosthetic socket. The prosthetist notes the individual characteristics of the residual limb, takes specific measurements of both the residual limb and the other leg and may either cast the residual limb according to established construction principles or complete a special computer form noting specific measurements. At this point, the socket may be fabricated on-site or the measurements (and cast) may be sent to one of several central fabrication companies. The central fabrication company may make just the socket or may put the whole prosthesis together. The socket itself may be fabricated by a computer (CAD/CAM) or may be made by a machine that molds a sheet of plastic di-

FIGURE 7.3

Transtibial prosthesis on an alignment instrument. A small wrench is used to loosen the four screws under the socket and move the socket as desired.

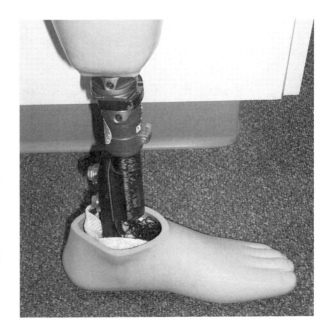

rectly over the positive model of the residual limb using a vacuum system. A test socket may be fabricated first and tried on the patient to ensure comfort and provide for appropriate weight-bearing and stabilizing pressures. A test socket is more frequently made for the transfemoral socket. (There are a number of Web sites describing central fabrication activities. Most can be reached by searching on "central fabrication" from the orthotics and prosthetic Web page: *www.oandp.com.*)

The socket is connected to the appropriate components with an alignment instrument between the socket and knee mechanism (transfemoral) or pylon (transtibial) (Fig. 7.3). Once the prosthesis is assembled, the prosthetist performs a **static alignment** while the client stands. The alignment allows the prosthetist to set the proper length and to ensure that the components are properly aligned with each other to maximize comfort and control. Depending on the client's ambulatory ability, **dynamic alignment** may also be performed at the same time. New clients often need gait training before final dynamic alignment can be set (see Chap. 8).

ANKLE/FOOT MECHANISMS

The prosthetic foot is the foundation of all prostheses except partial foot amputations. Ideally, it should duplicate all the activities of the normal foot. The normal foot accommodates to a great variety of terrains and surfaces, providing stability in all planes of motion. It also provides dynamic response in a wide range of situations such as running, walking, and jumping. If the prosthetic foot is to replace the normal foot, it should serve the following functions:

1. Joint motion and muscle activity simulation. The normal foot allows dorsiflexion/plantar flexion, inversion/eversion, and a smooth roll over from heel contact to toe off.
2. Muscle activity simulation. The anatomic foot and ankle have a complex neuromuscular structure that allows for considerable control of mobility activities such as running, jumping, balancing on narrow surfaces, or standing on one foot.
3. Shock absorption. The foot needs to absorb the forces generated at heel contact while allowing a smooth progression to foot flat and toe off. Prosthetic feet for transtibial or lower levels need to allow the knee flexion to occur during early stance phase.
4. A stable base of support. The foot must stabilize the body during the stance phase of gait.

Although prosthetic feet have improved markedly over the years, modern technology does not yet provide a foot that excels in both accommodation and response. Prosthetic feet can be divided into two major categories, the dynamic response or energy-conserving type and the nondynamic response feet. Dynamic response feet can be further divided into articulated or nonarticulated.[1] Feet are manufactured in a wide variety of juvenile and adult sizes. Some incorporate a footlike appearance, including toes, whereas others require a foot cover to achieve that appearance.

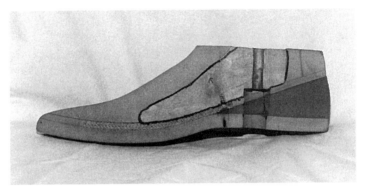

FIGURE 7.4
Cutaway of one type of solid ankle cushion heel (SACH) foot.

Nondynamic Response Feet

SACH (Solid Ankle Cushion Heel)

The SACH foot is a nonarticulated device with solid wood or aluminum keel, sponge rubber heel wedge, and molded cosmetic forefoot with or without individual toes (Fig. 7.4). Plantar flexion is simulated by compression of the heel wedge that is adjusted to the client's weight and activity level. There is no dorsiflexion, eversion, or inversion. It used to be the most common foot used throughout the world and may still be in most Third World countries. In Western countries it has been supplanted in popularity by the dynamic response foot.

Single-Axis Foot

The old single axis foot was made of wood with rubber bumpers that allowed limited dorsiflexion and plantar flexion. At heel contact, the plantar flexion bumper compresses, offering a true plantar flexion motion. The rapid foot flat increases knee extension moment and therefore prosthetic stability on stance. The dorsiflexion bumper that is a little firmer than the plantar flexion bumper limits dorsiflexion at midstance and terminal stance. The firmness of the bumpers is determined by the client's weight and activity level. Research comparing the function of the SACH and single axis foot reveals little gait difference other than slightly increased knee stability with the single axis foot.[2–4] Some of the design components of the single axis foot have been incorporated into single-axis and multiaxis dynamic response feet.

Dynamic Response (Energy-Conserving) Feet

Dynamic response feet were developed initially for clients who wanted to be active and perform such activities as running and jumping. Now they have become the main type of feet used with prostheses. A great variety of dynamic response feet are now available. Some are essentially single-axis feet providing for compression and shock absorption at heel contact and releasing some or most of the energy at terminal stance. Some are multiaxis, providing movement in more than one plane. Although space does not allow for discussion of all dynamic response feet, several that illustrate major functional categories will be discussed specifically.

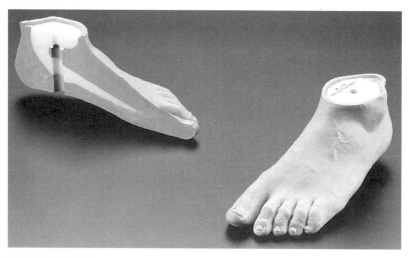

FIGURE 7.5
The Seattle Foot. (From the M+IND Corporation with permission.)

Soft Keel

Feet with mechanisms incorporated into a soft foam shell have an elastic keel that compresses on heel contact, controlling, to some extent, the rate of plantar flexion and the speed of movement to midstance. Inversion and eversion are minimally simulated by the cushioning of the rubberized heel. These feet are said to provide some adaptation for uneven ground. However, it must be noted that all these movements are minimal because no joint or articulation other than plantar flexion and return is involved.[5]

The Seattle Foot[6] (M+IND Corp.) (Fig. 7.5) incorporates a shock-absorbing tapered leaf spring that absorbs energy at heel contact and releases it in terminal stance, thereby aiding in propulsion. The faster the cadence, the more the time on the forefoot, and the more the distortion of the leaf in dorsiflexion. This increases the amount of energy that is absorbed and then released at terminal stance. The degree of spring also varies by the thickness of the leaf and its material. To some extent, the degree of spring can be varied according to the person's size, weight, and level of activity.[6, 7] The Seattle Light foot (M+IND Corp.) is a lighter and more streamlined version of the original foot. The basic principle of energy storing and release is incorporated in a number of different feet, although materials differ. Some feet use one or more carbon graphite leaves attached to a rigid keel incorporated into a foam foot.

Among the newest soft keel feet are the TT multiflex ankle (Fig. 7.6) and the Dynamic Response 2, manufactured by Endolite (*www.endolite.com*). Both ankle/foot units use a ball and stem assembly and a firm carbon fiber keel to provide energy return from heel strike through toe off. There is control of dorsiflexion and spring assist at toe off to provide support on uneven ground. Stiffness of the keel may be adjusted manually by the patient. The TT multiflex ankle incorporates a telescoping torsional pylon as part of the assembly. Shock absorbing pylons are discussed later in this chapter. There are a number of other feet that would fit within this category. They are similar in function.

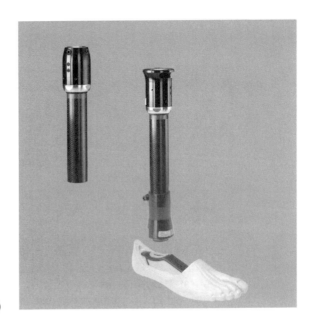

FIGURE 7.6
Endolite TT Multiflex Ankle and foot.
(Courtesy of Endolite USA with permission.)

Carbon Graphite Shanks

The Flex-Foot (Össur; *www.flexfoot.com*) uses a flat one-piece carbon fiber shank and foot, a carbon fiber heel, and a split toe forefoot.[8,9] The split toe forefoot provides for some degree of accommodation on uneven ground, but the foot provides more response (Fig. 7.7). There are a number of different feet within the Flex-Foot line. All can be classified as dynamic response and nonarticulated, and all provide varying degrees of response with little accommodation characteristics. Some are specially designed for active individuals who participate in athletics and a very active lifestyle. Others are designed for less active individuals. The amount of return ranges from about 30 to 90 percent of the input depending on a number of factors. The foot may be covered by a foam mold that simulates the normal foot, although many athletes choose to use the foot without cosmetic cover to obtain maximum dynamic return.

Multiaxis Feet

There are a number of multiaxis feet currently available. In addition to providing some degree of dynamic response, these feet also provide varying de-

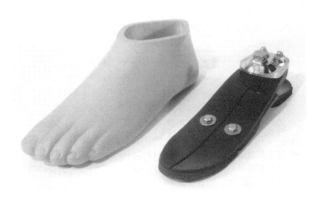

FIGURE 7.7
Flex-Foot Allurion and Flex-Foot foot cover. (Photograph courtesy of Össur.)

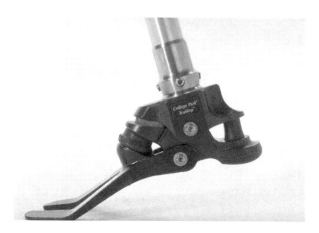

FIGURE 7.8
College Park multiaxis foot. (From College Park Inc. with permission)

grees of mediolateral movement or stability. The True Step foot (Fig. 7.8) manufactured by College Park Industries (*www.college-park.com*) incorporates plantar flexion and dorsiflexion bumpers made of hard rubber and a three-point weight transfer system that uses a forefoot bone with a split toe for mediolateral stability on both level and uneven surfaces. The ankle joint allows some transverse rotation and some accommodation. The dynamic response system is designed to provide a smooth transition from midstance through toe off. Multiaxis feet are heavier than many other feet, increasing the amount of energy required for ambulation. The extra weight is at the distal end of the prosthesis; the prosthesis acts as a long lever arm putting the weight at a distance from the axis of control at the knee joint. The weight of multiaxis feet limits their value for many individuals.

There were some early studies comparing dynamic response feet to each other and to the SACH foot. Generally, results indicated that clients spent more time wearing a prosthesis fitted with a dynamic response foot; they reported having more energy and not tiring as quickly. Athletes also favor dynamic response feet. However, no significant differences were found in oxygen uptake when the client walked at a client determined pace.[5–12] In a recent study involving one teenaged patient with bilateral transtibial amputations, a variety of gait parameters were studied when she was wearing bilateral patellar-tendon bearing (PTB) prostheses fitted with SACH feet than bilateral PTB prostheses filled with Flex feet. The results indicated a significant increase in cadence, sagittal plane power absorption, ankle range of motion and energy efficiency while wearing the Flex feet.[13]

Another problem with most prosthetic feet regardless of category is their inability to alter foot alignment when the client wears shoes of different heel heights. The prosthetist selects the foot configuration and aligns the prosthesis with the shoe given by the patient (see Chap. 8). Changes in heel height alter the relationship of foot to socket and may create abnormal forces on knee, hip, and back, leading to gait deviations and possible pain. Dynamic response feet can adapt to small changes in heel height, and some manufacturers advertise that alignment changes of up to ½ inch can be made with a small tool. The importance of being able to change the foot configurations for shoes of different heel height may influence the selection of a particular foot. PTs need to consider this when exploring the lifestyle needs of the client and share the information with the prosthetist. Table 7.2 outlines the advantages and disadvantages of different classes of feet.

TABLE 7.2 PROSTHETIC FEET

Component	Advantages	Disadvantages
Single axis foot	Enhances knee stability for individuals with transfemoral prostheses in which balance and knee control are problematic. Low cost, low maintenance.	Not indicated for transtibial or lower-level prostheses or individuals who are active walkers. Faster plantarflexion increases knee extension, slowing push off and gait speed.
SACH Foot	Low-cost, low-maintenance cosmetic foot that comes in many sizes and heel heights. Can be used with all levels of amputations including Syme's. Most frequently used prosthetic foot.	No propulsion at terminal stance. Cannot vary heel height without changing foot.
Dynamic response feet	Provides propulsion at terminal stance, enhancing the client's ability to walk long distances, run, and jump. Some are light weight and reduce fatigue.	Expensive. Some may provide too much spring for the slow and hesitant walker.

PARTIAL FOOT AND ANKLE DISARTICULATION

The major functional consequences of single-digit, ray, or partial foot amputations are related to loss of push off at terminal stance. Individuals with single-digit or ray amputations may encounter problems of shoe fit but usually do not bother with prosthetic replacement. Shoe fillers of soft foam or cloth can be used. Individuals with transmetatarsal amputations have lost forefoot mobility and support in terminal stance. The loss of the forefoot lever arm results in a premature initiation of swing phase and a shorter step with the non-amputated foot. Additionally, skin irritation can occur at the distal end of the **residuum** from pressure generated at toe off. A molded shoe insert can be constructed to provide a firm support surface for terminal stance and to distribute pressure. A full-length carbon graphite plate forms the foundation of the toe filler with a molded foot support over it. Carbon graphite plates are very thin and come in varying densities to accommodate differences in weight and activity level. Some include an arch plate for additional support. The finished molded support includes a filler for the distal part of the shoe and fits into the shoe.

Ankle Disarticulation (Syme)

The ankle disarticulation prosthesis is composed of a socket and a foot; suspension is inherent within the socket because of the configurations of the residual limb.

Sockets

The Syme prosthesis provides for a weight-bearing surface at the distal end (see Chap. 4) as well as along the shaft of the tibia and somewhat at the patella tendon. It is molded over the shaft of the fibula and the medial flares of the tibia for stabilizing pressure. A window is cut along the medial wall of the socket to allow the bulbous end, created by the tibial condyles, to slide down to the end-bearing part of the prosthetic foot. The window is covered by

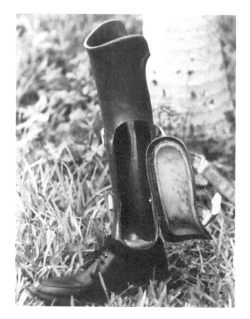

FIGURE 7.9
The conventional Syme prosthesis.

a panel that fits snugly into the opening and is secured by two straps (Fig. 7.9). The decrease in limb circumference proximal to the bulbous end enables suspension by virtue of the irregular contours of the socket itself. The standard Syme prosthesis is functional but not very cosmetic with a thick distal end and straps. The medial window also reduces the mechanical strength of the prosthesis. On occasion, the window is cut posteriorly rather than medially.

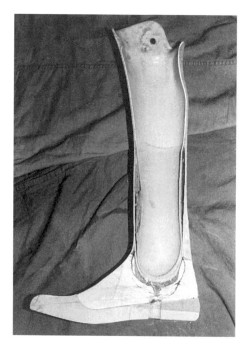

FIGURE 7.10
Cutaway of a closed expandable Syme prosthesis.

However, the prosthesis is considered to be structurally stronger with a medial rather than a posterior window.

The closed, expandable-socket Syme prosthesis was developed for the modified Syme amputation described in Chapter 4. The smaller distal end created by shaving the malleoli eliminates the need for a window. The prosthesis is fabricated with a liner attached to the inner wall of the socket. The liner is made of flexible plastic and extends from the distal end of the socket to a point where the diameter of the proximal leg equals the bulbous end distally. A space is created between the inner socket and the outer laminate, and the liner stretches as the end of the residual limb is inserted into the socket. The liner closes around the length of the residuum to maintain total contact and aid in suspension (Fig. 7.10).

Foot

Ankle disarticulations result in the loss of all ankle-foot motions. The length of the residual limb precludes the use of some of the prosthetic feet described in Table 7.2. However, several companies make dynamic response feet particularly for the Syme level. They provide a place for the distal end of the residual limb.

TRANSTIBIAL PROSTHESIS

The Socket

The PTB socket is the standard transtibial socket. It is a laminated plastic socket fitted with or without a liner (Fig. 7.11). Pressure tolerant areas include the patellar tendon, a relatively pressure insensitive area and the major

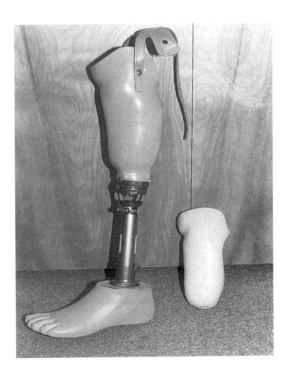

FIGURE 7.11
Patellar tendon bearing socket with liner on side.

weight-bearing area in this socket. Other pressure-tolerant areas include the flares of the tibial condyles, the areas just above the femoral condyles, the shaft of the fibula, and the popliteal fossa. Some pressure may be tolerated at the distal end of the residual limb. Stabilization is provided by molding the socket over the relatively flat flares of the proximal tibia and the shaft of the fibula if it is long enough. The head of the fibula with the peroneal nerve, the distal end of both the tibia and the fibula, and the sharp crest of the tibia are pressure-insensitive and must be relieved within the socket. The socket is shaped to configure to these demands and to the function of the knee joint. The optimum level for the posterior brim is the popliteal crease, but it must be low enough to allow the client to sit with knee flexed at least 90 degrees yet high enough to prevent undue bulging of flesh over the brim. The proximal edge is rounded to prevent sharp pressure on the back of the knee; grooves are provided at the medial and lateral corners for the hamstring tendons. The medial groove is deeper because the semitendinosus inserts more distally than the biceps femoris. The anterior wall reaches to mid-patella level and includes the shelf that increases weight bearing on the patella tendon. The medial and lateral walls reach approximately to the level of the adductor tubercle and control rotation of the residual limb (Fig 7.12). Total contact at the distal end is required for proprioceptive feedback and proper support of the residual limb.

Liners

Most PTB prostheses are constructed to be used with some sort of liner, an interface between the residual limb and the hard walls of the prosthesis. There are a great variety of liners currently available. Some may be made of polyethylene foam, urethane, silicone, or mineral oil-based gel. Some liners fit directly against the skin, and some require a cotton or wool sock between the skin and the liner (see Chap. 8). The liner absorbs some of the compressive and shear forces generated during ambulation. The liner cushions and protects the residual limb; however, the liner may deteriorate over time, may need more frequent replacement than the socket, and may still require the use of socks as the residual limb decreases in size.

In some instances, patients are fitted without a liner, using only one or more socks as an interface between the residual limb and socket. The major advantage is a more intimate fit because pressure and relief can be placed more exactly. The major disadvantage is that the socket must fit with great accuracy and does not adapt to changes in residual limb size. It also does not provide any shock absorption or cushioning.

Some liners are fabricated at the same time as the socket, following the same configurations. These are made of various materials such as silicone or polyethylene foams (see Figs. 7.11 and 7.12). These liners are lightweight, durable, and less expensive than gel liners. They have minimal shock absorption or shear absorption capabilities and require the use of stump socks between the residual limb and liner.

There are a great variety of gel liners now available on the market. Some are fabricated of silicone materials, others of mineral oil-based gels. The Alps Corporation (*www.easyliner.com*) (Fig. 7.13) fabricates some liners that are thin, flexible, and do not have a cloth covering on either surface. Other liners, such as the Alpha liner fabricated by Ohio Willow Wood Corp. (*www.owwco.com*)

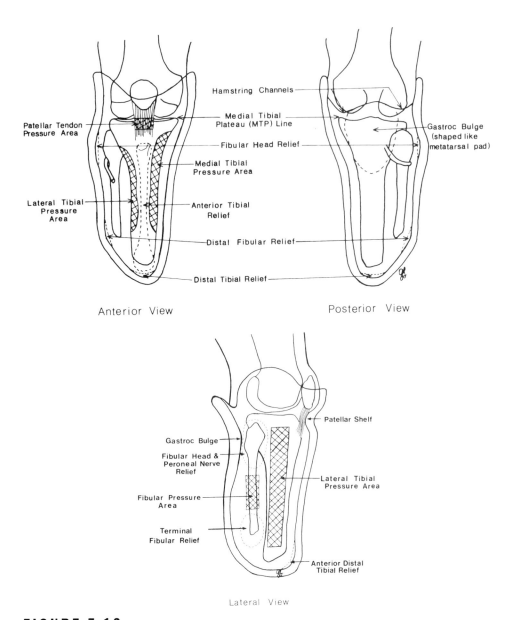

FIGURE 7.12

Pressure and relief areas for the patellar tendon bearing socket prosthesis. (Artist: Gloria Sanders)

are made of mineral oil-based gel and covered with a spandex-like fabric (Fig. 7.14). All come in a variety of sizes. The Alpha liners come in 3, 6, and 9 mm thicknesses. Liners such as the Alpha are modified for the individual patient by heat-molding over a positive mold of the residual limb.[14] The early Total Environmental Control liners (TEC Corp.; *www.Tecinterface.com*) required that a lubricant be applied to the skin prior to donning; current TEC urethane liners no longer require a lubricant. TEC liners are slightly heavier than other gel liners but are reported to have a flow characteristic that makes them particularly comfortable for short residual limbs.

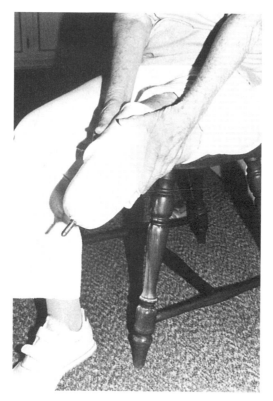

FIGURE 7.13
Donning a transtibial roll on shuttlelock socket.

Gel liners are more expensive than silicone or polyethylene foam liners and generally not as durable. However, they fit more intimately and provide greater shear reduction and cushioning. Gel liners require careful maintenance. They need to be cleaned nightly with a damp cloth and replaced on the stand provided with the liner to maintain their shape. Alpha liners are provided in pairs so the patient can wear one on alternate days, making sure it is dry and clean. Over time, all liners will lose some of the resiliency and may tear in areas of heavy wear. Most gel liners can be used either as a stump/ socket interface only or as part of a shuttlelock and pin or suction suspension system. These liners have made it possible to fit individuals with scarred, bony, deformed residual limbs as well as residual limbs with adhered skin, skin grafts, and other areas prone to abrasion from the shear forces generated within the socket during ambulation. Not all patients need or are suitable candidates for gel liners. Although most are fabricated of hypoallergenic materials, on rare occasions an individual will encounter irritability with the liners. Individuals with very fleshy residual limbs or those that are shrinking rapidly may do better with a foam liner initially.

The constantly changing variety of liners and materials makes it impossible for any PT to recommend one particular liner over the other. Different liner materials have different characteristics in terms of shock absorption, flow patterns, and stiffness. A recent study compared four different liner materials and human tissue and determined that none of the artificial materials was as resilient as human tissue but suggested that urethane might provide somewhat more shock absorption and flow characteristics on impact.[15] The

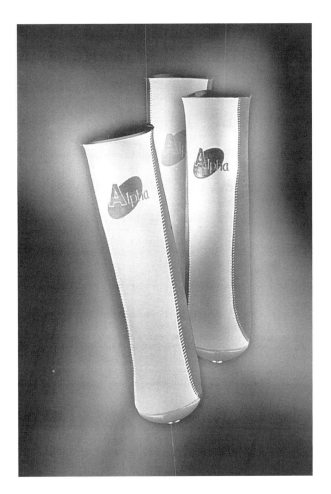

FIGURE 7.14
Alpha liners come in different thicknesses. (Courtesy of Ohio Willow Wood Corp.)

prosthetist who actually works with the materials is most competent to make specific recommendations. However, the PT needs to understand the demands of the different types of liners to provide accurate information about the patient's needs and to properly educate the patient in the care of the appliance.

Suspension

Table 7.3 describes the advantages and disadvantages of different suspension mechanisms.

Supracondylar Cuff

The supracondylar cuff may be made of leather or Dacron webbing. It is attached via studs to the proximal part of the socket in the posteromedial and posterolateral areas (Fig. 7.15). It encircles the thigh just above the femoral condyles and patella. The cuff suspends the prosthesis during swing phase. It is designed to hold the prosthesis over the patella and not circumferentially around the supracondylar aspect of the thigh but accurate suspension is difficult to obtain. The supracondylar cuff is not frequently used today.

TABLE 7.3 PTB SUSPENSION MECHANISMS

Suspension	Advantages	Disadvantages
Supracondylar cuff	Allows normal knee motion. Easy to don and remove. Relatively inexpensive. Durable and easily replaced.	Does not eliminate all pistoning. No mediolateral knee stability. May interfere with circulation of the distal thigh in obese clients. May cause pinching in distal thigh when sitting.
Waist belt	Provides auxiliary suspension. Some weight bearing on iliac crests.	May be uncomfortable, particularly for obese people. Uneven suspension on swing. Fork strap does not resist knee extension. More difficult to don. Uncosmetic.
Sleeve	Better suspension than all but suction. No circumferential constriction.	Increased perspiration and heat. No mediolateral stability. Not as durable as cuff. More expensive than cuff.
Supracondylar suprapatellar	Improves cosmesis. No circumferential constrictions. Aids in mediolateral stability. Better suspension for short residual limbs.	Enclosed patella can limit kneeling. Difficult to suspend over heavy thighs.
Suction	Reduces pistoning. Minimizes shear forces on residual limb. Does not limit knee flexion.	May be difficult to don. Increased perspiration and heat. Most expensive of all suspensions.

Sleeve

Latex rubber, neoprene, or polyurethane sleeves (Fig. 7.16) come in a variety of sizes and fit over the proximal part of the socket and the distal thigh. The sleeve holds the prosthesis firmly on the residual limb eliminating **pistoning** during swing phase. Suspension occurs secondary to a negative pressure during swing phase and the longitudinal tension in the sleeve itself. To function,

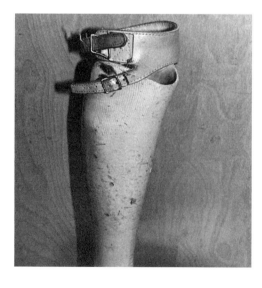

FIGURE 7.15
The supracondylar cuff suspension on well-worn prosthesis.

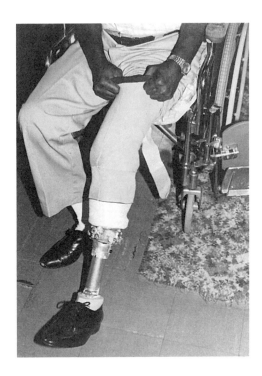

FIGURE 7.16
Sleeve suspension.

the sleeve must terminate above the socks to contact the skin. Some sleeves have latex and are contraindicated for individuals who are latex-sensitive. Some neoprene sleeves incorporate a 2-inch-wide circumferential band that fits around mid thigh to help with suspension, particularly for individuals with large, fleshy, conically shaped thighs. Figure 7.16 shows the band open and hanging on the suspension sleeve. The band does increase suspension but may also cause problems with edema and muscle bunching in the distal thigh. Patients have a tendency to secure the band too tightly.

Suprapatellar Supracondylar

The proximal brim of the prosthetic socket is extended over the patella and femoral condyles with suspension pressure exerted over the patella and the medial femoral condyle (Fig. 7.17). Suprapatellar suspension is created by an indentation of the socket brim over the soft tissue of the patellar. A cup is created for the patella ensuring that there is no pressure on the patella itself. Pressure over the medial femoral condyle is created by inserting a wedge in the medial portion of the proximal socket. Prostheses with suprapatellar-supracondylar suspension may be referred to as patellar-tendon supracondylar (PTS) although the more correct title would be PTBSPSC.

Shuttlelock System

A cup and pin may be inserted at the end of any gel liner to secure attachment of the socket on the liner and hence on the residual limb. The pin locks into a receptacle built into the bottom of the socket as the patient places weight into the prosthesis. It is released by pushing on a button placed on the medial part of the shank of the prosthesis (Fig. 7.18). The liner fits intimately on the

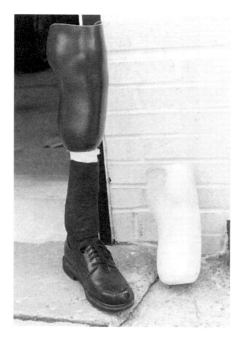

FIGURE 7.17

Suprapatellar supracondylar suspension on a patellar tendon bearing socket prosthesis with liner.

residual limb creating a suspension of the liner on the residual limb. By attaching to the socket, the whole prosthesis becomes an intimate part of the person. There is no movement between residual limb and liner or between liner and socket. The total contact fit creates greater proprioceptive feedback and enhances integration of the prosthesis. However, the patient must be sure the pin is properly aligned with the receptacle to obtain an proper lock. As the residual limb shrinks, the intimate fit can be maintained by adding socks between the liner and the socket. There are now commercially available socks with the hole for the pin knitted into the sock, hopefully reducing the chances of threads jamming the pin mechanism. Some individuals have reported distal end discomfort and the development of a distal end bursa created by the milking action within the residual limb created during the swing phase of gait. The shuttlelock holds the liner in place as the client takes the weight off the prosthesis. The liner adheres to the skin, holding the skin securely. As the client takes weight off the limb in swing phase, the tibia and fibula pull slightly away from the distal end, but the tissue remains adhered to the liner creating a slight tissue distraction. Although this is not a problem for most individuals, it can cause distal end problems with some people.

Suction Socket

A one-way expulsion valve is laminated into the bottom of the socket; as the patient pushes the residual limb and gel liner into the socket, air is expelled and does not reenter. A lightweight airtight sleeve is also used with this system. This creates a negative pressure that maintains the prosthesis. The one-way expulsion valve does not require as much space below the end of the liner, nor does it require accurate alignment of the pin with the receptacle. Some prosthetists have reported using the suction sleeve without the expulsion valve quite successfully. The mechanism is not as durable and requires careful maintenance.

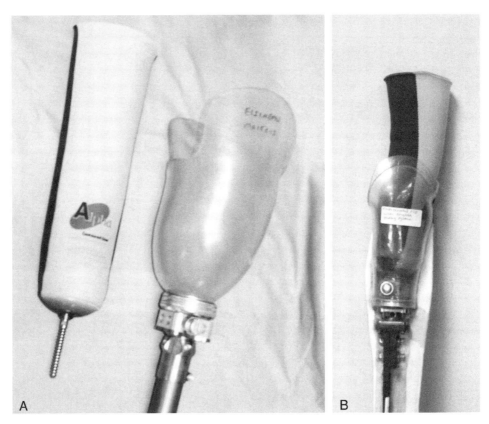

FIGURE 7.18
(A) Shuttlelock system. Note pin at end of liner and release button on socket. (B) Liner locked in socket.

Thigh Corset

The leather thigh lacer is used very rarely. It may be necessary when complete mediolateral stability is necessary or if a very short or painful residual limb cannot be suspended any other way. The leather corset attaches by metal side bars and hinged knee joints to the socket. It fits around the distal half of the thigh or may extend to the proximal thigh. It reduces weight bearing in the socket, limits knee motion and increases the weight of the appliance. It is also not cosmetic whether worn under or over clothing and is difficult to don.

Pylons

Pylons are the metal pipes that connect the foot to the socket. They are usually made of lightweight carbon graphite materials with a socket connector that allows aligning the socket on the foot (see Chap. 8). Some pylons are made of two telescoping pipes to provide additional shock absorption particularly with high level activity. Flex-Foot (*www.flexfoot.com*) has created the ReFlex VSP composed of a carbon fiber compression spring and telescoping tubes. It cushions the impact on high activity. It allows individuals to jump, run, and go up and down stairs step over step, without discomfort. It also stores and releases energy to allow the user to walk comfortably, efficiently, and naturally (Fig. 7.19). Other companies make similar products. Shock absorbing and rotational pylons are for active individuals. The PT, patient, and prosthetist must

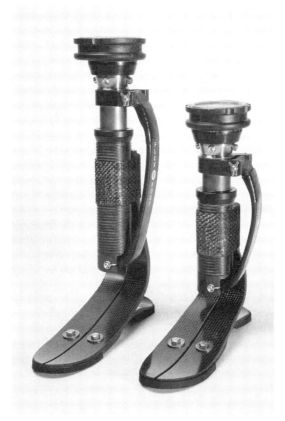

FIGURE 7.19
Flex-Foot Re-Flex VSP and Flex-Foot Low Profile
Re-Flex VSP. (Photograph courtesy of Össur.)

consult to determine if any of these devices is suitable for the individual person. Not all third-party payers reimburse for all of these components.

TRANSFEMORAL PROSTHESIS

Sockets

Three socket designs are in general use for transfemoral prostheses: the quadrilateral, the ischial containment, and the contoured ischial containment sockets. Modification of socket designs for the transfemoral level of amputation has focused on increasing mediolateral and rotational stability. Although the transtibial residual limb generally has areas that allow for contouring and stabilization, the transfemoral residual limb with its single bone well buried in muscle and soft tissue does not. The less the stabilization and rotational control, the greater the energy required for ambulatory activities, and the less is the proprioceptive feedback. Each socket design reflects attempts to provide better prosthetic control in locomotion and increased comfort in sitting.

The Quadrilateral Socket

The quadrilateral socket (Fig. 7.20) was developed in the late 1950s and is named for the four walls that each have a specific function. Distally the

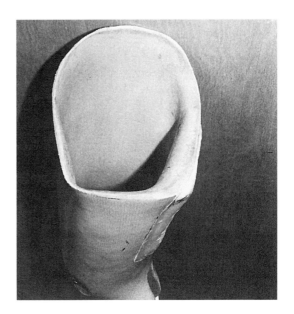

FIGURE 7.20
Transfemoral quadrilateral socket, viewed from above.

socket is contoured to provide total contact for the residual limb. The posterior wall provides the major weight-bearing area; the ischial tuberosity and some gluteal muscle rest on top of the wall that is thicker medially than laterally. Internally, the wall is contoured for the hamstring muscles, whereas externally, it is flat to prevent rolling in sitting. If the socket is made of rigid plastic, the exterior is padded to absorb sounds and protect clothing. The height of the posterior wall is determined by the position of the ischial tuberosity.

The anterior wall rises about 5 cm (2.5 inches) above the height of the posterior wall and, medially, provides stabilizing pressure to help keep the ischial tuberosity securely on the seat by molding over the femoral triangle. The anterior wall is convex laterally to allow space for the bulk of the rectus femoris muscle. The lateral wall is as high as the anterior wall and inclines medially to set the residual limb in about 10 degrees of adduction, thereby aiding pelvic control in stance. A relief channel is built into the corner of the medial and anterior walls for the adductor longus tendon. The quadrilateral socket provides minimal mediolateral and little rotational stability. It is not often prescribed today as the first socket; however, individuals who have worn a quadrilateral socket for many years may be loath to try a different design.

The Ischial Containment Socket

The ischial containment socket (Fig. 7.21) was developed in the late 1980s and early 1990s and is shaped differently from the quadrilateral socket. Improved pelvic control in stance, comfortable weight bearing, and a smoother swing phase are the major objectives of the ischial containment socket. The term "ischial containment" describes the major characteristic. The ischium and the ascending ramus are enclosed within the socket, and weight-bearing forces are distributed through the medial aspect of the ischium and the ramus as well as surrounding soft tissue. Compared to the quadrilateral socket, more of the residual limb is contained within the ischial containment socket, al-

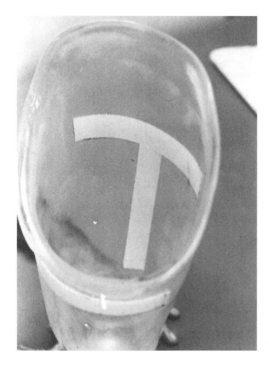

FIGURE 7.21
The ischial containment socket.

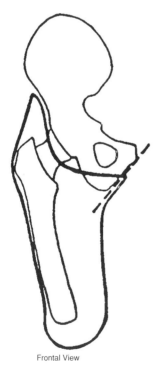

Frontal View

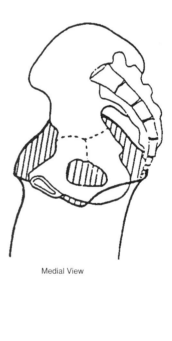

Medial View

FIGURE 7.22
(*Left*) Frontal view of the femur and pelvis in the ischial containment socket. (*Right*) Medial view of the pelvis in the ischial containment socket.

lowing for greater distribution of weight-bearing and stabilizing ⟨..
narrow mediolateral dimension and molding over the femoral shaft help keep
the ischium and the ramus against the posteromedial wall of the socket as
well as contribute to rotational stability. The lateral wall is extended well
over the greater trochanter to add to stance-phase stability of the pelvis. The
socket is contoured for total contact throughout. Figure 7.22 schematizes the
relationship of the socket walls to the bony structures.

Contoured Ischial Containment

In 1985, John Sabolich[16] published a description of the ischial containment
socket that was contoured around muscle compartments to increase the
mediolateral stability of the transfemoral residual limb in the socket. Since
that time, there has been considerable interest within the prosthetic community in trying to improve the mediolateral and rotational stability of the
transfemoral amputation level. The contoured ischial containment socket
has been modified and the concept purchased and further modified by different companies. The current version is the Hanger ComfortFlex socket (*www.
hanger.com*) (Fig. 7.23). The socket is contoured to lock the pubic ramus and
ischium within the socket and provide channels for functioning muscle
groups such as the hip adductors and extensors. The socket itself is made of
soft plastic that is meant to fit directly over the residual limb. However, a gel
liner or stump sock interface may be used, although such an interface lessens
the degree of proprioceptive feedback. The socket is designed to encourage
the individual to use remaining musculature actively within the socket during locomotion. The design is enhanced by such muscle activity that also
serves to maintain the tone of the residual limb (see Chap. 8 on prosthetic
training). The socket is usually placed within a carbon graphite frame (Fig.
7.24) that has the property to tighten during muscle activity and relax during
nonactive periods. The designer reports that this provides better rotational
and mediolateral control of the prosthesis. The socket is reported to be functional for all transfemoral prostheses and all activity levels.[17]

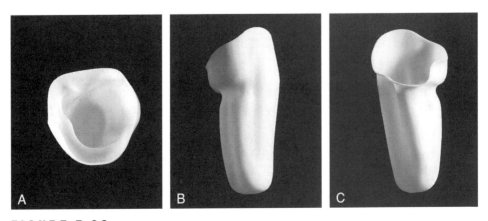

FIGURE 7.23
Three views of the Hanger ComfortFlex Socket. (*A*) Top view; (*B*) Lateral view; (*C*) Medial view. (Courtesy Hanger
Prosthetics & Orthotics, Inc.)

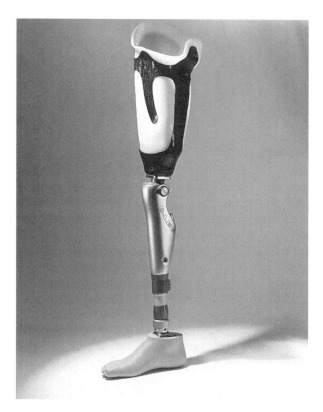

FIGURE 7.24
Hanger ComfortFlex socket attached to a Bock "C" leg. (Courtesy Hanger Prosthetic & Orthotics, Inc.)

Flexible Sockets

Flexible sockets incorporate a malleable thermoplastic socket supported in some type of rigid or semirigid frame. The frame can be of quadrilateral or ischial containment design, although the latter is more frequently used. Flexible sockets are reported to provide better proprioception, better suspension and be more comfortable.[18–20]

Advantages or Disadvantages

The literature does not report any specific advantages or disadvantages to any socket design. If an individual has been using a particular socket successfully, it is beneficial to continue with that design. Schuch,[21] summarizing the recommendations of several authors, suggested that the quadrilateral socket is most successful if the residual limb is long and firm with strong adductor muscles, whereas the ischial containment is more successful than the quadrilateral for short and flabby residual limbs. He further suggested that the ischial containment socket might be more beneficial for individuals who are very active. Gottschalk[22] and associates reported that socket configuration did not affect femoral adduction. However, the ischial containment socket overall is reported to provide greater mediolateral stability during activity and to be preferred by individuals with bilateral transfemoral amputations as well as the majority of individuals with transfemoral amputations.[23] Otherwise, it is probably a matter of client and prosthetist preference.

Suspension

Each of the following suspension methods may be used with any transfemoral socket. The advantages and disadvantages of each method of suspension are outlined in Table 7.4.

Suction

The suction socket (Fig. 7.25) is worn with the residual limb in direct contact with the socket without a sock. The process of donning the socket pushes all the air out of the valve hole at the medial distal end of the socket creating negative pressure within the socket. The valve prevents air from reentering the socket. During the swing phase of gait, negative pressure within the socket, augmented by muscle tension, holds the socket on the residual limb. Donning the socket (Fig 7.26) involves putting on a thin sock, standing, and pushing the residual limb into the socket while pulling the sock out of the valve hole. The client can palpate the end of the residual limb to ensure that it is well into the socket. An alternative method of donning involves spreading a thin layer of lotion over the residual limb. The lotion is absorbed into the skin and suction is maintained.[11] The client then pushes the residual limb fully into the socket and secures the valve. On occasion an elastic bandage may be used to pull the residual limb into the socket. The elastic bandage must not be wrapped circumferentially around the limb but rather started over the medial tissue brought down over the end of the limb and up to the lateral tissue and then dropped through the valve hole. The person pushes the residual limb into the socket as far as possible and then pulls the elastic bandage through the hole to pull in all the proximal tissues.

If a flexible socket is used, it is simply rolled over the residual limb and then inserted into the supporting frame. Suction provides an intimate suspension and good proprioceptive feedback, and allows full hip motion. It is difficult to maintain adequate suspension with suction alone if limb volume fluc-

TABLE 7.4   TRANSFEMORAL SUSPENSION MECHANISMS

Suspension	Advantages	Disadvantages
Suction	Allows full freedom of hip motion. Good proprioceptive feedback through its intimate fit.	Difficulty obtaining good fit. Suction can be lost through perspiration. Potential for skin shear and abrasions. Potential for skin irritation in a closed medium. Requires good balance and coordination for donning.
Silesian bandage	Lightweight additional suspension. Provides some rotational control.	Difficult to keep clean unless it is detachable. Can irritate the waist.
Total elastic suspension	Provides excellent suspension. Adjusts to the size of the individual. Generally comfortable. Adds less weight than the pelvic belt. Provides for rotational control.	Retains body heat, which may lead to skin irritations and discomfort. Wears out easily. Difficult to keep clean.
Pelvic belt	Easy to don. Provides rotational control. Provides mediolateral pelvic stability.	Adds weight to the prosthesis. Is usually not very comfortable.

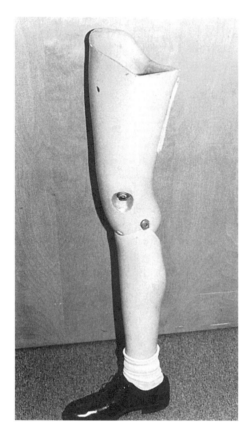

FIGURE 7.25
A transfemoral suction prosthesis with quadrilateral
socket and constant friction knee mechanism.

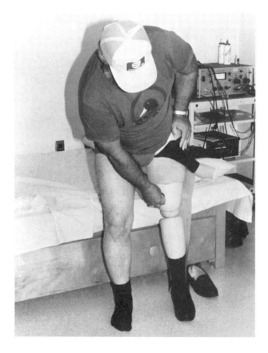

FIGURE 7.26
Donning a transfemoral prosthesis with suction
suspension.

tuates or if perspiration accumulates on the residual limb; many clients choose to add an auxiliary suspension.

Suction is indicated for individuals with firm, mature, and generally smooth residual limbs of medium to long length. The individual must have the balance and coordination to don the prosthesis properly.

Silesian Bandage

The Silesian bandage (Fig. 7.27) is a soft webbing strap that is attached to the lateral socket wall, encircles the pelvis, and connects with a strap on the anterior wall (Fig. 7.27A). The Silesian bandage aids in suspension and provides some control of rotation. The bandage is indicated as an auxiliary to suction suspension. There is also a 3-point Silesian band (7.27B) that may be used as

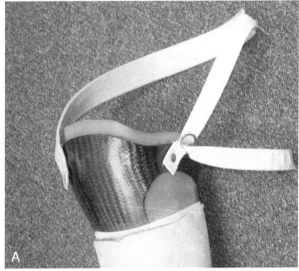

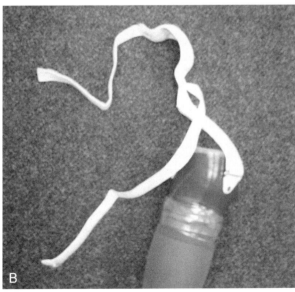

FIGURE 7.27
(A) Traditional single belt Silesian band;
(B) Three-point Silesian band with
ischial crest cup.

the major suspension with the ischial containment socket. This band has a cap sewn into the lateral part that fits over the crest of the contralateral ilium. It has a second small strap that runs from the middle of the back and connects to the contralateral side of the band anteriorly.

Total Elastic Suspension

The total elastic suspension (TES) is a wide neoprene band lined with nylon tricot material that is similar to the neoprene sleeve of the transtibial prosthesis (Fig. 7.28). The belt fits around the proximal part of the socket and then goes around the waist and pelvis to suspend the prosthesis. It can be used with suction or as a primary suspension mechanism.

Pelvic Belt

The pelvic belt (Fig. 7.29) is made of leather and metal and is connected to the prosthesis by a metal or nylon hip joint fastened to the superolateral aspect of the socket. The belt suspends the prosthesis and enables the wearer to don the limb in the sitting position. It is particularly useful if the client's weight fluctuates widely. It also provides some mediolateral stability and is useful for individuals with weak hip abductors. It adds weight to the prosthesis and may be uncomfortable against the trunk, particularly in sitting.

Knee Mechanisms

The prosthetic knee has several functions. It allows for sitting, kneeling, and similar activities; allows for a smooth and controlled movement of the shank

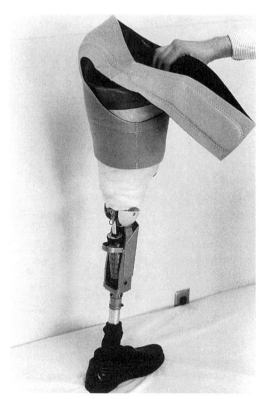

FIGURE 7.28

Total elastic suspension (TES) on transfemoral prosthesis.

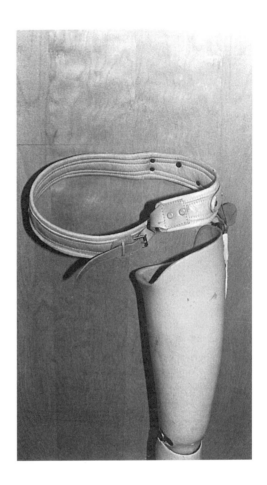

FIGURE 7.29
Pelvic belt suspension.

and foot during swing phase at any gait speed and on any type of surface; and provides stability during stance phase. A wide variety of knee mechanisms are on the market today. They perform a great variety of functions, range in complexity from very simple to highly complex and computerized, and vary in price from a few dollars to many thousand dollars. It is beyond the scope of this text to review all available knee mechanisms. We will consider representative mechanisms by major function and characteristics. The reader is encouraged to work with regional prosthetists to determine the specific knee mechanisms in use locally. Generally, knee units may be divided into three categories: those that are only mechanical in control, those that have hydraulic or pneumatic controls, and those that are computerized or controlled by a microprocessor. Functionally, they can be further subdivided into those that provide control only over stance phase of gait, those that provide control of swing phase, and those that provide control of both swing and stance phase.[24]

Knee Control

Knee units may function in stance, in swing, or during both phases of gait. Stability in stance is a function of the way the knee joint is aligned in the prosthesis (**alignment stability**) and the client's ability to keep the knee in extension (voluntary control). (See Chap. 8 for a discussion of knee control.) The most appropriate knee mechanism is one that requires the least amount of alignment stability yet offers adequate security in stance. The effort required to initiate swing phase is increased as more alignment stability is built into a prosthesis, thus affecting gait. The amount of alignment stability needed is inversely related to the length and strength of the residual limb. The amount of alignment stability needed is also determined by the type of knee mechanism used.

Stance phase control refers to the degree of stability when standing on the prosthesis. Stance stability is generally provided by alignment and the voluntary action of the client. In most knee mechanisms, failure to extend the knee fully prior to heel contact will cause the prosthetic knee to flex suddenly when weight is applied. Some knee mechanisms provide additional stability during stance, particularly if the client does not bring the knee into full extension before putting weight on the prosthesis. Obviously, stance phase control, whether provided by alignment, client function, knee mechanism, or a combination, is the most important aspect of knee function. If the client cannot be confident that the knee will remain stable throughout stance, regardless of the activity, then the individual will never be an effective walker.

From toe off to heel contact, the shank and foot of the prosthesis swings forward like a modified pendulum. If not controlled by the prosthetic knee, the shank and foot would function just like a pendulum, coming forward at a rate determined by the force exerted at toe off. For the foot to be in proper position for heel contact, the knee mechanism must exert some control over the rate of knee movement in swing phase. This is referred to as swing phase control. Swing phase control may be constant, that is, the foot comes forward at the same rate each step regardless of the speed of gait; or it may be variable, responding to the forces generated by the walking speed of the individual. Most knee units are manufactured for both endoskeletal and exoskeletal constructions. Advantages and disadvantages of the major types of knee joints are outlined in Table 7.5.

Mechanical Knee Mechanisms

Although it is true that all knee mechanisms are mechanical, for ease of discussion, this category is reserved for all the knee units that do not have hydraulic or microprocessor mechanisms. Knee joints may have one or more axes of motion. Units with one axis of motion are referred to as single-axis knee joints, others, as polycentric or multiaxis.

The constant friction knee (Fig. 7.25) is a single-axis knee that provides constant swing-phase control. Some friction is set into the mechanism by adjusting two small screws in front or in back of the knee mechanism. The rate stays the same regardless of the speed of gait. It does not provide any stance-phase control. It is one of the oldest knee mechanisms in use and rarely used in the Western world today. However, one will occasionally find an individual who has been using a constant friction knee for many years and does not want to change.

Polycentric knee joints are usually four-bar linkage systems. They have multiple axes of rotation that change during knee motion. These knees provide some response to changing gait speeds and some swing-phase control by shortening the shank during flexion to allow for better toe clearance. They offer some stance-phase control by varying stability through the different

TABLE 7.5   KNEE MECHANISMS

Knee Mechanism	Advantages	Disadvantages
Constant friction	Simple. Durable. Low-maintenance.	Only constant swing phase control. No stance control.
Multiaxis	Varying stability through stance. Shortens shank during swing for better toe clearance. Allows shank to rotate under knee when sitting.	Increased weight and bulk. Complex mechanism, less durable.
Pneumatic control	More responsive to changes in walking speed than constant friction.	Higher cost. Requires more maintenance. Heavier.
Extension aids	Increases speed of terminal extension. Used with many sliding friction knee mechanisms.	Constant rate of extension.

Sliding friction
    stance control
	Braking mechanisms if weight applied with knee
	    flexed 0–20 degrees.
	Helpful to slower clients.
		Requires regular maintenance.
		Not very responsive for active walker.

Manual lock	Total stability in stance phase.	No swing phase flexion, resulting in stiff knee gait.
Hydraulic swing control	Responds to changing gait speeds.	Higher cost than any other unit. Heavy.
Hydraulic swing and stance control	Responds to changing gait speeds. Has a braking mechanism for stance phase control.	Higher cost than any other unit. Heavy. May need more maintenance.

axes. Most prosthetic companies make one or more versions of the polycentric knee with varying characteristics. In general, the polycentric knee is particularly useful for individuals with long residual limbs or knee disarticulations, or for individuals who do not change walking speed a great deal. They are not the best knee mechanisms for active community ambulators or athletes.

Stance-control mechanical knee mechanisms may be a manual lock knee or a weight-activated mechanism (Fig. 7.1). A brake is activated at heel contact and remains active throughout the stance phase. There is some variability regarding how much weight is necessary to engage the mechanism and the range of knee flexion in which the brake will operate. Generally the mechanism operates within the first 20 degrees of knee flexion. If the knee is not fully extended as the client puts weight on the prosthesis, the knee will not buckle. These stance-control knees are sometimes referred to as "safety" knees, a misnomer that may be misleading to the client. Unlike the manual lock knee, the stance-phase control knee functions as a brake rather than an absolute lock. The stance-phase control knee is useful for the individual who walks mostly within the home, does not change gait speed, walks generally on level ground, and may have difficulty with a regular step-over-step gait. It may also be used for individuals with very short residual limbs who require the additional stance-phase control.

The manual lock knee provides absolute stance-phase control but does not swing because the knee remains locked in extension throughout the gait cycle. Manual lock knees have a locking mechanism that is activated by the client when standing and disengaged when he or she is ready to sit. They are occasionally used for individuals with bilateral amputations or extremely feeble individuals who require absolute stance-phase control and only walk with assistance for limited distances.

Pneumatic or Hydraulic Knee Mechanisms

Pneumatic-control knee mechanisms utilize an air-filled cylinder housed within the upper part of the shank to provide variable swing-phase control. Knee flexion forces air through a cylinder then through a port that can be adjusted for size. The smaller the opening, the more the resistance to swing phase. The amount of friction varies with the speed of walking, providing a swing-phase control that is responsive to the client's speed of gait. The range of response varies with the particular unit, although most provide moderate response. The major problem with pneumatic-control mechanisms is that they tend to leak air, and the range of adjustments is somewhat limited. They are not used frequently by themselves although some are used in computerized legs.[21,24,25]

Hydraulic Knee Mechanisms

Hydraulic knee mechanisms are similar to pneumatic systems except that the resistive medium is a silicone oil rather than air. The greater viscosity of the silicone oil increases the range of responses and is not subject to changes with extreme temperatures. There is a great variety of hydraulic mechanisms available today. Some provide only swing-phase control whereas others provide both swing- and stance-phase control. Some units have an additional manual locking system for individuals working around a bench or climbing a ladder. Hydraulic mechanisms provide a normal heel rise and forward swing appropriate to the client's speed of walking. Some, for example, allow separate adjustments for heel rise and terminal swing and provide a high degree of resistance to knee flexion when weight is borne on the prosthesis. The hyperextension moment at the knee that occurs as the individual rolls over the foot disengages the stance-control mechanisms allowing a smooth heel off and knee flexion for swing phase. Many that provide some form of stance control, usually resistance to sudden flexion that allows a slow deceleration, allow the athletic client to walk downstairs step over step. Cost and weight are directly related to the complexity of function. Some are very light, whereas others add some weight to the prosthesis. Usually the more functions the unit can perform, the heavier it is. Hydraulic knee mechanisms are appropriate for any individual capable of walking step over step with varying cadence. The specific knee selected for a client will depend on the projected activity level of the client.

Microprocessor Knee Units

There are several knee units that incorporate a microprocessor. The onboard computer chip provides a more fluid response to changes of cadence. The Endolite intelligent prosthesis (*www.endolite.com*) incorporates a knee mechanism with a wide range of stance- and swing-phase control, a lightweight socket, and a multiflex ankle system designed to support a wide range of activities (Fig. 7.30). The Otto Bock C-leg (*www.ottobockus.com*) (Fig. 7.24) features an onboard sensor that reads and adapts to the changes in the person's

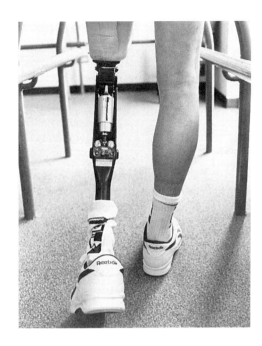

FIGURE 7.30
Endolite Intelligent Knee Control System. (From the Endolite Corporation of North America with permission.)

gait cadence. It also incorporates stance-phase control by providing resistance to knee flexion at appropriate times. The sensors read and respond to changes up to 50 times a second. Fine-tuning is done by the prosthetist using a computer and specially designed software. The client can move on flat terrain at different gait speeds with confidence as well as maneuver over slopes, stairs, and uneven surfaces.[23] Computerized knee mechanisms are very expensive. They represent the most advanced knee units available to date and are suitable for any individual capable of step-over-step ambulation at varying speeds and over uneven ground. They are ideal for community ambulators who have an active lifestyle. They have enabled athletes to improve performance and to set new world records at recent Paralympic Games.

Other Components

In previous years, individuals wearing transfemoral prostheses were limited by the rigid linear relationships of socket to knee to foot. Many activities in daily life are best performed with the knee partially flexed and with some degree of rotation. Golf is one such activity requiring a combination of knee flexion and body rotation. Torsion adapters are now available that allow such combination movements. The Otto Bock 4R485 and 4R486 Torsion Adapters (*www.ottobockus.com*) allow up to 20 degrees of internal and external rotation with individually adjustable ball bearings. These adapters also provide some torque absorption to minimize rubbing between the socket and residual limb.

Many individuals, particularly in Asian cultures, sit crosslegged on the floor or on cushions. Other people like to rotate their leg and place the foot on the opposite knee. There are rotator mechanisms that can be inserted below the socket that allow full rotation of the knee and shank. A small locking mechanism below the socket allows the individual, while sitting, to unlock the limb and rotate the lower leg at least 90 degrees.

HIP DISARTICULATION/TRANSPELVIC

Hip disarticulations and transpelvic prostheses are quite similar in component and alignment. The only difference is the socket. Rejection rates for
these prostheses are high because the gait cadence is slow and energy-
consuming. Wearers find the prostheses heavy and uncomfortable.[26–27]

The Sockets

The hip disarticulation socket is made of plastic, encloses the ischial tuberosity for weight bearing, and covers the iliac crest for stability in swing phase
(Fig. 7.31). It encircles the pelvis with an anterior slit to allow ease of donning
and removal. The medial aspect is cut to provide clearance for the other leg
and genitalia. Relief is provided over the anterior and posterior iliac spines.
Variations in socket construction include a lateral-opening diagonal socket
and a full socket similar to the transpelvic that encloses both iliac crests for
stability.

The transpelvic socket is similarly made except that it must include the
contralateral iliac crest for proper stabilization and suspension (Fig. 7.31).
Weight bearing is primarily on the remaining soft tissue and the contralateral
ischium. Care must be taken when constructing both sockets that no excess
pressure exists on bony prominences or in the perineum.

Both sockets can be made of rigid or flexible materials and padded for increased comfort on weight bearing. The socket may also be constructed of
flexible silicone rubber in a rigid frame to provide a softer, more intimate fit
that increases range of motion and comfort.[27]

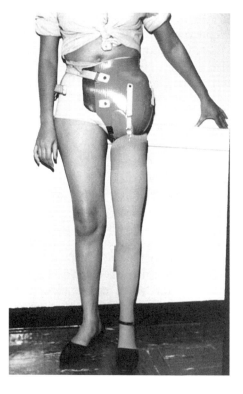

FIGURE 7.31
Endoskeletal hemipelvectomy prosthesis.

Hip, Knee, and Foot

The single-axis unlocked hip joint is attached to the anterior aspect of the socket to provide stance-phase stability and ease of swing phase (see Chap. 8 for details of alignment). A spring-assist mechanism may be incorporated for young active clients to aid in initiating swing phase. Hip and knee motion are controlled by extension straps and alignment (Fig 7.32).

Any knee joint can be used in the hip disarticulation prosthesis. A light-weight polycentric knee or stance-control unit is often utilized to keep the weight of the prosthesis low. Any of the feet discussed at the beginning of this chapter can be used.

BILATERAL AMPUTATIONS

Bilateral Transtibial Amputations

An individual with two transtibial amputations uses the same components as an individual with one transtibial amputation. The person may require feet with somewhat softer heels for increased stance stability.

Bilateral Transfemoral Amputations

Ambulation with bilateral transfemoral prostheses is energy-consuming, slow, and awkward, and most older individuals prefer to use a wheelchair rather than attempt ambulation. It is often unwise to try to fit individuals who do not exhibit considerable strength, endurance, balance, and good range of motion of both hips with prostheses. Younger, fit individuals should be fitted but

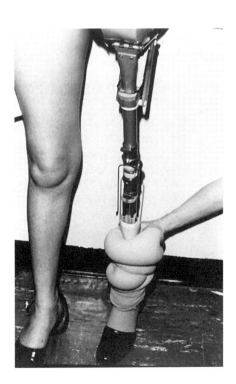

FIGURE 7.32
Endoskeletal components of the hemipelvectomy prosthesis. Note the elastic band posteriorly from socket to upper thigh in control swing phase.

will also need a wheelchair for times when they are not wearing their prostheses. To be functional with bilateral transfemoral prostheses, the individual should be able to ambulate step over step with no more than one cane for external support. The components are essentially the same, although most are fitted with ischial containment sockets for better hip control. The person should be able to don the prostheses in a sitting position. Some recommend fitting an individual with bilateral transfemoral prostheses with one manual locked knee. This is rarely advisable because it is hard to come to standing with a locked knee. Hydraulic knee mechanisms with some form of both stance and swing-phase control are more functional. Some individuals who use a wheelchair full-time request cosmetic prosthesis. These are usually foam construction, nonfunctional cosmetic limbs that can attach to the wheelchair.

Stubby prostheses are generally prescribed only for individuals who are motivated to ambulate but are not candidates for fitting with full-length prostheses. They may also be used as temporary prostheses. Stubbies are transfemoral prosthetic sockets set on rockers or prosthetic feet and are used to help the individual move around in an upright position. Many people find stubbies cosmetically unacceptable because of the extreme reduction in height. Ambulation in stubbies obligates exaggerated trunk rotation. Short canes or crutches are usually needed. Sitting in a chair and stair climbing are very difficult because of the shortness of the prostheses. The limbs also protrude in front of the chair when the person is sitting because of the lack of knee joints. If the individual becomes proficient in walking with stubbies, then the question of whether to have full-length prostheses can be raised. Although the person may be very stable when walking with stubbies, the lack of height will likely be a source of embarrassment. Factors to be weighed in the consideration of longer legs are the increased demand on the cardiovascular system and the decrease in balance and stability by virtue of raising the center of gravity and providing knee joints. If good balance, endurance, and motivation are present, then standard limbs may be considered.

RESEARCH AND DEVELOPMENT

New designs, materials, and fitting procedures are being developed and tested. Improved international communications have led to greater sharing of information, research, and technology.[28-29] Major prosthetic companies have research and development arms, and information can be found by starting at the Web site *www.oandp.com*. Through this Web site, one can search company advertisements and reports, research articles, and the *Journal of Prosthetics and Orthotics*, the publication of the American Academy of Prosthetics and Orthotics. Much of the current research is focused on improvement of materials and the function of already available components.

The Össur Company (*www.ossurusa.com*) recently reported on a research project to develop and improve TSB sockets. The principle is to distribute socket pressures throughout the residual limb rather than use selected points for pressure. The benefit of using quasi-hydrostatic weight-bearing principles is that the peak pressures on the skin are lower because the load is spread more uniformly across the residual limb.[30] The principles apply to both transtibial and transfemoral sockets and are being used, to some extent, in transfemoral sockets today.

In a similar area, the Össur Company reported on the initial development of a sensor socket designed to wirelessly transmit information about the residual limb to the prosthetic shop. The socket can be applied after surgery and throughout the healing phase as well as after the person has been fitted with a definitive prosthesis. The purpose is to reduce the number of trips to the prosthetic shop and to maintain up-to-date information about residual limb changes.

On the negative side, complex components are expensive and are usually not reimbursed by third-party payers. Government support of prosthetic research has also dwindled, increasing the cost of research and development and subsequently the cost of the components. Cost-containment measures will probably affect the development of new, more complex, and more functional components. It behooves the therapist working with clients who have lost a limb to stay abreast of new developments to help educate the client regarding available components.

Summary

The field of prosthetic components is rapidly changing, and the PT and PTA need to work closely with local prosthetists to help select the most functional components for each client. Much of the information gathered during the postsurgical period is helpful in component selection.

Glossary

Alignment stability	Stance-phase knee extension and stability created by aligning the knee joint posterior to the vertical knee axis line.
Components	The parts of a prosthesis.
Dynamic alignment	The slight movement of the foot or knee component in relationship to the socket to provide the client with an optimum gait. Can only be done after the client has learned how to walk with the prosthesis.
Endoskeletal	A lightweight metal tube to connect the components. The shank is covered by a soft foam cover that matches the color and configuration of the other leg.
Exoskeletal	Wood or rigid polyurethane covered with a rigid plastic lamination.
Myoelectric	The stimulation of muscle action by electric current.
Pistoning	The dropping of the prosthesis away from the residual limb during swing phase of gait. Usually occurs with inadequate suspension.
Residuum	Residual limb.
Shank	The part of the prosthesis corresponding to the lower leg of the unamputated limb, or the part that connects the foot

	to the socket (transtibial) or knee unit (transfemoral). The shank includes the pylon and cosmetic cover of the endoskeletal and is the finished part of the exoskeletal.
Socket	Component into which the residual limb is inserted.
Static alignment	Placing the prosthetic components in proper relationship to each other in the standing position. The socket, knee component (if used), and foot are placed to duplicate the trochanter, knee, and ankle relationships of the nonamputated leg.
Voluntary knee control	Stance-phase stability of the transfemoral prosthesis that is controlled by the client's extension of the residual limb against the posterior wall of the socket.

References

1. Romo, HD: Specialized prostheses for activities: An update. Clinical Orthopaedics and Related Research 361:63–70, 1999.
2. Culham ET, Peat M, Newell E: Analysis of gait following below-knee amputation: A comparison of the SACH and single-axis foot. Physiother Can. 36:237–242, 1984.
3. Brouwer BJ, Allard P, Labelle H: Running patterns of juveniles wearing SACH and single-axis foot components. Arch Phys Med Rehabil. 70:128–134, 1989
4. Winter DA, Sienko SE: Biomechanics of below-knee amputee gait. J Biomechanics 21:361–367, 1988.
5. Fergason J: Prosthetic feet. In Lusardi MM, Nielsen CC: Orthotics and Prosthetics in Rehabilitation. Butterworth Heinemann, Boston, 2000.
6. Burgess, EM, et al: The Seattle prosthetic foot—A design for active sports: Preliminary studies. J Prosthetic Orthot 37:25–31, 1983.
7. Kapp, S, and Cummings, D: Transtibial amputations: Prosthetic management. In Bowker, JH, and Michael, JW (eds): Atlas of Limb Prosthetics: Surgical, Prosthetic, and Rehabilitation Principles. Mosby Yearbook, St. Louis, 1992.
8. Czerniecki, JM, et al: A comparison of the power generation/absorption characteristics. Arch Phys Med Rehabil 68:636, 1987.
9. Czerniecki, JM, and Gitter, A: Impact of energy-storing prosthetic feet on below-knee amputation gait (Abstract). Arch Phys Med Rehabil 71, 1990.
10. Macfarlane, PA, et al: Gait comparisons for below-knee amputees using a Flex-Foot versus a conventional prosthetic foot. J Prosthet Orthot 3: 150–61, 1991.
11. Wirta, RW, et al: Effect on gait using various prosthetic ankle-foot devices. J Rehabil Res Dev 28:13–24, 1991.
12. Childress, DS, and Knox, EH: Dynamic response prosthetic feet and their role in human ambulation. Paper presented at the 8th World Congress of the International Sociaety for Prosthetic and Orthotics, Melbourne, Australia, April 1995. Published on the World Wide Web.
13. White, H, et al: Bilateral kinematic and kinetic data of two prosthetic designs: A case study. J Prosthet Orthot 12(3):97–100, 2000.
14. (No author listed). Alpha Liner offers alternative roll-on suspension. American Prosthetic & Orthotic News 5(2), Fall 1999. (*www.oandp.com/facilities/ia/amp/fall99*)
15. Covey, SJ, et al: Flow constraint and loading rate effects on prosthetic liner material and human tissue mechanical response. J Prosthet Orthot 12:15–32, 2000.
16. Sabolich, J: Contoured adducted trochanteric-controlled alignment method (CAT-CAM): Introduction and basic principles. Clin Prosthet Onhot 9: 15–26, 1985.
17. Carroll, K: Personal communications. March 2001.
18. Pritham, CH: Biomechanics and shape of the above-knee socket considered in light of the ischial containment concept. Prosthet Orthot Int 14:9–21, 1990.
19. Haberman, LJ, et al: Silicone-only suspension (SOS) for the above-knee amputee. J Prosthet Orthot 4:76–85, 1992.
20. Valenti, TG: Experiences with Endoflex: A monolithic thermoplastic prosthesis for below-knee amputees. J Prosthet Orthot 3:43–50, 1991.

21. Schuch, CM: Prosthetic management. In Bowker, JH, and Michael, JW (eds): Atlas of Limb Prosthetics: Surgical, Prosthetic, and Rehabilitation Principles. Mosby Year Book, St. Louis, 1992.
22. Gottschalk, FA, et al: Does socket configuration influence the position of the femur in above-knee amputations? J Prosthet Orthot 2:94–102, 1990.
23. Schuch, CM, and Pritham, CH: Current transfemoral sockets. Clin Orthop 361:48–54, 1999.
24. Michael, JW: Modern prosthetic knee mechanisms. Clini Orthop 361:39–47, 1999.
25. Mooney, V, and Quigley, MJ: Above-knee amputations, section II, prosthetic management. In American Academy of Orthopedic Surgeons: Atlas of Limb Prosthetics. Mosby Year Book, St. Louis, 1981.
26. Jensen, JS, and Mandrup-Poulsen, T: Success rate of prosthetic fitting after major amputation of the lower limb. Prosthet Orthot Int 7:119–122, 1983.
27. Shurr, DG, et al: Hip disarticulation: A prosthetic follow-up. Orthot Prosthet 37:50–57, 1983.
28. van der Waarde, T, and Michael, JW: Prosthetic management. In Bowker, JH, and Michael, JW (eds): Atlas of Limb Prosthetics: Surgical, Prosthetic, and Rehabilitation Principles. Mosby Year Book, St. Louis, 1992.
29. Pritham, CH: Emerging trends in lower-limb prosthetics: Research and development. In Bowker, JH, and Michael, JW (eds): Atlas of Limb Prosthetics: Surgical, Prosthetic, and Rehabilitation Principles. Mosby Year Book, St. Louis, 1992.
30. Michael, JW, and Bowker, JH: Prosthetics/orthotics research for the twenty-first century: Summary of 1992 conference proceedings. J Prosthet Orthot 6:100–07, 1994.
31. Michael, J: John Michael's Corner. November 2000, *www.oandp.com*.

CHAPTER EIGHT

Lower Extremity Prosthetic Management

OBJECTIVES

At the end of this chapter, all students are expected to:

1 Describe the factors that mitigate against prosthetic fitting.
2 Describe major gait deviations that may be exhibited by individuals walking with a transtibial or transfemoral prosthesis.
3 Describe the critical components of the prosthetic training program.
4 Compare and contrast the training program for an individual with one or two transtibial prostheses.

In addition, physical therapy students are expected to:

1 Outline the steps in transtibial and transfemoral prosthetic evaluations.
2 Establish functional goals for an individual with a transfemoral or transtibial prosthesis.
3 Develop a plan of care for any individual with a transfemoral or transtibial prosthesis.

The first step in the prosthetic management of individuals with lower extremity amputations is to determine who is and is not a candidate for prosthetic fitting. The decision may be made by an amputee clinic team or an individual physician, or it may be initiated by a physical therapist (PT). The PT or physical therapist assistant (PTA) working in home health or a rehabilitation center is in a particularly good position to make a referral to a local clinic or to discuss prosthetic fitting with the surgeon.

Case Studies

Each of our clients has been referred to the amputee clinic for prosthetic evaluation today. Prior to clinic, each client is evaluated by a PT. The information is used by the clinic team in its decision making.

Diana Magnolia: It is now 12 weeks since her discharge from the hospital. Ms. Magnolia has been referred to the amputee clinic by the home health PT. See Figure 8.1 for the preclinic examination.

Ha Lee Davis: It is now 8 weeks since his surgery. He is wearing a removable postsurgical prosthetic socket with 10 ply of stump socks. This socket has a foot and pylon attached and can be removed for inspection of the residual limb. He is referred by the outpatient PT. See Figure 8.2 for his preclinic examination.

Benny Pearl: It is now 5 months since his discharge from the hospital. Following discharge he went to a rehabilitation center for 2 weeks and then went home. He has been referred to the amputee clinic by the vascular surgeon. See Figure 8.3 for his preclinic examination.

Betty Childs: Betty underwent a series of chemotherapy and radiation therapy treatments following surgery. She has now completed all **adjuvant therapy** and is referred to an amputee clinic at the request of the orthopedic surgeon who performed the amputation. It is 3 months since amputation. See Figure 8.4 for her preclinic examination.

■ *Case Study Activities*

Explore your beliefs about the statement, "Everyone is entitled to be fitted with a prosthesis." What conditions have to exist for a patient not to be a prosthetic candidate? What does the research literature reflect on long-term prosthetic use?

PROSTHETIC FITTING DECISIONS

No general rule can safely be applied to all clients when deciding to fit or not to fit the person with a prosthesis. The client is part of the decision-making process, but wanting a prosthesis is not sufficient. Many people are not aware of the physiological demands of prosthetic ambulation, particularly at transfemoral levels. The development of lightweight prostheses, stabilizing knee mechanisms, and hydraulic systems have made it possible to successfully fit more individuals than in the past; however, some consideration for not fitting is necessary.

Energy Expenditures

Individuals with transtibial amputations reach a higher level of function and use less energy for ambulation than individuals with transfemoral amputations.[1,2,3] Walking speed affects energy utilization: the faster one walks, the more energy one expends. Most individuals select a walking speed that maintains a comfortable level of oxygen consumption. Individuals with transtibial amputations are reported to expend significantly less energy when walking with a prosthesis at a self-selected speed than when walking on crutches without a prosthesis. The difference in energy expenditure for individuals using a transfemoral prosthesis or walking on crutches is not statistically significant.[4] Studies of energy expenditure between individuals using a transtibial or a transfemoral prosthesis vary if walking speed is client-selected or externally imposed. A comparison of a matched group of normal subjects and of individuals with a unilateral transfemoral prosthesis revealed no significant difference in oxygen consumption when the clients selected their own walking speed. However, the people with transfemoral prostheses walked at a

Interview: Patient stated she would like a "leg" so she can walk and "take care of her kids." Stated she was not sure she could go back to work. Stated she had gone on Medicaid when her ulcer had forced her to quit work.

Hx: As previously reported.

Tests and Measures:

Pain: Patient reports occasional burning pain in left (phantom) foot.

ROM:
        Left lower extremity:
                Active & passive knee flexion = 120 deg; extension = −10 deg;
                Active & passive hip flexion = 130 deg; active extension = −13 deg; passive =
                    −9 degrees
                Active & passive hip abduction/adduction and rotation: WNL
        Right lower extremity:
                Active ankle: dorsiflexion = +5 deg; passive = +10 def; active & passive plantar
                    flexion = 22 degrees
                Active & passive knee: flexion = 120 deg; extension = 0 deg
                Active & passive hip: flexion = 130 deg; active extension = −10 deg; passive =
                    −5 degrees

Muscle Strength:
        Left lower extremity:
                Knee flexion & extension: G−(4−/5)
                Hip: All musculature grossly good to good + range (4 to 4+/5)
        Right lower extremity:
                Ankle: dorsiflexion = G−(4−/5); plantar flexion = G+ (4+)
                Knee & hip grossly good + (4+/5)

Residual Limb:
        Residual limb length = 15.5 cm
        Circumferential measurement: L   R

	L	R
At tibial tubercle	13 3/4"	14"
1" below	13 1/8"	13 3/8"
2" below	12 7/8"	13 3/8"

        Appearance: Well-healed nonedematous residual limb, independent mobility skills and is
             ready for prosthetic fitting.

Vascular Status:
Right lower extremity: Toes are cool to touch, with severe clubbing of toe nails. Hairless throughout lower extremity. Patient has small beginning ulceration just behind the heel, which is being dressed by family and home health nurse. Decreased sensation to touch in right foot and ankle to malleoli, more pronounced on plantar surface of foot and over toes. Cannot consistently discern dull and sharp on plantar surface of foot and dorsum of toes.

ADL: Patient can ambulate independently in the parallel bars and with a walker. Reports being independent in self care and around the house except getting in and out of the bathtub. Needs assistance with cooking, cleaning and household activities.

Home Health Report: Therapist report confirms above measurements. Pt has been using the walker around the house and outside but complains of cramping in right lower extremity after about 90 feet. Patient's teenage son has been helping her wrap the residual limb over the shrinker since the residual limb has decreased in size. She verbalizes a desire and need for a prosthesis. Social services have been contacted regarding obtaining proper shoes and an individually designed shoe insert for the right foot.

*Examination results have been limited to key data only to conserve space. Some psychosocial and medical information was provided in previous chapters. Students may hypothesize congruent additional information if necessary.

FIGURE 8.1
Preclinic examination for Diana Magnolia.

Interview: Ha Lee stated that he has gone back to school; complains that he cannot work; states he wants to get a "real" leg now. Mr. Davis lives with his parent and two younger siblings. He is finishing his last year of high school and has private insurance under his family plan. He was working part time in a fast food restaurant and did not have specific vocational or educational plans prior to the accident. He has been referred to the Department of Vocational Rehabilitation for evaluation.

Hx: As previously reported.

Tests and Measures:

Pain: No report of specific pain; pt has phantom sensation, particularly at night.

Residual Limb:
　　　　Length: 18 cm; well-healed, nonsensitive, nonedematous
　　　　Circumference:
　　　　　　　Medial tibial plateau (MTP) level = 31 cm;
　　　　　　　 5 cm = 33 cm;
　　　　　　　10 cm = 33 cm;
　　　　　　　18 cm = 32 cm

ROM and muscle strength:
　　　　Right hip and knee within normal limits
　　　　Left lower extremity within normal limits
　　　　Right hand and wrist exhibit normal strength, ROM and function

ADL: Wearing a removable postoperative prosthesis with pylon and Flex Foot and 10 ply of stump socks. Walks with one forearm crutch because not allowed full weight bearing. Independent in all mobility activities with crutches and prosthesis.

*Examination results have been limited to key data only to conserve space. Some psychosocial and medical information was provided in previous chapters. Students may hypothesize congruent additional information if necessary.

FIGURE 8.2
Preclinic examination for Ha Lee Davis.

slower and less efficient speed.[5] Most studies of energy expenditure indicate that the higher the level of amputation, the greater the oxygen uptake values. It is summarized that individuals with a single transfemoral amputation use at least 49 percent more oxygen than someone without an amputation, and individuals with bilateral amputations use up to 280 percent more oxygen than individuals without an amputation. Additionally, individuals with amputations exhibit a decrease in walking speed and walking efficiency commensurate with the level of amputation.[6,7] Individuals with unilateral transfemoral amputations are more likely to stop using the prosthesis than individuals with unilateral transtibial amputations. Associated medical problems such as coronary artery disease and hypertension, limited premorbid function, and level of amputation have the most influence on long-term outcomes.[8,9] It may be helpful to remember that the higher the level of amputation, the heavier the prosthesis and the more artificial joints the person must control to achieve a smooth, energy-efficient gait.

Transtibial Levels

Most individuals with transtibial amputations can be fitted with a prosthesis. Flexion contractures, scars, poorly shaped residual limbs, and adherent skin are not necessarily contraindications, even though such problems create diffi-

Interview: Mr. Pearl states that he would like to be able to walk; the family states that he needs a leg to be able to get around. They indicate that he spends most of his time in the wheelchair. He complains that his stump just aches all over.

Mr. Pearl presents as a somewhat obese individual, dependent on family for his care other than self-care. He is on Medicare with a supplemental insurance.

Tests & Measures:

Pain: Pt reports nonspecific residual limb pain of 3 on 10-pt scale. Reports phantom sensation with occasional cramping pain in right foot.

ROM:
    Right hip (Active):
        Flexion = 125 deg; active extension = -17 degrees;
        Abduction: = 25 deg; adduction = 5 degrees

    Right hip (Passive)
        Flexion = 140 deg; extension = -12 degrees
        Abduction = 25 deg; adduction = 5 degrees

    Left Lower Extremity
        Active & passive hip flexion = 125 deg; active hip ext = -14 deg; pass = -9 deg
        Abduction, adduction, and rotation within functional limits
        Active & passive knee flexion = 135 deg; extension -5 deg
        Active ankle dorsiflexion = 4 deg; passive = 9 deg; active & passive plantar flexion = 28 deg

    Muscle Strength
        Right hip: flexion: G+ (4+/5); extension: F (3/5) (measured sidelying; cannot get prone)
          Abduction = G+ (4+/5); adduction = G+ (4+/5)

        Left Lower Extremity:
          Ankle dorsiflexion = G (4/5); plantar flexion = G+ (4+/5 NWB)
          Knee extension = G+ (4+/5); flexion (sidelying) = G+ (4+/5)
          Hip flexion = N (5/5); extension (sidelying) = F+ (3+/5)
          Hip abduction = G (4); hip adduction = G (4)

Residual Limb: Residual limb is well healed but still slightly edematous with no change in measurements for the past 3 weeks. No specific areas of tenderness. Patient had some difficulty with wrapping and was fitted with transfemoral shrinker, which he states he wears all the time.

Vascular Status: Left lower extremity is hairless below the knee with evidence of dysvascularity in the foot. It is relatively thin with evident dryness of skin. Patient states it will swell when he sits all day; occasionally wears an elastic stocking on the leg. He complains of some night cramping. He states he occasionally has some cramping if he stands or walks too much. No evidence of ulcerations. Sensation appears present throughout, and Mr. Pearl can differentiate sharp and dull on foot.

Functional Status: Mr. Pearl is independent in all wheelchair transfer activities; generally uses a wheelchair at home except that he uses the walker to go to the bathroom. He is independent in all self care except for bathing, as he cannot get into the bathtub.
    Mr. Pearl is able to ambulate independently in the parallel bars and can use a walker within the department with contact guard.

*Examination results have been limited to key data only to conserve space. Some psychosocial and medical information was provided in previous chapters. Students may hypothesize congruent additional information if necessary.

FIGURE 8.3
Preclinic examination for Benny Pearl.

culty with socket fit and prosthetic **alignment.** Circulatory problems in the nonamputated extremity, unless so severe as to preclude ambulation, are indications for fitting at the earliest possible time because bipedal ambulation reduces stress on the remaining extremity. Additionally, the individual who has learned to ambulate with one prosthesis is more likely to be able to ambulate with two. There are few contraindications to fitting someone with a prosthesis after a transtibial amputation other than contraindications to ambulation itself. Individuals who were nonambulatory prior to surgery for rea-

Interview: Betty indicated that she was glad to be finished with chemotherapy. "It made me so weak." Betty stated she stopped wearing the shrinker in the past 2 weeks since she lost weight and it did not fit well. Betty has continued to attend school sporadically since her amputation. She received home teaching services when necessary and returned to school on a full-time basis last week. She lives with her family and has some coverage from her family insurance, but they are not sure it will pay for a prosthesis. She and her family are anxious for her to get a prosthesis and return to a normal life. Prior to her amputation, Betty was a reasonably active individual although she was not particularly involved in sports activities.

Tests & Measures:

Pain: Betty does not report any specific pain other than phantom sensation on occasion.

Residual Limb: Well-healed, conical, no edema.
　　　Length from greater trochanter to end of limb = 32 cm
　　　Circumference:
　　　　　At ischial level = 40 cm
　　　　　　5 cm = 38 cm
　　　　　　8 cm = 29 cm
　　　　　　13 cm = 26 cm
　　　　　　28 cm = 26 cm

Strength: Gross muscle strength right hip is within normal limits; gross muscle strength of the left lower extremity appears well within normal limits.

ROM: Active ROM normal in all ranges of both legs except active and passive right hip extension prone is possible only to about 5 degrees.

ADL: Independent on crutches in all ambulation, elevation and self-care activities.

*Examination results have been limited to key data only to conserve space. Some psychosocial and medical information was provided in previous chapters. Students may hypothesize congruent additional information if necessary.

FIGURE 8.4
Preclinic examination for Betty Childs.

sons other than the problems leading to the amputation will probably not be ambulatory after an amputation. However, individuals who were nonambulatory and debilitated because of infection, loss of diabetic control, and ulcers may well regain the necessary strength and coordination for ambulation after the diseased limb has been removed. The increased energy requirements of ambulating with two prostheses may preclude fitting individuals with cardiac disease and limited respiratory reserves. Generally, individuals requiring nursing or custodial care will not be able to use a prosthesis; often, equipment sent to a nursing home becomes lost, and fitting such individuals may be a waste of limited resources.

Transfemoral Levels

Many people with a unilateral transfemoral amputation can become functional prosthetic users with or without external support. The physiological demands of walking with a transfemoral prosthesis are considerably higher than walking with a transtibial prosthesis, and not all individuals have the necessary balance, strength, and energy reserves. The transfemoral prosthesis is heavier than the transtibial, and control of the artificial knee joint requires considerable balance and coordination. Severe hip flexion contractures, weakness or paralysis of hip musculature, poor balance and coordination, or severe organic brain syndrome may mitigate against successful ambulation. The person's level of activity and participation in the postsurgical program help determine potential for prosthetic ambulation. The individual who is willing to learn to ambulate on the remaining extremity and shows the ability to expend the necessary energy to participate in an active postsurgical program is a candidate for fitting. However, an individual content to sit in a wheelchair except during scheduled therapy sessions probably will not become a successful prosthetic user. A temporary prosthesis is a good assessment tool, although cost must be considered. Family may demand that their family member be fitted, hoping that prosthetic replacement will make caregiving easier. Unfortunately, family motivation does not translate into patient motivation. The PT must ascertain the patient's motivation to expend the necessary level of energy to use a transfemoral prosthesis.

Most individuals amputated at hip level are young and learn to use a prosthesis relatively easily. Although early fitting is physically and psychologically beneficial, active involvement in chemotherapy or radiation therapy may delay fitting. Radiation therapy often burns the skin, making fitting impossible until the skin has healed. Clients undergoing chemotherapy are often ill, lose weight, and may not have the stamina to participate in a prosthetic training program. The postsurgical program is individually adjusted and supportive until chemotherapy is complete. If the person has lost considerable weight, fitting will have to be delayed because it is difficult to adjust the prosthesis for the eventual increases in weight.

Individuals with Bilateral Amputations

Fitting or not fitting someone with bilateral amputations is a difficult decision. Individuals with good balance and coordination are generally good candidates for prosthetic fitting. Most people with bilateral transtibial amputations can become quite functional with prostheses. Essentially, the same criteria are applied as with someone with one amputation although greater energy expenditure is necessary for ambulation with two transtibial prostheses. Individuals with bilateral transtibial amputations reach a higher level of independent function than individuals with one transfemoral and one transtibial amputation or individuals with bilateral transfemoral amputations.[3,10,11]

Ambulation with one transfemoral and one transtibial prosthesis takes considerably more energy than ambulation with bilateral transtibial prostheses. Individuals with transfemoral and transtibial amputations have a better chance of becoming ambulatory if the first amputation was at the transfemoral level, and if the person successfully used a transfemoral prosthesis before losing the other leg. Most older individuals with two transfemoral amputations do not become successful prosthetic wearers because of the energy and balance requirements. The person who has lost both lower extremities needs more strength, better coordination, better balance, and greater cardiorespiratory reserves than the person who has lost one lower extremity. The decision to fit or not to fit is made after careful individual evaluation of the person's total potential and needs. The person's level and extent of participation in the postsurgical exercise program is a critical source of information; however, the ability to move independently without prostheses on a mat table does not translate into being able to use two transfemoral prostheses or even one transfemoral and one transtibial prosthesis. The best evaluation is the use of temporary prostheses or even training prostheses that have a hinged knee mechanism.

Factors Affecting Prosthetic Wear

Residual limb problems delay prosthetic rehabilitation. Skin problems, such as dermatitis, **furuncles,** cysts, and infections, usually require avoidance of the prosthesis, care in skin hygiene, and, occasionally, medication. Soap residue left on the skin can become an irritant, and the client must be taught to rinse the residual limb, socks, socket, and liner well after washing.

Clients with vascular disease must be alert to pressure on the residual limb from the prosthetic socket. Necrosis of distal tissue can occur even after wound healing. Individuals with diabetes who may have decreased sensation need to learn to carefully inspect the residual limb after each wearing to note any areas of redness or pressure. If some of the skin around the incision adheres to the distal end of the bone, the forces created by prosthetic wear may cause pain or abrasions and even open sores. Occasionally, skin grafts necessary for healing in some traumatic amputations may adhere to distal bone, may be insensitive, and may be the source of prosthetic pain or abrasions. Although care must be taken during the healing period to prevent adhesions by careful massage and movement of the skin around the bone, not all can be avoided. Modern gel liners and socks and the more intimate fit of the prosthetic socket make fitting such residual limbs easier; the patient must be aware of the greater risk for skin breakdowns.

Occasionally, an individual wearing a gel liner with a shuttlelock system may complain of pain distally and may develop a small bursa or bruised area distally. The gel liner adheres to the skin aiding in suspension, but the prosthesis pulls away from the limb a small amount on every swing phase. That pulling action may create a milking effect of superficial issue on subcutaneous tissue, particularly in individuals who have somewhat fleshy residual limbs. Although the problem does not occur frequently, the therapist must be alert to complaints of pulling or pain distally. In those instances, another type of suspension is indicated. Occasionally, bone spurs develop, causing excessive pressure on the overlying skin. Children are subject to problems created by bone growth through the skin at the end of the residual limb (see Chap. 11).

Pain, from whatever source, is the single biggest deterrent to prosthetic wear and the major issue of patients with amputations. In a survey of 114 individuals with lower extremity amputations, issues related to the fit of the socket were a primary concern of respondents.[12] In another study of 148 individuals who responded to a questionnaire, the presence or absence of pain in the residual limb was the most important of the factors affecting perception of the results of amputations. Other factors included the condition of the contralateral limb, the comfort and function of the prostheses, and social issues.[13] Pain may be from physiological or psychogenic origins and often encompasses elements of both. Chronic pain is difficult to treat. A painful phantom can be extremely resistant to treatment, as discussed in Chapter 5. In a recent study, 74 percent of respondents reported some pain in the residual limb or other body areas, and 72 percent reported having had some phantom pain; the majority indicated that the pain was episodic and of low disability.[14]

A neuroma is a natural sequellae of the transection of a nerve. The size and location of the neuroma is the critical issue; if small and situated in soft-tissue well above the distal end of the residual limb, it will usually not interfere with prosthetic wear. Large superficial neuromas may be compressed between the socket wall and the bone and cause pain. Sometimes, relieving the socket wall at the site of the neuroma resolves the problem. Injecting the neuroma with an analgesic or steroid formula may be necessary, and, because the relief is only temporary, may need to be repeated several times. In more stubborn instances, surgery to excise the neuroma may be indicated. Centrocentral anastomosis or inserting a nerve graft at the neuroma in an end-to-end connection has been reported to eliminate neuroma pain in a small sample of clients.[15] The use of ice or electrotherapy measures has been successful on occasion and should be tried first.

Pain during or following wearing of the prosthesis may be due to a problem with the prosthetic socket. Minor impingement of the socket in areas of superficial tendons or excessive soft tissue may only cause problems after prolonged wearing. Careful inspection of the stump-socket interface is necessary to make sure that the pain is not due to changes in socket pressure, excessive socket pressure in one area, or from changes in residual limb size or overall weight.

THE PROSTHETIC EVALUATION

The first step in prosthetic management is to make sure that the prosthesis fits properly and that it is as prescribed by the clinic team. Figures 8.5 and 8.6 depict forms that may be used to evaluate the prosthesis. If the client is a new prosthetic wearer, only the initial parts of the evaluation are performed; evaluation of gait is delayed until the person has learned to walk with a consistent gait pattern. Gait deviations are explored later in this chapter.

The evaluation is designed to ensure that the prosthesis fits appropriately and that the wearer has adequate stability and is satisfied with the device. In many clinics, the prosthetist initially delivers the appliance on the alignment instrument. Beginning evaluation and training are performed while the prosthesis is easily adjustable. It takes time for the person and the residual limb to adjust to the prosthesis. Once optimal alignment and fit have been obtained, the prosthesis can be finished. Although alignment changes are easier with endoskeletal limbs, it is still a good practice to have the prosthesis initially unfinished. When the prosthesis is delivered directly to the client without review by a clinic team, the prosthetist may finish the limb, making alignment changes difficult, particularly with exoskeletal limbs. Whenever possible, the therapist needs to ensure that initial evaluation and training are performed while the limb is still unfinished. Although the prosthetist performs a static and dynamic alignment prior to delivering the prosthesis, an integrated plan of prosthetic evaluation and gait training usually results in the optimum fit.

■ *Case Study Activity*

Individually or in groups, review each item in the transfemoral and transtibial evaluation forms, preferably those involving a prosthesis.

1. Is the prosthesis as prescribed?

2. If fitted with a shuttlelock system, does the lock and release pin operate smoothly and easily?

3. If fitted with suction sleeve, does the mechanism operate properly?

Standing:

4. Does the client have any pain or discomfort when bearing weight in the prosthesis?

5. Is the knee stable? Does the patient have to resist to prevent the knee from being forced into flexion or extension?

6. Is the pelvis level when weight is borne equally on both feet?

7. Is the pylon vertical when weight is borne evenly on both feet?

8. Does the sole of the shoe maintain even contact with the floor?

9. Are tissue rolls around the trim line of the socket excessive?

10. Is there any gapping at the brim of the socket?

11. Is there evidence of total contact?

12. If wearing a gel liner, does it fit properly and smoothly?

13. Is suspension maintained as the foot is lifted off the floor?

14. If using a sleeve suspension, does the sleeve extend over the limb socks?

Sitting:

15. Is the person comfortable while sitting with the sole of the shoe flat on the floor?

16. Is there adequate flaring of the posterior trim line to accommodate the hamstring tendons?

17. Are the tissue rolls in the popliteal area excessive?

18. Is the residual limb forced out of the socket excessively?

19. Can the patient sit comfortably with knees flexed to at least 90 degrees without excessive pressure on knees?

20. Are the knees level?

21. Are the color and contour of the prosthesis similar to the sound leg?

Walking:

22. Is the gait satisfactory? If the gait is not satisfactory, check the deviations.

At Heel Contact:

Ball of foot more than one inch from the floor
Knee extended   Unequal stride length

From Heel Contact to Foot Flat:

Knee flexes jerkily   Knee flexes abruptly
Maintains knee extension

(continued)

FIGURE 8.5
Transtibial prosthetic checkout.

At Midstance:

Lateral trunk bending exceeds 5 cm

Lateral displacement of socket exceeds 1/2 inch

Shoe not flat on the floor

No lateral or medial socket displacement

Midstance to Heel Rise:

Drop off

Prosthesis drops away from stance

Knee flexes jerkily

At Heel Rise:

Knee goes into extension

During Swing Phase:

Vaulting

Circumduction

Toe drags on floor

Check with Prosthesis Off:

23.   Is the skin free of any abrasions, blisters or excessive redness or areas of pressure?

24.   Is there any discoloration or discomfort?

FIGURE 8.5 (CONTINUED)

Explain why each item is important, and discuss the effect on the client if the item does not meet standards. Be as specific as you can; pain is not an adequate answer—rather state where the pain would be felt and how it would affect function.

TRANSTIBIAL EVALUATION

Before any gait training can be instituted, the fit of the prosthesis must be evaluated. Areas to be examined include socket fit, suspension, comfort, leg length, and static alignment (Fig. 8.7). Table 8.1 depicts the key items of evaluation in the transtibial prosthesis and possible problems that may occur with misalignment. Contemporary fabrication methods, especially computer-generated sockets fabricated from digital measurement of the residual limb, reduce static alignment problems. The fabrication process usually also includes check sockets that further improve accuracy of fit. However, it is critical to check for socket comfort, initial socket flexion, **total contact,** and proper height prior to initiating gait training. If the prosthesis is not comfortable, the client will not be able to learn a smooth, step-over-step gait. Pressure areas may also lead to skin breakdowns that can jeopardize the status of the residual limb.

The Knee in Normal Gait

In each cycle of normal gait, the knee flexes and extends twice. Just before heel contact, the knee is extended or nearly so; it flexes to about 15 degrees at

Check Prosthesis before Donning:

1.   Is the prosthesis as prescribed?

2.   Is the inside of the socket smoothly finished?

3.   Do all joints move freely and smoothly?

Comments on items 1–3:

Sitting:

4.   Is the socket securely on the residual limb?

5.   Does the length of the shin and thigh correspond to the shin and thigh of the unamputated leg?

6.   Can the client sit comfortably without burning or pinching?

7.   Is the client able to lean forward and reach her/his shoes?

Comments on items 4–7:

Standing:

8.   Does the socket fit properly and comfortably?

9.   Is the knee stable when weight is placed on the prosthesis?

10.   Is the pelvis level when weight is borne evenly on both legs?

11.   Is the client bearing weight properly for the type of socket?

12.   Does the socket maintain good contact with the residual limb on all sides as the client shifts his weight?

13.   Is there an adductor roll?

14.   Is there pressure on the pubic ramus?

Comments on items 9–15:

Walking:

15.   Is suspension maintained during swing phase?

16.   Is the socket stable against the lateral shift of the residual limb?

17.   Is there optimum swing-phase control?

18.   Is level walking free of gait deviations? If not, check the deviation observed.

Heel Contact to Foot Flat:

Forceful heel strike   Knee instability
Excessive external rotation of prosthesis

Midstance:

Lateral trunk bending toward prosthetic side   Abducted gait
Lateral gapping of socket

FIGURE 8.6
Transfemoral prosthetic checkout.

Midstance to Toe Off:

Premature heel rise   Pelvic rise (climbing a hill)
Drop off: delayed swing
Excessive lumbar lordosis

Swing Phase:

Circumducted gait
Lateral heel whip   Medial heel whip
Terminal swing impact   Lack of knee flexion
Excessive heel rise

Comment on gait

After Ambulation:

19.   Prosthesis can be removed easily?

20.   Residual limb is free of any abrasions or red areas.

FIGURE 8.6 (CONTINUED)

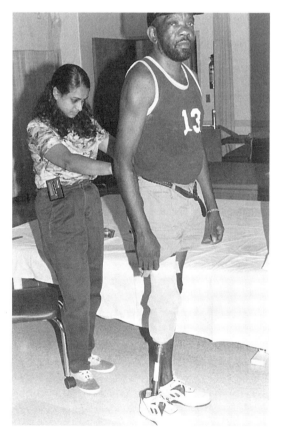

FIGURE 8.7

Checking the length of the prosthesis by
checking for a level pelvis.

TABLE 8.1   STATIC TRANSTIBIAL PROSTHETIC CHECKOUT

Checkout Item	What to Check	Possible Problem
Sitting		
Is the person comfortable while sitting with the sole of the shoe flat on the floor?	Check for excessive pressure between residual limb and socket.	Excessive pressure can lead to skin abrasions.
Is there adequate flaring of the posterior trim line to accommodate the hamstring tendons?	Check for pressure on the hamstrings when sitting.	Client will keep leg outstretched when sitting to reduce pressure.
Are the tissue rolls in the popliteal area excessive?	Check the posterior wall of the socket.	Too much tissue may indicate inadequate AP dimensions.
Is the residual limb forced out of the socket excessively?	The stump will rise out of the socket a little when sitting.	May indicate a socket that is too small or the client is wearing too many socks.
Can the patient sit comfortably with knees flexed to at least 90 degrees without excessive pressure on knees?	The residual limb tends to move up a little when person sits; sleeve or liner need to stretch adequately to prevent excessive pressure.	May push residual limb to bottom or front of socket excessively; client will keep leg outstretched to reduce pressure.
Does the cuff suspension, if worn, tend to loosen when the amputee sits?	The cuff suspension should loosen slightly when sitting.	Too tight or loose a cuff will lead to inadequate suspension.
Are the knees level?	The length of the shank should correspond to the other side.	May lead to gait deviations.
Are the color and contour of the prosthesis similar to the sound leg?	The finished prosthesis should match the other leg.	Poor cosmesis may lead to nonwearing.
Standing		
Does the client have any pain or discomfort when bearing weight on the prosthesis?	Check limb/socket interface particularly bony prominances.	Excessive pressures can lead to skin problems.
Is the knee stable? Does the patient have to resist to prevent the knee from being forced into flexion or extension?	PTB socket aligned in 5–8 degree of flexion.	Too much flexion will lead to counterknee extension and anterior distal pressure. Too little flexion can lead to end bearing.
Is the pelvis level when the amputee bears his weight equally on both feet?	Palpate the iliac crests with client standing evenly on both feet.	A long or short prosthesis will lead to gait deviations.
Is the pylon vertical when weight is borne on the prosthesis?	On weight bearing check the pylon connecting the socket and foot.	See medial- and lateral-leaning pylons on gait deviations.
Does the sole of the shoe maintain even contact with the floor?	Check that the foot is fully on the floor on weight bearing.	May lead to excessive knee pressures on gait.
Are tissue rolls around the trim line of the socket or the cuff suspension minimal?	Check the edges of the stump at the socket line.	Excessive rolls may indicate a socket that is too tight proximally.
Is there gapping at the brim of the socket?	Check the edges of the stump at the socket line.	Gapping may indicate a socket that is too large proximally.
Is there evidence of total contact?	Put a little ball of playdough at the end of the socket and then have the client bear weight. The displacement of the playdough indicates the extent of total contact.	Too little contact can cause distal end skin problems and a stretching pain. Too much can cause excessive pressure at the end of the stump and pressure pain.
If wearing a gel liner, does it fit properly and smoothly?	The liner should be smooth, free of wrinkles, worn areas, or holes.	Gel liners have a limited life span; wrinkles, holes, or worn areas create skin abrasions.
Is suspension maintained when clients lifts leg off the floor?	Check that there is not excessive movement of the prosthesis away from limb when weight is removed. On weight bearing, make a small pencil mark at the anterior socket brim, or if sleeve or shuttle lock suspension, place a finger lightly at edge of socket.	Too much movement between residual limb and socket creates abrasions and can lead to toe drag on swing.
Does the sleeve extend over residual limb socks (if worn)?	The sleeve should be in direct contact with the skin for at least 2 in above any socks.	Failure to have skin to sleeve contact will lead to loss of suspension and pistoning.

midstance extending back to neutral or 5 degrees of flexion by terminal stance. The knee flexes again in early swing, then extends in terminal swing prior to the next heel contact. From heel contact to midstance, the quadriceps are active to decrease and control knee flexion whereas the hamstring muscles are quiet. Quadriceps action reaches its peak about midstance. Knee flexion in swing occurs mostly from momentum, and the hamstrings function mainly to decelerate hip flexion and prevent knee hyperextension in terminal swing.[16]

Socket Evaluation

The PTB socket is aligned in 5 to 8 degrees of knee flexion to allow for better weight bearing on the patella tendon and to simulate normal gait. Excessive socket flexion creates knee instability; the client extends the knee to counteract the instability and drives the anterior distal end of the tibia that is close to the skin against the wall of the socket, causing pain and possible abrasion (Fig. 8.8). Insufficient socket flexion reduces the weight-bearing potential of the patellar tendon and medial tibial flares, causing the residual limb to press too hard on the bottom of the socket. Insufficient socket flexion can also decrease the effectiveness of quadriceps motion.

Total contact provides for good kinesthetic feedback during ambulation and enhances venous return at the distal end of the residual limb. A space left between the end of the residuum and the socket may lead to the skin becoming callused and rough. Lack of total contact can also lead to distal edema. The intimate fit of modern prostheses, particularly those incorporating gel liners and either suction or shuttlelock suspension, reduces problems with lack of total contact. However, problems can be created if the patient does not put the liner and prosthesis on properly.

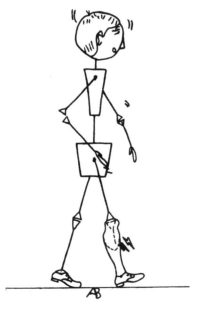

FIGURE 8.8

Heel contact to foot flat: extension force on knee creating anterior distal pressure. (Artist: Angie Britt)

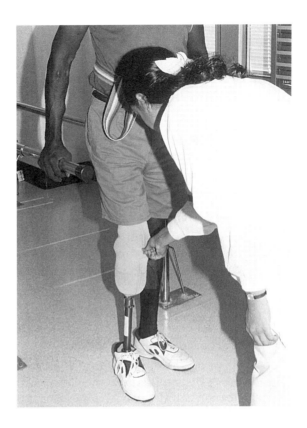

FIGURE 8.9
Checking for pistoning with sleeve
suspension.

The prosthesis must be held firmly on the residual limb by the suspension mechanism. Suspension is not a major problem with shuttlelock and suction suspension mechanisms but may occur with sleeve or supracondylar cuff suspension. Proper suspension is checked with the client standing. If the client is wearing other than sleeve suspension, a light pencil mark is made on the sock at the level of the anterior brim. The client is then asked to lift the prosthesis straight off the ground without bending the knee. The prosthesis should not drop down more than about 1 cm. If the client is wearing a sleeve suspension, the therapist can place a finger at the anterior brim and have the client perform the same movement (Fig. 8.9). Any drop can be palpated.

The foot should be flat on the floor with the body weight evenly distributed between the heel and toe of the prosthetic foot when the client is standing erect with weight equally on both feet. If the prosthesis is on the alignment instrument, the pylon connecting the foot to the socket should be perpendicular to the floor when the feet are a comfortable distance apart. The pylon will not be perpendicular if the client is bearing more weight on the unamputated leg.

TRANSTIBIAL GAIT ANALYSIS

Normal Prosthetic Gait

Gait analysis is best done when viewing the client walking both from an anteroposterior (AP) and a lateral (prosthetic side) point of reference. The therapist needs to obtain an overall impression of the gait and then focus on each part of the body individually to ensure a thorough analysis.

The client with a transtibial amputation walking with a well-fitting and well-aligned prosthesis exhibits a smooth, step-over-step pattern, with little trunk sway and with symmetrical arm movements. The gait requires a minimum amount of energy.

Heel Contact, Lateral View

The knee is slightly flexed, and the ball of the prosthetic foot is no more than 4 cm from the floor. The pelvis and trunk are erect, with the body weight transferring from the intact to the prosthetic leg.

Heel Contact to Foot Flat, Lateral View

Progressing toward foot flat, the knee flexes smoothly 10 to 15 degrees as the foot comes gently to the floor. The heel of the prosthetic foot may be seen to compress 1.5 to 2 cm, depending on the person's weight and type of foot. This compression is not as evident with the Flex or similar foot, but the progression through the stance cycle must be smooth. The trunk remains balanced over the point of support.

Midstance, AP View

At midstance the client bears full weight on the prosthesis. The pelvis and upper body remain balanced over the prosthesis with no more than 2.5 cm of head or trunk sway toward the prosthetic side. The overall gait base is no more than 5 cm wide. There is minimum lateral socket displacement. On the alignment instrument, the pylon is perpendicular to the floor. The foot is flat on the floor.

Midstance, Lateral View

The prosthetic foot is flat on the floor; the knee is flexed 10 to 15 degrees and stable.

Midstance to Toe Off, Lateral and AP Views

Weight progresses smoothly from the amputated to the intact side with little head, trunk, or pelvic sway or drop. The knee flexes smoothly, and there is no more than 5 cm between the two feet.

Swing Phase, Lateral View

The knee flexes easily and allows the toe to clear the floor. The socket remains securely on the residual limb. Step length is the same on each side.

Swing Phase, AP View

The shank and foot swing in the line of progression, and the pelvis remains level.

Transtibial Gait Deviations

Gait deviations may be due to an improperly fitting socket, a poorly aligned prosthesis, a painful residual limb, or poor walking habits. Gait deviations increase energy consumption, can cause discomfort in the residual limb, and limit functional use of the prosthesis. It is desirable to identify gait deviations as early as possible so they can be remedied before problems become permanent. A client wearing a prosthesis with a supracondylar cuff may exhibit a slight lateral thrust of the proximal brim of the socket during midstance; however, this is usually not seen with other forms of suspension unless the residual limb is quite short. Lateral thrust is the result of the adduction of the femur and the slight valgus position of the normal knee. Normal floor reaction forces create a slight varus movement of the knee at midstance. As long as the movement is slight and does not affect comfort or stability, it is considered normal. It is also not seen with individuals wearing closed patella-tendon supracondylar suprapatellar (PTSCSP) prostheses.

Heel Contact to Foot Flat

Excessive Knee Extension

In the normal gait pattern, the knee flexes smoothly 8 to 12 degrees from heel contact to midstance. Flexion reduces the excursion of the body's center of gravity, allows for absorption of the floor reaction forces generated at heel strike through the joints of the lower limb, and reduces the amount of energy required in gait. Keeping the knee extended increases the amount of energy expended in walking; the deviation can best be seen from the side by observing the prosthetic knee from weight acceptance to midstance (Fig 8.8). The client reports a sense of walking uphill. Maintaining an extended knee with a socket aligned in flexion may lead to anterior distal pain and skin abrasion. Extension also increases pelvic displacement; it may look as if the prosthesis is too long.

The two major prosthetic causes of excessive knee extension are a **toe lever arm** that is too long and a heel support that is too soft. The two deviations can be differentiated from each other by watching the heel-from-heel contact to midstance. Knee extension may also be the result of inadequate gait training or weakness of the quadriceps.

1. **Too Soft Heel Support.** A heel wedge or plantar flexion bumper that is too soft for the client's weight will allow the prosthetic foot to plantar flex too fast. This premature contact of the foot with the floor tends to keep the knee in extension rather than allow normal rolling over the foot.

2. **Too Long Toe Lever Arm (Posterior Displacement of the Socket over the Foot).** Posterior displacement of the socket (Fig. 8.10) brings the center of gravity line posterior, thereby increasing the length of the anterior segment or toe lever arm. If the foot is set too far anterior under the socket, the length of the toe lever arm is increased and that of the heel level arm decreased. As the client progresses from heel contact to foot flat, the center of gravity very quickly moves anterior to the axis of rotation of the knee, forcing the knee into hyperextension. The client feels as if he is walking up a hill as the length of the anterior support component is increased.

Other possible causes include:

1. **Shoe with a Lower Heel.** In normal walking, contact of the sole of the foot with the floor coincides approximately with the end of knee flexion and the beginning of knee extension. If the prosthetic foot is in an attitude of excessive plantar flexion, foot flat will occur prematurely, preventing normal knee flexion after heel strike.

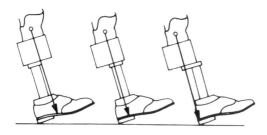

POSTERIOR SOCKET DISPLACEMENT

FIGURE 8.10

An overlong toe lever arm is caused by placement of the socket too far posterior on the foot. The first placement is correct. The other two are different degrees of incorrect placement.

2. **Weakness of the Quadriceps.** If the quadriceps are not strong enough to control the knee at heel strike, the client may compensate in much the same way as he would with anterodistal discomfort. These gait maneuvers tend to force the knee into extension and thereby lessen or eliminate the need for quadriceps activity.

3. **Habit.** Individuals who have established a pattern of walking with the knee held in extension after heel strike may continue to walk in the same manner when they are making the transition to a new transtibial prosthesis. Usually, a brief period of instruction with early follow-up will suffice to establish a satisfactory walking pattern.

Knee Instability

Knee stability is critically important to a smooth, energy-efficient gait. A client who does not feel stable and fears the knee will buckle will be loath to trust the limb. Knee instability can be seen at initial or terminal stance depending on the prosthetic cause (Fig. 8.11). Two major prosthetic causes of knee instability are a toe lever arm that is too short and a heel support that is too long. The short toe lever arm is described under terminal stance.

1. **Too Long Heel Support; Dorsiflexed Foot, Higher-Heel Shoe.** The compressibility of the prosthetic foot, the density of the plantar flexion bumper, or the rigidity of the dynamic response foot is determined by the size, weight, and activity level of the client. If the foot characteristics do not match the patient, the necessary amount of plantar flexion and shock absorption will not take place, and the knee on the prosthetic side will be forced into excessive flexion from heel contact to midstance. Knee instability and buckling may result. The client may try to maintain knee stability by extending the knee against the flexing forces, thereby creating excessive pressure at the anterior distal end of the residual limb and, possibly, the posterior proximal brim of the socket. Excessive anterior distal pressure can lead to abrasions and skin breakdowns because the distal end of the tibia is quite close to the socket wall.

Midstance

Excessive Rising or Dropping of the Hip on the Prosthetic Side

1. **Too Long Prosthesis.** If the prosthetic leg is longer than the sound leg, the client will raise the center of gravity over the support joint during stance phase. The deviation can best be seen from the rear by watching the prosthetic hip and shoulder during midstance. The client may also have diffi-

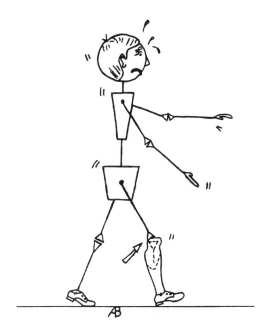

FIGURE 8.11
Heel contact to foot flat: knee instability.
(Artist: Angie Britt)

culty bringing the prosthetic leg forward in swing and will either bend the knee excessively or raise the body up on the toe of the sound leg to allow room to clear the prosthetic foot. The latter deviation is called vaulting.

2. **Too Short Prosthesis.** If the prosthetic leg is shorter than the sound leg, the person will seem to be walking in a hole on the prosthetic side (Fig 8.12). The hip and shoulder on the amputated side drop at the beginning of stance phase. The deviation can best be observed from the rear by watching the hip and shoulder at midstance. Some individuals prefer the prosthetic leg to be just slightly shorter than the sound leg, especially those who have had discrepancy in leg lengths for their whole lives. Although ideally the legs should be the same lengths, comfort and function must be the guide in determining appropriate length alignment. This deviation is sometimes confused with "drop off" that occurs at terminal stance. In drop off, the prosthetic knee may have a tendency to buckle; this buckling usually does not occur with a prosthesis that is too short.

Wide-Based Gait

If the base of support is moved laterally, support is lost medially during single foot stance (Fig. 8.13). The client attempts to move the pelvis laterally to reach the support point and exhibits a wide-based gait with the hips and the shoulders dropping laterally during stance phase. Excess pressure will be felt at the proximal lateral brim of the socket and the medial distal end of the residual limb. Two prosthetic causes of wide-based gait are an outset foot and a medial leaning pylon. Both deviations can best be seen in the front or rear view, particularly evident in the movements of the trunk and shoulders in stance. The outset foot can be differentiated from the medial leaning pylon by looking at the pylon at midstance. The gait deviation may sometimes be noted if the person does not shift the weight properly over the prosthesis on stance. This training problem can be differentiated from a prosthetic

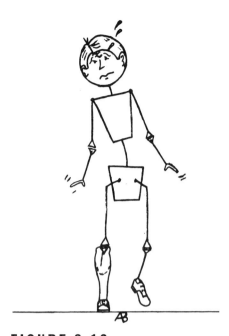

FIGURE 8.12
Midstance: prothesis too short. (Artist: Angie Britt)

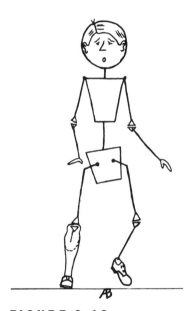

FIGURE 8.13
Midstance: wide-based gait. (Artist: Angie Britt)

problem by looking at the pylon at midstance and noting the width of the gait base.

1. **Outset Foot.** Dynamically, the foot is usually set 1 cm medial to a line from the center of the posterior wall to the floor. If the foot is set too far lateral to the line, the client will lose support medially during stance. The sole of the shoe usually remains flat on the floor when the foot is outset.
2. **Medial-Leaning Pylon.** Proper dynamic alignment places the pylon perpendicular at midstance. If the top of the pylon is medial to the bottom (Fig. 8.14), the pylon is said to lean medially. The client exhibits a wide-based gait and seems to lose support medially as in an outset foot, but if the problem is a medial-leaning pylon, the foot will have more pressure on the medial side.

Narrow-Based Gait and Excessive Lateral Thrust of the Prosthesis

A narrow-based gait and thrust of the prosthesis laterally away from the knee at midstance often occur together and derive from the tendency of the prosthesis to rotate around the residual limb (Fig. 8.15). If the base of support (the prosthetic foot) is moved medially, support is lost laterally during single foot stance. Because there is no support for the pelvis in its normal alignment, it drops. In an attempt to maintain the pelvis level, the client may overcompensate and lean away from the prosthetic side on stance or may allow the drop to take place and lean laterally over the prosthesis on stance. In both instances, there is excess movement of the pelvis and shoulder either toward or away from the prosthesis. This gait deviation simulates a weak gluteus medius gait. The client will report increased pressure at the medial proximal and lateral distal end of the socket. The socket may be seen to move laterally at midstance, opening a gap between the residual limb and the top of the socket. A slight lateral thrust of the knee on stance is considered normal; an

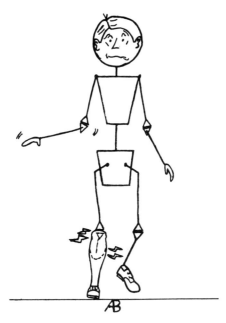

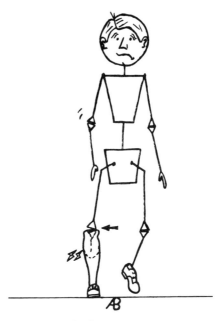

FIGURE 8.14
Midstance: Medial leaning pylon results in excessive pressure on the proximal lateral and distal medial areas of the residual limb. (Artist: Angie Britt)

FIGURE 8.15
Midstance: Lateral-leaning pylon results in excessive pressure on the proximal medial and distal lateral areas of the residual limb. (Artist: Angie Britt)

excessive lateral thrust can cause injury to the knee joint. Two major prosthetic causes of this deviation are an excessively inset foot and a lateral-leaning pylon. Both deviations can best be seen from the rear. In all deviations involving the alignment of the pylon, it is important to note the position at midstance and not at any other part of the **gait cycle.**

1. **Improper Mediolateral Tilt of the Socket (Lateral-Leaning Pylon)** (See Fig. 8.15). If the socket is set in abduction and the top of the pylon is more lateral than the bottom at midstance, the pylon is said to lean laterally. This increases pressure at the medial brim. In addition, the prosthetic foot is not flat on the floor and the weight is borne on the lateral border of the foot. These circumstances can be remedied by adducting the socket.

2. **Inset Foot.** An inset foot results when the prosthetic foot is placed too far medially to the dynamic alignment line. At midstance, the sound extremity is swinging through the air so that all the body weight is supported by the prosthetic foot on the floor. If this supporting foot is too far medial to the line of action of forces transmitted through the socket, a force couple is created that tends to rotate the socket around the stump. In almost all instances, this lateral thrust can be minimized or eliminated by "out-setting" the prosthetic foot slightly.

Terminal Stance

Knee Instability

Short Toe Lever Arm (Drop Off)   The toe lever arm provides support from midstance to terminal stance and allows the client to roll over the foot in a smooth manner (see Fig. 8.16). The **heel lever arm** provides support from heel

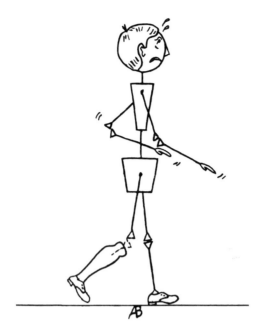

FIGURE 8.16
Terminal stance: drop off. (Artist: Angie Britt)

strike to midstance, allowing smooth descent of the prosthetic foot and controlled knee flexion. Just prior to heel off during normal gait, the knee is extending. At heel off or immediately thereafter, knee flexion begins. This change from extension to flexion coincides with the passing of the center of gravity over the metatarsophalangeal joints. If the body weight is carried over the metatarsophalangeal joints too soon, the resulting lack of anterior support allows premature knee flexion or drop off. If the foot is placed too far posteriorly under the socket, the toe lever arm will be shortened and the client will not be supported in the terminal stance phase (Fig. 8.17). This premature loss of support causes the prosthetic knee to flex and the hip to drop sharply just before the end of stance. This deviation is called "drop off." It can best be seen from the lateral viewpoint by watching the hip and knee in terminal stance.

Knee Extension; Vaulting
Long Toe Lever Arm If the body weight is carried forward over a long toe lever arm, the knee joint remains in extension during the latter part of the stance phase and the client complains of a "walking uphill" sensation, because the center of gravity is carried up and over the extended knee (Fig. 8.18). This prosthetic problem may best be seen laterally.

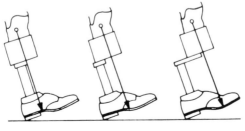

ANTERIOR SOCKET DISPLACEMENT

FIGURE 8.17
Too short toe lever arm is caused by placement of the socket too far forward on the foot. The first placement is correct. The other two are different degrees of incorrect placement.

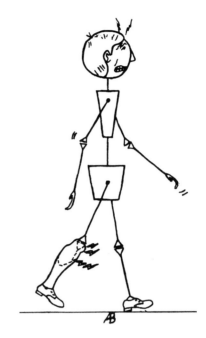

FIGURE 8.18
Terminal stance: a too long toe lever arm causes an extension moment. (Artist: Angie Britt)

Swing Phase

Pistoning (Loss of Suspension)

If the suspension mechanism is loose or inadequate, the prosthesis will slip as the foot leaves the ground for swing phase (Fig. 8.19). The toe of the prosthesis

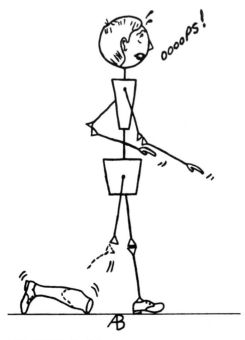

FIGURE 8.19
Swing phase: loss of suspension. (Artist: Angie Britt)

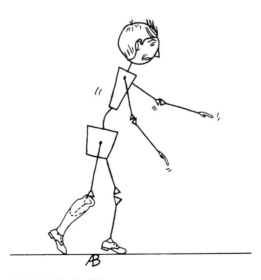

FIGURE 8.20
Swing phase: loss of suspension causes stubbing of the toe on the floor. (Artist: Angie Britt)

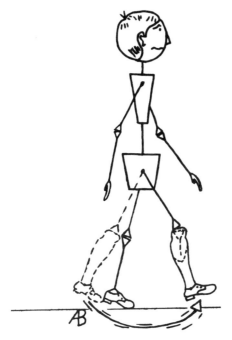

FIGURE 8.21
Swing phase: circumduction of the prosthesis.
(Artist: Angie Britt)

can catch on the ground, or the movement of the socket against the skin may cause abrasions (Fig. 8.20).

Uneven Step Length

Clients may develop the habit of taking a long prosthetic step and a short step with the unamputated leg. This may be the result of a poorly fitting socket causing pain, fear of putting weight on the prosthesis, or a prosthesis that is too long.

Circumduction

Circumduction is described as a semicircular swing of the prosthesis to the side during swing phase (Fig. 8.21). It may be seen if the prosthesis is too long, the suspension is inadequate, or the person has difficulty flexing the hip and knee.

TRANSFEMORAL PROSTHETIC EVALUATION

Table 8.2 depicts the key items to check initially with a transfemoral prosthesis. In addition to the socket fit, suspension, comfort, leg length, and static alignment that are similar to the transtibial level, knee stability is an important consideration in the transfemoral limb. Two parts of knee control are alignment (involuntary control) and active hip extension (voluntary control). In most instances, the knee is placed in a line or slightly posterior to a line drawn from the trochanter to the ankle axis (**TKA line**) as shown in Fig. 8.22. This placement allows the body weight line to fall anterior to the knee to create an extension moment on weight bearing. If the knee axis is on or anterior to the line, the body weight will fall behind the knee, creating a flexion or unstable moment. This alignment changes somewhat with multiaxis knee

TABLE 8.2   STATIC TRANSFEMORAL PROSTHETIC CHECKOUT

Checkout Item	What to Check	Possible Problem
Before Donning		
Is the prosthesis as prescribed?	Compare to prescription and residual limb.	Changes in prescribed components need to be justified.
Is the inside of the socket smoothly finished?	Feel the inside of the socket.	Roughness can cause skin abrasions.
Do all joints move freely and smoothly?	Check particularly the hip and knee joints. Check stance: support knees by putting weight on them with the knee in slight flexion.	Too stiff or loose joints can cause gait deviations. Failure of stance support can lead to falls.
Sitting		
Is the socket securely on the residual limb?	Pull on the socket slightly.	Suspension should be maintained in all positions.
Do the length of the shin and thigh correspond to the shin and thigh of the unamputated leg?	Check to see that the knees are level when the client is sitting with the knee flexed to 90 deg.	A high prosthetic knee could indicate a misaligned knee joint and lead to poor swing through.
Can the client sit comfortably without burning or pinching?	Check the posterior wall, particularly the pressure of the posterior brim against the seat and residual limb.	A sharp posterior wall can cause sciatic nerve pressure.
Is the client able to lean forward and reach her/his shoes?	Check the anterior wall height when sitting.	The anterior wall may impinge on the abdominal area.
Standing		
Does the socket fit properly and comfortably?	Ask the client if he/she is comfortable.	Areas of discomfort can cause gait deviations, nonwearing, and skin problems.
Is the knee stable when weight is placed on the prosthesis?	The knee joint is initially aligned on or just behind a line dropped from the trochanter to the knee axis. If the knee is in front of the line, it will be unstable.	An unstable knee can lead to an insecure gait.
Is the pelvis level when weight is borne evenly on both legs?	Palpate both iliac crests with the client standing with weight equally distributed on the two legs.	Too long or short a prosthesis will lead to gait deviations.
Does the socket maintain good contact with the residual limb on all sides as the client shifts his weight?	Check the brim of the socket as the client shifts his weight.	Too loose or too tight a socket may lead to skin abrasions and discomfort.
Is there an adductor roll?	Check high in the groin for excessive tissue around the medial wall.	An adductor roll can be pinched between the top of the medial wall and the pubic ramus, leading to pain and an abducted gait.
Is there pressure on the pubic ramus?	Ask the client.	Pain can lead to an abducted gait.

mechanisms with moving centers of gravity. What is important is for the client to have a stable knee during stance phase yet be able to flex the knee smoothly in terminal stance to initiate swing phase. In the prosthesis fitted with single axis or stance control knee mechanisms, the client must learn to extend the residual limb against the posterior wall of the prosthesis to maintain the knee in extension from heel strike to midstance. This may not be as important in hydraulic knee mechanisms, although active muscles in ambulation provide for better kinesthetic feedback and control of the prosthesis. Normally, the prosthetist will align the socket in about 5 degrees of flexion to increase the client's ability to extend the hip without excessively arching the back and to match normal femoral alignment. In clients with a hip flexion contracture, the socket must be set in flexion 5 degrees more than the limits

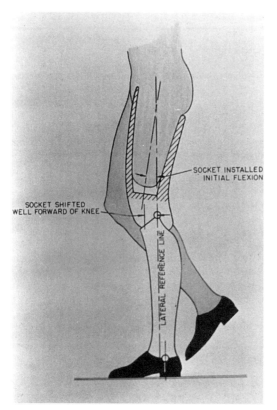

FIGURE 8.22
The trochanter knee ankle line (lateral reference line).

of the contracture. The greater the contracture and the longer the residual limb, the more problems of socket construction are created. There is a balance between involuntary and voluntary knee control. The more involuntary knee control there is, the greater stability in stance there is, but the person will have more difficulty initiating knee flexion on swing. Active individuals require a minimum of involuntary knee control to maintain as much voluntary control of knee action as possible. It is important for the therapist to understand the proper alignment and use of the client's knee mechanism. Close communication with the prosthetist and regular review of the manufacturer's description of specific knee mechanisms is a valuable activity for therapists.

TRANSFEMORAL GAIT ANALYSIS

Normal Gait

Heel Contact to Midstance, Lateral View

The knee is in extension from heel contact to midstance as the foot descends smoothly to the floor and the weight of the body progresses easily to a balanced point over the support leg. The body moves forward and slightly laterally to achieve this position.

Midstance, Anterior View

There may be a slight pelvic drop, not more than 5 degrees and no more than 2.5 cm of lateral bending of the trunk. The individual exhibits good mediolateral stability and balance on the prosthesis as the contralateral foot is picked up for swing phase. The width of the gait base should not exceed 5 cm.

Midstance to Toe Off, Lateral View

There is smooth heel rise as the weight is brought forward over the prosthetic forefoot. The hip extends without lumbar lordosis, and the knee begins to flex as the toe leaves the ground.

Swing Phase, Lateral View

The foot leaves the ground, and the prosthetic knee bends smoothly. The hip and knee flex as the prosthetic leg swings forward in the line of progression. Heel rise is adequate for the prosthetic toe to clear the floor but is not excessive. The shank swings smoothly and quietly forward, and the knee is extended just prior to the next heel contact. The stride length is equal on both sides.

Transfemoral Gait Deviations

Heel Contact to Midstance, Lateral View

Knee Instability
Knee instability is the major problem that can occur from heel contact to midstance (Fig. 8.23). It is essential for the knee to be extended for the client to feel secure.

Causes of knee instability include:

1. If the knee axis is placed anterior to the TKA line, the line of body weight falls behind the knee, creating a flexion moment. The knee can be poorly aligned if the socket is placed too far anteriorly (long heel lever arm).
2. Knee instability can also be caused by lack of adequate socket flexion, limiting the client's active hip extension.

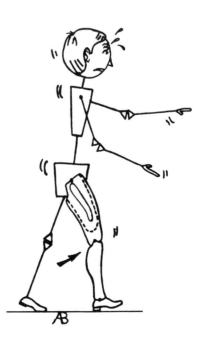

FIGURE 8.23
Heel contact to midstance: knee instability. (Artist: Angie Britt)

3. Heel support that is too hard and does not accept body weight may also create a flexion moment at heel strike.
4. A severe hip flexion contracture not accommodated in the socket makes it difficult for the client to control the knee.

Terminal Impact

Terminal impact refers to a rapid forward movement of the shank that allows the knee to reach maximum extension with too much force before heel strike. It occurs most frequently with constant friction knees because the individual uses the sound to indicate that the knee is ready for heel contact. It is a difficult habit to change. The impact, if severe, can cause bruising of the distal end of the residual limb. It does not occur with well-functioning hydraulic knee mechanisms or most multiaxis or stance control knee units.

Foot Slap

If the forefoot descends too rapidly it will make a slapping sound as it hits the floor (Fig. 8.24). Foot slap may be caused by plantar flexion resistance that is too soft or a heel lever arm that is too short. The client may also be driving the prosthesis into the walking surface too forcibly to ensure extension of the knee. It is not a frequent problem.

Midstance, AP View

Lateral Trunk Bending

All individuals walking with a transfemoral prosthesis exhibit some lateral bending from the midline to the prosthetic side because the prosthesis cannot fully compensate for loss of skeletal fixation to the ground (Fig. 8.25). Excessive bending may have several causes:

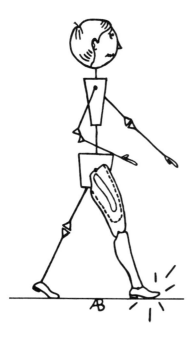

FIGURE 8.24
Heel contact to midstance: foot slap. (Artist: Angie Britt)

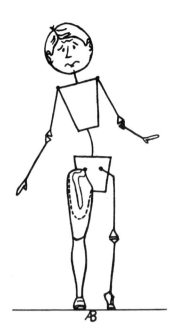

FIGURE 8.25
Midstance: lateral trunk bending to prosthetic side. (Artist: Angie Britt)

1. The lateral wall of the socket is designed to provide mediolateral stability by holding the limb in adduction. If there is a short residual limb or inadequate adduction of the socket, there will be lateral trunk bending at midstance. The ischial containment socket was designed in part to provide better mediolateral stability than the quadrilateral socket, and the Hanger Comfort Flex socket is designed to provide even more mediolateral stability through its grasp on muscular compartments (see Chap. 7).
2. A prosthesis that is too short will cause a hip drop at midstance along with lateral trunk bending.
3. If the medial wall of the socket is too high, the individual may bend laterally to avoid pressure on the pubic ramus.
4. The client may not have adequate balance to properly shift the weight over the prosthesis or may have a very short residual limb that fails to provide a sufficient lever arm for the pelvis.
5. The client may have weak abductors on the prosthetic side and be unable to control the body weight over the prosthesis.
6. This gait deviation may also be seen if the client has a painful residual limb.

Abducted Gait
An abducted gait is characterized by a gait base that is wider than 5 cm at midstance (Fig. 8.26). Causes include:

1. A prosthesis that is too long.
2. An improperly shaped lateral wall that fails to provide adequate support for the femur.
3. A high medial wall that causes the client to hold the prosthesis away to avoid ramus pressure.
4. An abduction contracture or poorly developed gait habit.

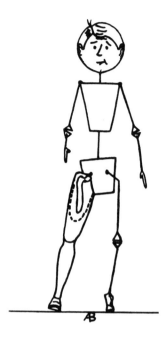

FIGURE 8.26
Midstance: abducted gait. (Artist: Angie Britt)

Extensive Trunk Extension

The client creates an active lumbar lordosis during stance phase (Fig. 8.27). This extensive trunk extension is caused by one of the following:

1. Insufficient initial socket flexion leads the client to extend the lumbar spine to obtain hip extension at heel contact.
2. The client may have a flexion contracture that cannot be accommodated prosthetically.
3. The client may have weak hip extensors and or weak abdominal muscles.

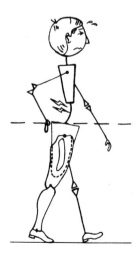

FIGURE 8.27
Midstance to toe off: lumbar lordosis. (Artist: Angie Britt)

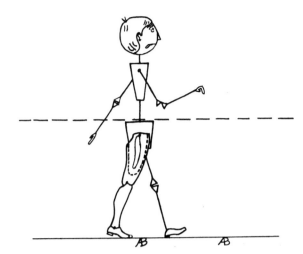

FIGURE 8.28
Terminal stance: drop off. (Artist: Angie Britt)

Midstance to Toe Off, Lateral View

Drop Off

As with the transtibial prosthesis, there is a sudden downward movement of the trunk as anterior support is lost prematurely (Fig. 8.28). The main reason is usually a short toe lever arm. It is an unstable deviation because it may cause the knee to buckle prematurally.

Inadequate Heel Off

If the client does not feel secure allowing the body weight to shift forward over the toe of the prosthesis, the heel may not come off the floor until the whole foot is brought forward. This deviation is associated with uneven steps as discussed later.

Swing Phase, AP View

Circumducted Gait

During a circumducted gait, the prosthesis swings laterally in an arclike manner during swing phase. Causes include:

1. A prosthesis that is too long.
2. A mechanical knee with too much alignment stability or friction in the knee, making it difficult to bend the knee in swing through.
3. The client may lack confidence for flexing the prosthetic knee because of muscle weakness or fear of stubbing the toe.
4. The stance phase control knee may not be functioning properly.

Vaulting

The client rises on the toe of the sound foot to swing the prosthesis through with little knee flexion. Some individuals use this maneuver temporarily to walk rapidly. Unwanted or continuous vaulting may be caused by:

1. A prosthesis that is too long.
2. Inadequate socket suspension.
3. Excessive stability in the alignment or some limitation of knee flexion.

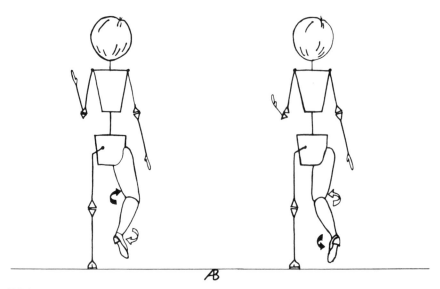

FIGURE 8.29

Swing phase: (*Left*) medial heel whip; (*Right*) lateral heel whip. (Artist: Angie Britt)

4. Fear of stubbing the toe or flexing the knee.
5. Discomfort.

Medial or Lateral Whips

Whips are best observed when the client walks away from the observer (Fig. 8.29). A medial whip is present when the heel travels medially on initial flexion at the beginning of swing phase; a lateral whip exists when the heel moves laterally. Prosthetically, whips are always related to the knee joint as follows:

1. Medial whips result from excessive external rotation of the prosthetic knee.
2. Lateral whips result from excessive internal rotation of the prosthetic knee.

Other causes may include a socket that is too tight, thus reflecting residual limb rotation, or the client may have donned the prosthesis in internal or external rotation.

Uneven Arm Swing and Uneven Timing

These two deviations go together. The arm on the prosthetic side is held close to the body, and the individual takes steps of unequal duration and length with a short stance phase on the prosthesis. The major cause is poor training and fear of putting weight on the prosthesis.

BASIC GAIT TRAINING

■ *Case Study Activities*

1   Design a prosthetic training program for each client. What do you already know how to do, and what do you need to learn?

2   Compare and contrast the prosthetic training program for an individual fitted with a transtibial prosthesis and someone fitted with a transfemoral prosthesis.

3   What parts of the training program are appropriately done by a PTA?

DONNING THE PROSTHESIS

Proper prosthetic **donning** is one of the first things to be learned. Teaching proper donning involves showing the client the appropriate reference points between the residual limb and the socket and the client's learning the correct feel of the prosthesis. Sockets that fit snugly such as some suction prostheses are more difficult to don.

Residual Limb Socks

Some prostheses are worn with a sock that fits directly over the residual limb and is applied before the limb is inserted in the socket. Socks come in different thicknesses or plys. A thin cotton sock is considered to be one ply; wool socks are made in either three or five plys. Some clients may choose to wear a thin nylon sheath under the cotton or wool sock to reduce skin friction during ambulation. There are also gel-impregnated socks that can be used as the first sock against the skin. Gel socks come in a variety of styles and thicknesses and provide some cushioning and protection of bony prominences or sensitive areas. Gel socks are equivalent to two to four ply, depending on construction.

Many individuals are fitted with gel liners that fit directly over the residual limb. They come in various thicknesses that are measured in millimeters. Check with the prosthetist to determine the actual thickness of the gel liner. As the residual limb shrinks, additional socks are added. Individuals fitted with gel liners will add socks over the liners. If the liner incorporates a shuttlelock pin, the sock must have a hole in the bottom to allow the pin to come through. Care must be taken that no lint, thread, or piece of sock remains around the pin because it is likely to jam the mechanism making it hard to remove. One-ply socks are added as the residual limb gets smaller. When the individual is wearing three one-ply socks, he or she can substitute a three-ply wool sock. By the time the individual needs a total of 10- to 15-ply socks, it is time to replace the socket. Socks and sheaths come in a variety of sizes and widths for both transtibial and transfemoral residual limbs. During initial training, the PT or PTA emphasizes that the sock must be pulled completely up the residual limb with the distal seam running parallel to the incision line in a mediolateral direction. Care must be taken that the sock is smooth and wrinkle-free. If the client is using a sleeve suspension, it is important to understand that the sleeve must come at least 2 inches higher than the top of the socks to properly suspend the prosthesis. The PT or PTA teaches the client how to adjust socks as the residual limb becomes smaller as will be discussed later in this chapter. Figure 8.30 illustrates several types of residual limb socks and sheaths. Figure 8.31 is a handout that can be given to clients.

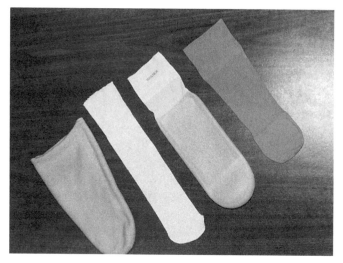

FIGURE 8.30

Residual limb socks and sheaths. From the bottom left: a five-ply wool sock; a one-ply cotton sock; a Silosheath (Silipos Corp.); and a nylon sheath.

Syme and Transtibial Prostheses

The residual limb fits snugly into the socket with the distal end touching the distal end pad in transtibial prostheses and with some weight bearing in the Syme leg. At both levels, the patellar bar presses the midline of the patella tendon. Some prostheses are designed to fit snugly, and the client may have to stand to get all the way into the socket. Care must be taken not to create any skin abrasions when donning the prosthesis. On occasion, clients may experience some difficulty donning a prosthesis with high medial and lateral walls; a slight turning of the residual limb as the prosthesis is being donned will ease the tibial condyles past the wings of the prosthesis. The suspension sleeve is rolled up over the socket and residual limb after the residual limb is well into the socket. If there is a urethane or silicone liner, it can be donned first and then the residual limb and liner inserted into the socket (Fig. 8.32). This process may be difficult for some clients with impaired balance or impaired vision, and fitting the liner and socket separately may increase the likelihood of an improperly donned prosthesis. It may be easier to teach the client to put the socket and liner on as one unit. When a gel liner is used, it is rolled on the residual limb first, and then the residual limb is inserted into the socket. The shuttlelock system requires that the individual fit the pin carefully into the receptacle and then stand to push the limb well into the socket until the lock is heard clicking into place. The limb is removed by pushing the small button built into the medial socket wall. The regular suction socket is donned in a similar manner.

Transfemoral Prostheses

When the client dons the ischial containment socket, he or she must take care to ensure that the socket is not rotated internally or externally. The lateral wall and foot position are guides to proper donning (Fig. 8.33). In the

If you are fitted with a polyurethane liner, you will wear one or more residual limb socks over your residual limb within the prosthetic socket. The sock is designed to increase the comfort of the prosthetic socket and to assist in control of perspiration. The socks allow you to maintain a close socket fit as your residual limb gets smaller.

Socks come in different lengths, widths, thicknesses, and materials. Your socks have been selected to fit your particular residual limb. No other type of residual limb cover will fit properly and only stump socks should be used over your residual limb when wearing your prosthesis. The thickness of the stump sock is called a "ply." Thin or cotton socks are considered 1 ply. Socks that contain a gel within the material may be equal to 2 or 3 ply. Your initial fit may be with 1 ply or a thin sock. Thicker socks are made of wool and are generally either 3 or 5 ply. Socks can come in other thicknesses for special needs. Your prosthetist will give you a supply of socks of varying plies with your initial prosthesis. As your socks wear out, you will need to purchase replacement socks from the prosthetist.

PUTTING ON THE SOCKS PROPERLY

The sock is pulled on firmly and without wrinkles. The seam at the end of the sock should run parallel to, not across the suture line. Clean dry socks should be put on each day because wet or dirty socks can cause injury to the residual limb. If you are wearing more than one sock over your residual limb, put each one on separately making sure it fits snugly and has no wrinkles.

SOCKS WITH GEL LINERS

If you are fitted with a gel liner, the liner will go directly over your skin. The gel liner must be rolled on smoothly making sure the end of your residual limb is in contact with the end of the liner. The liner is usually folded down so you can put the end of the liner directly against the end of your residual limb and then roll the liner up smoothly. If you need to use residual limb socks as your limb shrinks, they are added on top of the liner. Socks are never worn under a gel liner. If you are fitted with a liner that has the shuttlelock at the end, you will need socks with a hole at the end to allow the stem to be free to enter the receptacle at the bottom of the socket. Make sure that there is no lint or pieces of socks on the stem. Material caught in the shuttlelock system can jam the system and make it hard to remove.

FIGURE 8.31
Proper use of socks for residual limb.

CARE OF THE SOCKS

Wool socks are washed by hand with mild soap, rinsed well, and dried flat. They are not to be cleaned in the washing machine or dryer. Cotton socks and socks made from acrylic may be machine washed in cold water and dried at low temperatures.

Gel liners are washed with a damp cloth each night and allowed to dry on the stand provided. Gel liners should never be folded, stuffed into the prosthesis, or allowed to wrinkle and stay in a wrinkled position.

ADJUSTING SOCKS

A snug comfortable fit between the residual limb and the socket is necessary to prevent any injury to your residual limb. A good fit includes contact between your residual limb and the bottom of the socket. As your residual limb gets smaller (shrinks), you may feel you are going too deep in the socket and may feel excess pressure at the distal end or on a bony prominence at the top of the socket. The socket may also feel loose. If your socket feels loose or if you feel excess pressure at the bottom of the socket, add one thin sock. It may be necessary to add a second thin sock if the first does not relieve the symptoms. Be careful of adding too many socks and pushing your residual limb out of the socket. Add only one sock at a time and check the fit of the socket each time. You may substitute a 3-ply sock (with the yellow band at the top) for three cotton socks, or a 5-ply (with the green band at the top) for five cotton socks. Some people need to add a sock in the middle of the day after wearing the prosthesis for several hours.

If wearing a gel liner, add socks over the liner. Depending on the size of the liner, it may be possible to eventually obtain a thicker liner. Discuss this with your prosthetist.

SHEATHS

If you are not fitted with a gel liner, you may prefer to use a thin nylon sheath directly over the residual limb prior to donning the regular socks. Some people like the sheath to reduce possible friction between the socket and the residual limb and to provide a smoother interface. A gel-impregnated sheath is also available to provide additional cushioning.

REMOVING SOCKS

Some people gain weight after they have been fitted with a prosthesis or have fluctuations in the size of their residual limb. Wearing too many socks will push your residual limb out of the socket, and you will no longer be in contact with the bottom. After you have worn a prosthesis for several months, your residual limb will stabilize and you will not need to add or remove socks unless your weight changes or you have major fluctuations in body fluids. If you have any questions about proper use of socks, ask your prosthetist or physical therapist.

FIGURE 8.31 (CONTINUED)

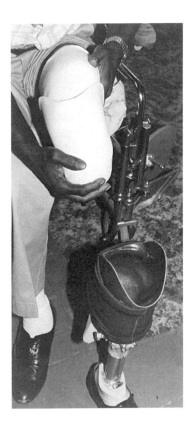

FIGURE 8.32
Donning the patellar socket-bearing liner before donning the
prosthesis. The residual limb is covered by a sock.

quadrilateral socket, the adductor longus channel at the anteromedial corner
of the socket and the ischial seat on top of the posterior wall are the major reference points. Transfemoral prostheses with pelvic band suspension are usually donned in the sitting position, whereas the suction socket is donned
standing.

The suction transfemoral prosthesis is worn without a sock; a stockinet
or elastic bandage is used to pull the residual limb into the socket and push
the air out of the socket at the same time. The skin of the residual limb must
be dry and free from abrasions. The "pull wrap" is put on the residual limb
smoothly and without wrinkles to the groin, and the end is placed through
the hole at the end of the socket. The client then stands and places the prosthesis slightly in front of the other leg while maintaining all weight on the
sound leg. The patient then flexes and extends the sound hip and knee while
pulling downward on the end of the wrap. In this manner the residual limb is
pulled into the socket, and the air is pushed out. The process is continued
until the residual limb is in the socket and the wrap has been removed. The
valve is then replaced, and any remaining air is expelled by shifting all of the
body weight into the prosthesis while holding the valve stem open. If a Silesian bandage is worn, it is secured at this time (see Chap. 7, Fig. 7.21). The patient learns to carry a pull wrap at all times in case the prosthesis is removed
for any reason. Donning a suction socket takes balance and coordination; not
all patients like the process. In warm, humid climates, perspiration makes
donning and maintaining suction difficult.

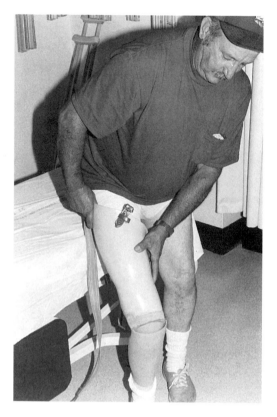

FIGURE 8.33

Donning a transfemoral prosthesis with an ischial containment socket suspended by a Silesian bandage.

Gel liners, soft sockets, and sockets requiring residual limb socks are donned in a similar manner as the transtibial prosthesis.

Hip Disarticulation and Hemipelvectomy Prostheses

Donning these prostheses can be done in either the sitting or standing position. Most of the body weight is borne on the sound side, and the socket is slipped into place. After standing, the client tightens the straps to adjust for comfort. The major reference points are the iliac crest and ischium on the amputated side for hip disarticulation or the contralateral iliac crest and ribs for the hemipelvectomy prostheses. Instead of socks, many clients prefer to sew the bottom of a T-shirt together on the amputated side and slide it over the residual limb. This maneuver limits bunching of fabric that can cause pressure points.

PROSTHETIC TRAINING

The major goal of prosthetic rehabilitation is for the client to attain a smooth, energy-efficient gait that allows him or her to perform activities of daily living and participate in desired employment and recreational activities. Mobility refers to the skills required to solve movement problems confronted during activities. The client is an integral part of the prosthetic training program including establishing expected goals. Clients who have functioned with a diseased limb for a considerable period of time frequently exceed their immediately premorbid levels of function.

Factors that contribute to a smooth, energy-efficient gait include the ability to (a) accept the weight of the body on each leg, (b) balance on one foot in single limb support, (c) advance each limb forward and prepare for the next step, and (d) adapt to environmental demands. Traditional prosthetic training has focused on breaking down the gait cycle into small steps and teaching each step. Normal gait is an integrated activity that may not be learned most efficiently through the practice of each part. Dennis and McKeough[17] developed a taxonomy of motor tasks based on the work of Gentile[18] that describes environmental conditions involved in regaining independent function. The taxonomy is easily applicable to the clinical setting and provides a reference point for organizing and sequencing patient activities.

Figure 8.34 is a schematic representation of the Dennis and McKeough taxonomy as a two-dimensional grid. One dimension (the horizontal axis of

		BODY STABLE		BODY TRANSPORT	
		Without Manipulation	With Manipulation	Without Manipulation	With Manipulation
CLOSED ENVIRONMENT	Without Intertrial Variability	Body is stable, arms and legs are still, the task does not change, the environment is fixed in time & space.	Body is stable, task does not change, environment is fixed in time & space, arms or legs are moving.	Body is moving, limbs moving in relation to movement task, task does not change, environment is fixed in time & space.	Body is moving, arms or legs moving independently of task, environment is fixed in time & space.
	With Intertrial Variability	As above but task changes require slight modification in motor plan from trial to trial.	As above but task changes require slight modification of motor plan from trial to trial.	As above but task changes require slight modification of motor plan from trial to trial.	As above but task changes require slight modification of motor plan from trial to trial.
OPEN ENVIRONMENT	Without Intertrial Variability	Body is stable, arms & legs are still, task is fixed, environment is changing in time and space.	Body is stable, task is fixed, arms & legs are moving independently of tasks, environment is changing in time and space.	Body is moving, task is fixed, arms and legs and synchronous with task, environment is changing in time & space.	Body is moving, arms or legs moving independently of task, task is fixed, environment changing in time & space.
	With Intertrial Variability	As above, but task changes each trial.	As above, but task changes each trial.	As above but task changes each trial.	As above but task changes each trial.

FIGURE 8.34

Taxonomy of motor tasks: dimensions of task difficulty. (Adapted from Dennis, JK, and McKeough, DM: Mobility. In May, BJ: Home Health and Rehabilitation: Concepts of Care, FA Davis, Philadelphia, 1993.)

the grid) represents desired outcomes, progressing from simple goals requiring body stability (e.g., sitting or standing) to more demanding goals requiring transporting the body through space and time (e.g., walking). Both classes of outcomes—body stability and body in motion—are subdivided into two further classifications: goals that do not require manipulation (e.g., sitting while someone combs his or her hair), and those that do (e.g., reaching for an object). The result is four categories of goals ranging along the horizontal axis and progressing from simple on the left to more demanding on the right. Similarly, the vertical axis of the grid represents variables in the environment, with the less demanding environmental situations at the top and the more demanding at the bottom. The two primary categories in the environmental dimension are closed and open. A closed environment, for example, a room with furniture but no people, is one that does not change during the performance of the desired goal. An open environment, for instance a room with a dog moving around, is one that changes during the task performance. Again, each major category is further subdivided into two variables: in one there is no change in the environment between trials (e.g., the space remains the same each time the client attempts the activity); in the other, more difficult variable, the environment changes between trials (e.g., furniture is moved closer together, the dog runs around the room). As with the horizontal axis, the categories on the vertical axis are arranged in order of increasing difficulty, the simplest at the top and the most challenging on the bottom. Each of the 16 cells on the resulting grid represents a separate level of task or goal difficulty, with the simple tasks in the upper left and the most difficult in the lower right.

These concepts can guide the therapist in planning the sequence of training activities. The training program starts in a closed environment with stability and then mobility activities, and progresses to the more complex, open environment. As success is achieved at one level, activities can be made more complex by varying the independent limb mobility or adding intertrial variability.

Teaching Prosthetic Control

Before an individual can develop a smooth, energy-efficient gait, he or she must be able to balance on the prosthesis long enough to bring the other leg forward in a controlled manner. Early training starts in a closed environment with little independent limb manipulation (i.e., simple motion problems). Gradually the movement problems become more complex. Goal-oriented activities that require side-to-side weight shifting, one-legged standing, reaching for objects in different directions, and forward-and-back stepping with one foot help the client learn basic prosthetic control and the "feel" of the prosthesis when the weight is shifted to different parts of the foot (Fig. 8.35). Reaching for an object in different locations helps the client shift weight on and off the prosthesis in a functional manner (Fig. 8.36). Individuals with transtibial prostheses must learn to let their knee flex slightly from heel strike to midstance in a natural gait pattern. Individuals fitted with transfemoral prostheses need to learn to control the prosthetic knee as part of the initial balancing activities. The PT or PTA can provide some kinesthetic feedback by pushing slightly on the back of the prosthetic knee with the client in the parallel bars. The client extends the residual limb against the posterior wall of the socket and begins to feel how to control the knee.

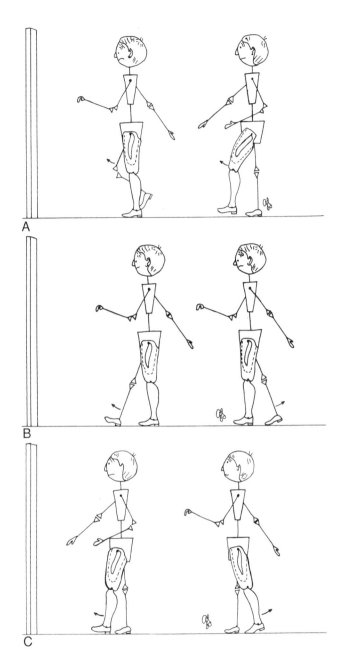

FIGURE 8.35

Early prosthetic training. (*A*) Weight shifting on and off the prosthesis to increase knee control. (*B*) Stepping forward and back with the sound leg increases weight bearing on the prosthesis. (*C*) Alternating stepping forward and back with the prosthesis can increase knee control in swing phase. (Kicking a soft ball enhances both activities shown in *B* and *C*.) (Artist: Gloria Sanders)

Clients often tend to look at the floor during initial training because they cannot feel the floor directly. A mirror helps the individual keep the head erect and focus on feeling the socket pressures change during the different parts of weight shifting (Fig. 8.37). Focusing on achieving the goals of an activity such as touching a ball or reaching into a cabinet helps prevent looking at

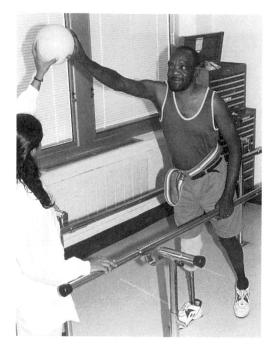

FIGURE 8.36

Reaching for an object promotes weight shifting on and off the prosthesis.

the feet. The ability to shift weight and balance on and off the prosthesis is critical to a satisfactory gait for all prosthetic wearers. Incorporating functional movements into the early training is critical to help the client integrate the prosthesis into total body movements. It is important for clients to focus on the goal and allow the prosthesis to become a part of their natural movements. A creative therapist can devise a wide variety of activities that facilitate such integration. Despite the pressure to curtail the number of visits to physical therapy, learning balance on the prosthesis and integration of weight shifting in a wide variety of positions and situations is the most critical element of gait training. Individuals who develop skill in this early integration are most likely to develop a smooth, energy-efficient gait pattern and become functional prosthetic users. If this first phase of training is curtailed and the patients are pushed to walk with external support before they are comfortable with the prosthesis, they are most likely to develop a slow and inefficient gait pattern. Throughout training, the client, as an integral part of the team needs to learn to give himself or herself feedback on the performance. Asking the client questions such as "How did that feel?" and "What would help you make the performance feel natural?" are helpful.

Initial Walking

Walking may be initiated in the safety of the parallel bars, in a secure area in the home, or in a closed environment with outside parallel bars or external support. The therapist's judgment based on the client's ability to weight shift and balance is key to this decision making. A person with good balance may quickly be able to function safely and properly outside the parallel bars. A mirror may help the person assume a better standing position with the weight well distributed over the feet. Figure 8.38 depicts an initial walking sequence

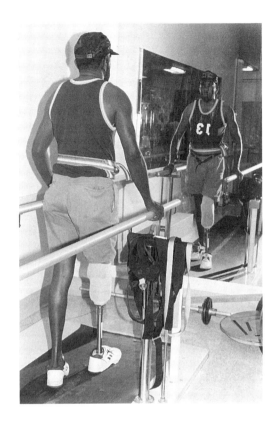

FIGURE 8.37
Training in front of a mirror reduces the tendency to look at the floor.

with a transfemoral prosthesis. The individual with a transtibial prosthesis follows a similar sequence but must be reminded to roll over the foot, allowing the knee to flex slightly from heel contact to midstance. Throughout the early training sequence, the client should be encouraged to put as little weight on the parallel bars as possible, particularly if independent ambulation without external support or only a cane is anticipated. During initial walking, the PT or PTA can provide feedback based on observation of the gait pattern, suggesting possible changes in movements that may improve the pattern. However, some people cannot benefit from suggestions regarding individual movements. They may develop an awkward gait pattern—such as a longer step with the unamputated leg that shifts weight over the prosthesis more—when trying to emphasize what has been suggested. In some instances, particularly with older people, suggesting that they try and walk "like you did before you lost your leg" is helpful. When the pattern is particularly smooth, asking them "How did that feel?" helps them reintegrate the normal movements into their activities. There is sometimes reluctance by PTs or PTAs to spend adequate time in balance and initial walking activities. The limited time allowed for rehabilitation by third-party payers sometimes drives the therapist to accept a less than desirable gait pattern or a greater level of support.

One of the more difficult parts of walking is learning to shift the weight on and off the prosthesis in a smooth pattern. The creative therapist finds many ways to lead the client to making this movement. Tapping on the side of the hip as the patient walks may help with sideways weight shifting. Occa-

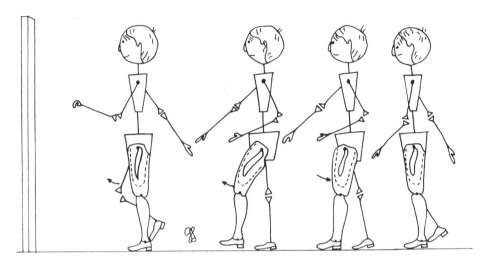

FIGURE 8.38
Learning to walk forward in a coordinated manner using minimal external support if possible. (Artist: Gloria Sanders)

sionally, having the client hold the bar or a cane on the amputated side for several steps may encourage weight shifting (Fig. 8.39). In the home setting, incorporating everyday activities such as reaching for something on a high shelf, making a bed, or wiping a counter all encourage prosthetic weight shifting in a functional pattern (Fig. 8.40). It is important for the client to make a direct transition from the parallel bars to the anticipated final external sup-

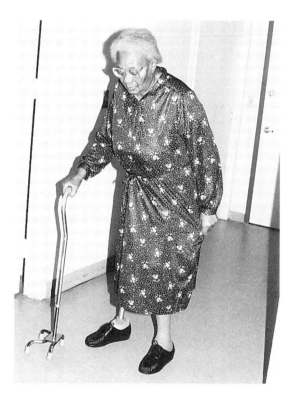

FIGURE 8.39
Sometimes using the cane on the prosthetic side helps the client learn to weight-shift to that side.

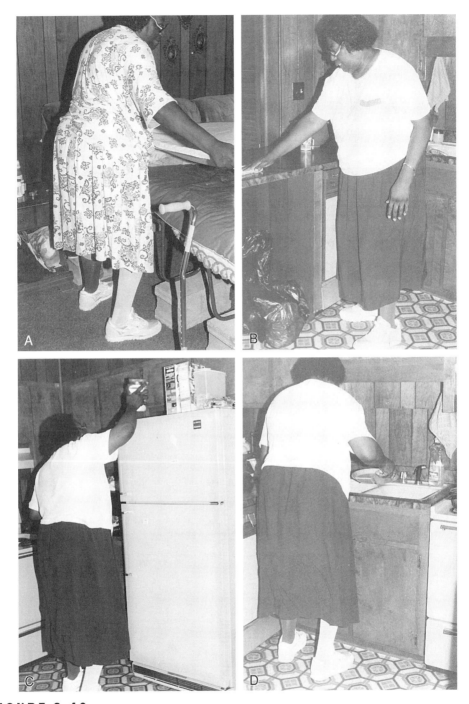

FIGURE 8.40

Prosthetic training in the home: Incorporating functional activities increases the internalization of prosthetic use.

port. Effective gait training encourages the least amount of external support necessary.

Integration of the prosthesis into a variety of gait situations is important, and learning to sidestep and walk backwards are helpful activities to provide for weight shifting, prosthetic control, balance, and function (Fig. 8.41). During the initial training period, the person must be taught a safe way to get up and down from a chair (Fig. 8.42). Figure 8.43 illustrates the use of the taxonomy to progress training activities for the patient.

Hydraulic Knee Mechanisms

Many different knee mechanisms are in use throughout the United States. The PT and PTA must be familiar with the devices used locally through regular contact with prosthetists. Training an individual fitted with a hydraulic knee mechanism may be a little different than training one fitted with a mechanical knee joint, and the therapist must know and understand the functional characteristics of the specific knee unit. In all models, the hydraulic

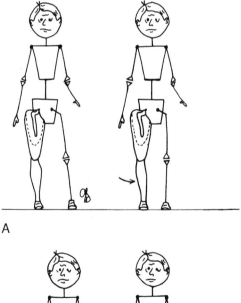

A

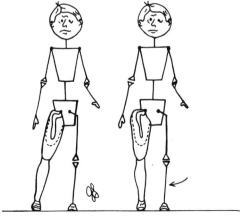

B

FIGURE 8.41
Prosthetic training: learning to step sideways.
(Artist: Gloria Sanders)

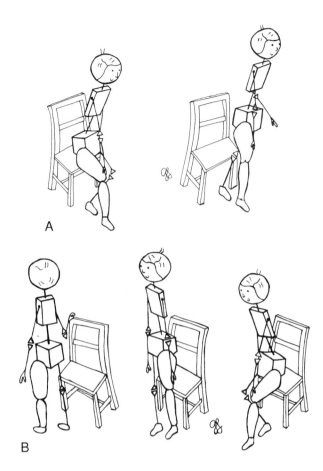

FIGURE 8.42

Prosthetic training: learning to stand up from and sit down on a chair is an early training activity. (Artist: Gloria Sanders)

mechanism is designed for swing-phase control and adjusts the swing of the shank to ensure that the foot is ready for heel strike at the appropriate time. Rather than increasing or decreasing hip flexion force to adjust shank swing, the person lets the hydraulic mechanism and the speed of the gait cycle do the job. The client needs to experience different cadences to fully understand the capabilities of hydraulic swing-phase control. For the system to be fully operational, the client must be taught to walk over the ball of the foot. Putting pressure on the ball of the foot allows the knee to flex naturally. Active individuals gain control easily, but more timid walkers may have difficulty initiating knee flexion. An active step-over-step gait is necessary to properly use the mechanisms of most hydraulic, some multiaxis, and most computerized knee mechanisms. Most of these units function best when the person develops a smooth, natural, step-over-step pattern, and training must emphasize that type of gait pattern.

Swing- and stance-phase control systems require different training for knee control. Some mechanisms provide both swing- and stance-phase control, allowing a slow deceleration if the patient puts weight on the prosthesis with the knee somewhat flexed. This deceleration allows time for the patient to regain balance and control. Some systems may also have an automatic knee extension moment if weight is taken off the prosthesis with the knee slightly flexed. This automatic knee extension allows the person to take small steps around a table

		BODY STABLE		**BODY TRANSPORT**	
		Without Manipulation	With Manipulation	Without Manipulation	With Manipulation
C L O S E	Without Intertrial Variability	Keeps balance standing while PT/PTA gently and predictably pushes on body.	Dons prosthesis in sitting or standing. Stands and reaches for object with 1 or 2 hands.	Rolling over in bed; sit to stand from bed or wheelchair using cane, crutches, or wheelchair.	Carries the same object from place to place using same pathway. Sit to stand with an object in hand (not a walking aid).
	With Intertrial Variability	Keeps sitting or standing balance on different surfaces e.g., carpet, tiler, straight chair.	Stands at a counter reaching for different objects placed in different positions. Sits, bends and reaches for object in different directions.	Sit to stand from different surfaces and different height chairs. Up and down curbs of different heights.	Carries objects of different size and weight from place to place using different pathways.
O P E N	Without Intertrial Variability	Keeps balance in a moving elevator or a moving platform.	Rearranges packages in a moving elevator. Handles several objects while standing on an unstable surface.	Walks down a hallway with the same person coming toward them.	Carries an object while walking down the hallway.
	With Intertrial Variability	Keeps balance while catching and throwing a ball.	Stands in a crowded room, eating or drinking from glass or plate in hand.	Community ambulation; walks through a busy gym.	Shops in a supermarket; goes to a room, picks up some objects, walks back through busy hallway.

FIGURE 8.43

Using the taxonomy of motor skills to prioritize training activities. (Adapted from Dennis, JK, and McKeough, DM: Mobility. In May, BJ: Home Health and Rehabilitation: Concepts of Care, FA Davis, Philadelphia, 1993.)

or bench and maintain knee control. Hydraulic knee mechanisms function best when the individual has the balance and stability to walk safely without external support or a cane at the most. But, as in all the other types of prostheses, gaining early confidence in bearing weight through the prosthesis and shifting smoothly on and off the limb will ensure a good gait pattern.

External Support

Energy expenditure is a major concern. It is directly related to the smoothness of the gait pattern and the use of external devices. Most desirable is training the client for functional ambulation without external devices. A single-point or quad cane is often needed by elderly people for use outside in the street. On occasion, crutches may be needed if the client has other medical conditions that preclude ambulating with less support. A four-point gait is usually taught unless the client needs to protect the unamputated leg from full weight bearing (Fig. 8.44). A walker is not indicated in most instances and should not be considered as an intermediate step between the parallel bars and a cane. A walker does not allow a smooth step-over-step pattern and reinforces a slow gait pattern characterized by uneven steps. This gait negates the principles of prosthetic design and alignment. The walker also reinforces for-

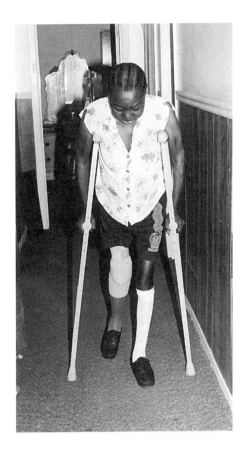

FIGURE 8.44
Some clients need to limit weight bearing on the sound leg. This can be done using the four-point gait with crutches.

ward flexion and eliminates the normal use of the arms in the gait pattern. Using the walker as a shortcut to allow the client to be discharged from treatment early or to use the prosthesis at home before a good gait has been achieved leads to gait deviations and a dependency on the walker that may never be overcome. A walker should be used only if it is obvious that the individual will not be able to use the prosthesis with any other form of external support. An unstable person who can go to the bathroom independently with a walker is easier to care for at home than one who may be wheelchair dependent. However, the walker should be used sparingly and only after careful evaluation of the individual's potential.

Advanced Training

■ Case Study Activities

1   Design a training program for Diana Magnolia and Ha Lee Davis that incorporates the progression from a closed to an open environment.
2   Identify at least two activities for each cell of the model that you would do in a rehabilitation center and in a home environment.

Changing the environment is an integral part of the gait-training program. It is hardly functional to have the client walk only in the sheltered and simple

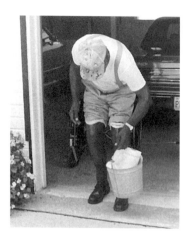

FIGURE 8.45

Learning to pick up an object from the floor requires balance and coordination.

environment of the physical therapy gym. Functional ambulation takes place in complex closed environments and in open environments. It is the PT's and PTA's responsibility to provide opportunities to practice these skills. Walking around furniture, through narrow doorways, on rugs, and around obstacles is very different from walking in the gym. Although this type of training is still

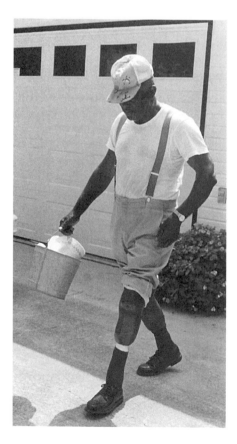

FIGURE 8.46

Carrying an item is an advanced activity requiring independent limb manipulation.

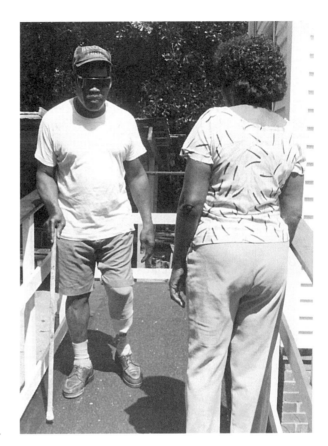

FIGURE 8.47
An open environment activity can be created by having a family member walk in front of the client while the client is ambulating in a familiar space.

in a closed environment because there are no moving objects requiring predictive ability, it is more complex than wide pathways without obstacles. Placing obstacles on the floor to step around or over or walking in a busy hallway of the treatment centers are progressive activities. The home environment is also replete with opportunities for such progression. Requiring the client to pick something up from the floor or carry an object in one hand is an example of an even more complex closed environment (Figs. 8.45 and 8.46). These activities require balance, coordination, and the ability to shift one's weight on and off the prosthesis while in different body positions. It becomes an open environment activity if there are people in the room or hall (Fig. 8.47).

During advanced training the client is taught a safe way to get up from and down to chairs of different heights and seat resilience, especially toilet seats.

CARE OF THE PROSTHESIS, RESIDUAL LIMB, AND SOCKS

Teaching the client proper care of the residual limb and how to adjust socks is an integral part of the training program. The PT and PTA should contact the prosthetist to learn proper care of the particular materials used in the prosthesis. Most plastic sockets and liners can be washed with a damp cloth and dried thoroughly. The socket should be washed at night to allow plenty of drying time. Likewise socks must be washed and changed daily. Wool socks require handwashing with a mild soap and flat drying. Learning to adjust socks for a shrinking residual limb or for an individual whose weight fluctuates is more complicated, but it is important that each client understand both the purpose and adjustment of socks. Figure 8.31 depicts instructions that can be given to clients on the care of the socks.

INDIVIDUALS WITH BILATERAL PROSTHESES

The basic gait training activities for a person with bilateral prostheses are similar to those used with patients who have one prosthesis. If the individual ambulated with one prosthesis prior to losing the other limb, the training process is easier. Most individuals with two prostheses need some form of external support, especially for elevation activities.

Considerable time needs to be spent on balance and weight-shifting activities because the individual no longer has any direct contact with the ground. Individuals with two prostheses use a somewhat wider base of support than those with one prosthesis, and many exhibit a tendency to roll a bit from side to side. Although these extraneous movements need to be minimized, they might not be completely eliminated. The client should progress directly from the parallel bars to whatever form of external support will be used at home. A walker is not the external support of choice. Functional outcomes are directly related to the balance, strength, and coordination of the patient and to the levels of amputation. The amount of energy expended must not preclude participation in other activities. The higher the levels of amputation and the more external support needed, the less functional the ambulation.[8]

Because all individuals with one prosthesis need support for times when they are not wearing the prosthesis, those with two prostheses need a wheelchair—one with offset wheels or anterior weights to counter the loss of weight in the front of the chair.

Summary

Training the individual to regain independence in mobility with a prosthesis is a sequential program of balance and basic and advanced gait activities. The discharge environment and the client's functional needs and expectations must be considered in planning an effective treatment program. The training program demands the PT's and PTA's creativity as well as an understanding of motor skills acquisition.

Glossary

Adjuvant therapy	The use of other forms of treatment in addition to the major treatment, usually surgery.
Alignment	The relationship between the different components or parts of the prosthesis in both linear and angular positions.

Doffing	Removing the prosthesis.
Donning	Putting on the prosthesis.
Gait cycle	The period between heel contact of one foot and the next heel contact of the same foot. Includes a period of single stance of each foot, a period of double stance, and a period of swing on each leg.
Furuncle	A boil.
Heel lever arm	The distance from the end of the prosthetic heel to midpoint of the shoe.
Toe lever arm	The distance from the middle of the prosthetic foot to the end of the toe.
Total contact	The residual limb is in contact with all parts of the socket with appropriate pressure.
TKA line	A line drawn from the greater trochanter through the knee axis to the middle of the ankle that is used to align the part of the prosthesis.

References

1. Siriwardena, GJA, and Bertrand, PV: Factors influencing rehabilitation of arteriosclerotic lower limb amputees. J Rehabil Res 28 (3):35–44, 1991.
2. Steen Jensen, J, et al: Prosthetic fitting in lower limb amputees. Acta Orthop Scand 54:101–03, 1983.
3. Traugh, GH, et al: Energy expenditure of ambulation in patients with transfemoral amputations. Arch Phys Med Rehabil 56:67–71, 1975.
4. Waters, RL, et al: The energy cost of walking of amputees—Influence of level of amputation. J Bone Joint Surg (Am) 58:42–46, 1976.
5. Jaegers, SMHJ, et al: The relationship between comfortable and most metabolically efficient walking speed in persons with unilateral above-knee amputation. Arch Phys Med Rehabil 74:521–25, 1993.
6. Waters, RL: The energy expenditure of amputee gait. In Bowker, JH, and Michael, JW (eds): Atlas of Limb Prosthetics: Surgical, Prosthetic and Rehabilitation Principles, ed 2. Mosby Year Book, St. Louis, 1992.
7. Thompson, N: Normal locomotion and prosthetic replacement. In Engstrom, B, and Van de Ven, C: Therapy for Amputees, ed 3. Churchill Livingstone, Edinburgh, 1999.
8. Pinzur, MS, et al: Functional outcome of below-knee amputation in peripheral vascular insufficiency: A multicenter review. Clin Orthop 286:247–49, 1993.
9. Muecke, L, et al: Functional screening of lower-limb amputees: A role in predicting rehabilitation outcome? Arch Phys Med Rehabil 73:851–58, 1992.
10. Nitz, JC: Rehabilitation outcomes after bilateral lower limb amputation for vascular disease. Physiother Theory Pract 9(3):165–170, 1993.
11. Nissen, SJ, and Newman, WP: Factors influencing reintegration to normal living after amputation. Arch Phys Med Rehabil 73:548–51, 1992.
12. Legro, MW, et al: Issues of importance reported by persons with lower limb amputations and prostheses. J Rehabil R & D 36(3):155–63, 1999.
13. Matsen, SL, et al: Correlations with patients' perspectives of the results of lower-extremity amputation. J Bone Joint Surg (Am) 82-A(8):1089–95, 2000.
14. Ehde, DM, et al: Chronic phantom sensations, phantom pain, residual limb pain, and other regional pain after lower limb amputation. Arch Phys Med Rehabil 81(8):1039–44, 2000.
15. Barbera, J, and Albert-Pampl, R: Centrocentral anastomosis of the proximal nerve stump in the treatment of painful amputation neuromas of major nerves. J Neurosurg 79:331–34, 1993.

16. Perry, J: Normal gait. In Bowker, JH, and Michael, JW (eds): Atlas of Limb Prosthetics: Surgical, Prosthetic and Rehabilitation Principles, ed 2. Mosby Year Book, St. Louis, 1992.
17. Dennis, JK, and McKeough, DM: Mobility. In May, BJ: Home Health and Rehabilitation: Concepts of Care. FA Davis, Philadelphia, 1993.
18. Gentile, AM: A working model of skill acquisition with application of teaching. Quest 27:3, 1972.

CHAPTER NINE

Long-Term Care

OBJECTIVES

At the end of this chapter, all students are expected to:

1 Discuss long-term adjustment to living with a prosthesis.
2 Describe methods of teaching activities of daily living (ADL) and instrumental activities of daily living (IADL).
3 Discuss recreational opportunities for individuals of all ages with protheses.
4 Develop a program to teach the client how to care for the prosthesis and residual limb on a long-term basis.

Case Studies

Diana Magnolia is now independent in ambulation with her prosthesis and one cane in the physical therapy department. She can go up and down steps with a handrail and can go up and down a curb as high as 8 inches. She has the prosthesis at home and is receiving therapy from a home health agency.

Ha Lee Davis is independent with his prosthesis and no external support. He was discharged from active therapy after 2 weeks and is going through a work evaluation program sponsored by the State Vocational Rehabilitation Agency. He comes by the physical therapy department one day to ask if he could learn to run competitively with his prosthesis. He states he is interested in getting involved in sports activities but does not know where to turn.

Benny Pearl has been inconsistent in attendance at the outpatient clinic. He spent 2 weeks in the local rehabilitation hospital and was discharged independent in donning and doffing the prosthesis and walking with limits around the house with a quad cane. He takes a long prosthetic step and a short step with his other foot. His wife reports that he needs help to go up and down the three steps outside his house even though there is a handrail; he cannot step down the one step into the screened porch that does not have a rail. She states that he also has difficulty getting up and down from the toilet that is low.

Betty Childs has returned to school with her prosthesis that she wears every-day for all activities. She is not in any active therapy program but returns to the amputee clinic for follow-up.

■ *Case Study Activities*

1 Discuss each of the client's possible long-term psychosocial and financial adjustments to the loss of a limb.
2 What problems might each person have to face to achieve full return to a meaningful life style?

Learning how to walk with a prosthesis is only one component of the rehabilitative process. Living with a prosthesis requires making some changes in lifestyle and daily habits. The individual must cope with new problems that range from learning how to go to the bathroom in the middle of the night to finding gainful employment. Return to a full active life is the goal: the dimensions of that life are differentially defined by each individual. For some it includes vigorous vocational and recreational activities; for others it may mean being able to putter in the garden and walk across the street to visit neighbors. Regardless of lifestyle, each person with an amputation must cope with many physical, psychological, social, and financial adjustments.[1,2]

PROSTHETIC CARE

A prosthesis, just as any mechanical equipment, requires maintenance. Clients also need to be monitored to ensure they are adding socks as the residual limb reduces in size (see Chap. 8). Prosthetists and amputee clinics establish long-term recheck appointments with their clients to ensure proper maintenance of the appliance. Generally, the first reevaluation following discharge from initial training takes place within 1 to 2 months of discharge from therapy. Residual limb shrinkage is likely to have occurred, and it is important to ensure that the client is adjusting socks appropriately. After the client has integrated prosthetic function into daily life and has stabilized medically and functionally, reevaluations can be scheduled on an annual basis.

Ideally the clinic schedule needs to allow time for a full examination by the physical therapist (PT) prior to review by the complete team. The examination allows time to explore any problems and obtain data comparable to previous visits. Table 9.1 outlines the major components of a long-term recheck. The specific tests and measurements vary with each client, the type of prosthesis and the cause of amputation. The first prosthesis usually lasts 1 to 2 years, depending on the amount of soft tissue in the residual limb at the time of initial fitting, the activity level of the client, and whether the client gains or loses weight. Weight gain is a major problem. Many individuals, particularly those who do not return to a premorbid level of activity, tend to gain weight from overeating and inactivity. Obviously the prosthesis does not expand with the residual limb, and the client may soon find that the residual limb no longer fits into the socket. Continued wear in such instances leads to skin breakdowns and abrasions.

The prosthesis itself needs to be checked to make sure all components are in good condition and functioning properly. Clients need to be encouraged to return to the prosthetist for repairs rather than employ a "do it yourself" approach (Fig. 9.1). Some individuals try to make small repairs themselves, such

TABLE 9.1   LONG-TERM REEVALUATION

Interview	Prosthetic wear pattern
	Number of days
	Length of time each day
	Reason for wear pattern
	Comfort level with prosthesis
	Activities performed with or without prosthesis
	Adequacy of sock supply
	General medical health
	Condition of other foot
Residual limb	Skin condition
	Circumference measurements
	Range of motion of proximal joint
	Muscle strength
Nonamputated leg (if dysvascular)	Condition of skin, particularly foot and ankle
	Presence of any sores or ulcers
	Presence of edema
	Gross range of motion of major joints, particularly foot and ankle
	Gross strength of major muscles
Prosthesis	Socket fit and number of plys worn
	Condition of:
	Socket and liner if used
	Suspension
	Joints
	Foot
	Shank or cosmetic cover
Gait pattern	Gait deviations
	Ancillary support used
	Changes since discharge from physical therapy (PT)
Other	Condition of shoe, particularly heel height
	Weight as compared to discharge from PT
	Specific tests required for particular disability

as taping a loose strap or crack or using regular socks rather than stump socks. It is advisable for the therapist to deter such action because the client may unknowingly cause more serious damage. Inculcating a positive attitude toward regular prosthetic maintenance will lead to better fit and a more functional prosthesis over a longer period of time. In time, the client will need a new prosthesis either because of residual limb shrinkage, component wear, or both. In a recent international study, it was reported that over a 10-year period clients needed an average of 5 new prostheses, 6 major refits, and 17 minor repairs. Individuals under the age of 60 required more refits and more minor repairs.[3]

Although many clients like to continue with the type of prosthesis they have used before, new components that may improve function or comfort should be considered by the PT and client. Individuals who have worn a prosthesis for many years need to be introduced to the many technological changes that have improved prosthetic fit, comfort, and function. One study recommended allowing the individual to try a new component for 1 week before making a final decision and that final alignment should not be made for 3 weeks to be sure the gait has stabilized.[4]

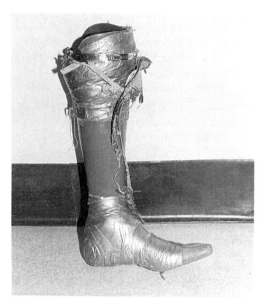

FIGURE 9.1
A "self-repaired" prosthesis as it was worn into the clinic.

VOCATIONAL ADJUSTMENT

Many individuals with amputations are able to return to their preamputation employment situation, although sometimes a change in assigned work within the same company is required. A change that leads to lower job status or a decrease in salary tends to increase the person's feelings of inadequacy. For some, a return to preamputation employment is not possible, and the individual must seek other vocational placement. Often it is the individual from lower educational and socioeconomic levels who has the most difficulty finding gainful employment after amputation. In all states, the Department of Vocational Rehabilitation (different states may have different names) use federal and state funds to help disabled individuals of working age return to the workforce. The help may include providing a prosthesis, rehabilitation, and job retraining and placement. The extent of help available is determined by many factors including available funds. Despite the American with Disabilities Act (ADA) that prohibits discrimination on the basis of disability, some employers are reluctant to hire handicapped individuals. Counselors from the Department of Vocational Rehabilitation can be educative to both clients and employers. Many factors affect the employability of individuals with amputations including the general economic status of the country and the attitudes of employers in the community.

Many individuals who sustain lower extremity amputation are retired either because of complex medical problems or because they have reached retirement age. The demands to be met in satisfactory adaptation to retirement are as many as to employment.

■ *Case Study Activities*

1 Assume you are part of a PT/physical therapist assistant (PTA) team working with Diana Magnolia at home. Discuss and practice the ac-

tivities you would teach her to help her reach full independence in all ADLs and IADLs.

2   How would you answer Ha Lee Davis' questions about running and sports activities? Explore special components, programs, and adapted equipment.

3   Assume you are part of a PT/PTA team working with Benny Pearl in the PT department of a hospital outpatient center. Discuss and practice the activities you would teach him to achieve the goals of getting in and out of his house and using the bathroom safely. Explore the need for any special equipment.

4   Explore the functional and social issues Betty might face as she enters the teenaged years.

ACTIVITIES OF DAILY LIVING

The individual must master many activities once basic walking and climbing stairs have been mastered. Basic ADLs include self-care and mobility in the home, such as walking, using the toilet, getting in and out of a bathtub, and the like. IADLs include activities necessary for broad functions such as going shopping, using the phone, cooking, and the like. Advanced activities usually occur in an open environment. Walking on sand, city streets, farmlands, and grass are very different from walking inside a house or therapy department. Learning to cross the street during the green or walk light can be an adventure. The ability to move from place to place independently is of paramount importance in today's lifestyle. Unanticipated barriers can sometimes lead to difficulty, and the wise PT or PTA anticipates such barriers and helps the individual learn to surmount them. For example, escalators can seem as difficult to surmount as mountains when the patient first encounters them. A person with relatively good balance can step on and off the escalator with the sound foot on both ascent and descent. Individuals who use crutches or whose balance is not secure are better advised to use elevators. Theater rows or church pews may represent other significant obstacles. The individual needs to be able to sidestep as well as step backwards securely before taking the prosthesis outside. Sidestepping, facing the already seated patrons, allows the individual to use back and arm rests for any unexpected loss of balance. There is also the issue of adequate knee flexion to allow the foot to be tucked under the seat and out of the way.

Advanced Activities

Individuals with an amputation below the knee generally learn advanced activities relatively easily. Regardless of the level of amputation, the PT or PTA needs to ensure that the client is able to perform each of these activities without the possibility of falling (Fig. 9.2. 9.3, 9.4, and 9.5). Depending on the client's physiological state, balance, and frailty, falling may or may not be practiced. The client needs to be advised to try to fall away from the prosthesis and to put the body weight on the uninvolved side. If the activity is practiced, it is a good idea to practice both forward and backward falling. Although it is not appropriate to practice falling with all clients, methods of self-protection should be discussed routinely. Many elderly individuals who are quite functional without external support in the home need a cane outside the home to ensure extra balance.

Some individuals with one transtibial prosthesis can go up and down stairs one step over the other, depending on the length of the residual limb, the height of the step, and the person's balance and coordination. Extending the knee, as is required by this activity, drives the anterior distal end of the residual limb into the anterior socket wall. Individuals with sensitive skin and poor balance should not attempt this maneuver. Some clients prefer to go up and down steps one step at a time, leading with the sound leg going up and the prosthesis going down. The amount of advanced training varies with the level of amputation and the balance and coordination of the client.

Most people with a transtibial prosthesis can walk on ramps and inclines with little difficulty. Many of today's dynamic response feet permit enough dorsiflexion to allow a step-over-step pattern on ramps and hills. More rigid keel feet and steeper hills may require more knee flexion or even a shorter prosthetic step. Individuals with limited balance and coordination need to be taught each of the advanced activities; the more active individuals quickly develop their own techniques after they have learned the basics and have had some practice.

Active clients with long transfemoral residual limbs and good balance and coordination can learn to go down steps one leg over the other, flexing (breaking) the prosthetic knee on alternate steps regardless of the type of knee. Many hydraulic knee mechanisms allow a controlled flexion moment, facili-

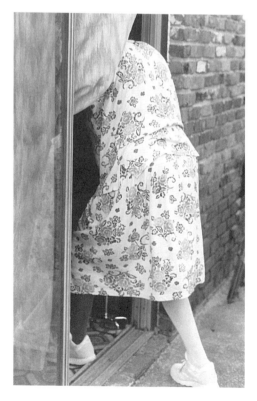

FIGURE 9.2

Independence requires the ability to get into and out of the home.

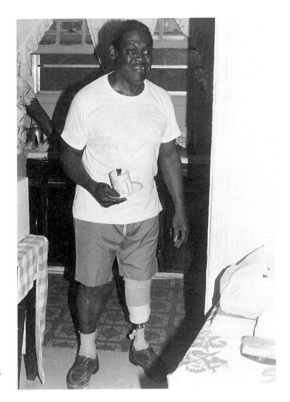

FIGURE 9.3
Carrying an object from room to room enhances balance and coordination training.

tating a step-over-step descent. The client must be taught to place the prosthetic foot only halfway on the step to create a flexion moment as the weight is shifted forward.

Stance-control knee units usually do not allow a step-over-step descent because the same mechanism that controls stance with the knee slightly flexed will interfere with the flexion action of going down a step. A step-over-step ascent is much more difficult unless the person has a long residual limb and the step is shallow. The activities outlined in Tables 9.2 and 9.3 are generally designed for individuals wearing single transfemoral prostheses but can be easily adapted for those with one transtibial or other prosthesis.

Ambulatory individuals with two transtibial or one transtibial and one transfemoral prostheses need to adapt the activities. Individuals with two prostheses use a wider base of support and external support such as a cane or crutches. Those with two transtibial prostheses usually lead with the longer residual limb going up the steps and the shorter limb going down steps (Fig. 9.6). Individuals with one transfemoral and one transtibial prosthesis must lead with the transtibial prosthesis going up steps and the transfemoral limb going down. One or two handrails or a handrail and a cane are usually necessary for independent stair climbing. It is unusual for an individual to regain functional ambulation with two transfemoral prostheses because of the excessive energy required.

Teaching advanced activities must be individualized, depending on the type of prostheses, type of knee control and agility of the individual. Those who ambulate with two transfemoral prostheses often have a manual or hydraulic knee lock on one side to provide needed stability for ACLs. Climbing

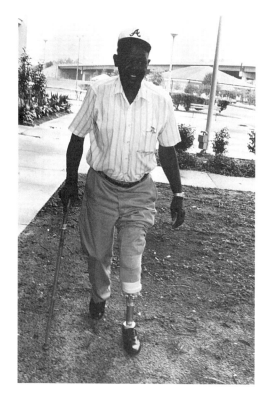

FIGURE 9.4
Learning to walk on uneven ground is part of prosthetic training.

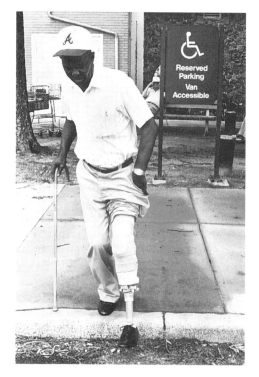

FIGURE 9.5
Crossing the street is a necessary advanced activity.

stairs, getting up and down from a chair, and getting up and down from the floor are very difficult activities for individuals with bilateral transfemoral prostheses or one transfemoral and one transtibial prosthesis. They can also be a challenge for individuals with bilateral transtibial prostheses, especially for individuals with any balance, coordination, or strength deficits.

Other Activities

For many people, independent mobility means driving a car. Depending on the side and level of amputation, adjustments to the automobile may or may not be necessary. For the client with a right-sided amputation, switching the gas or brake pedal for use with the left foot may be necessary. Individuals with bilateral lower extremity amputations need hand controls that allow safe operation of the accelerator and brake (Fig. 9.7). Most mechanics can install hand controls or make necessary adaptations to automobiles. Some individuals, particularly those with transfemoral or hip disarticulation amputations, may encounter difficulty getting in and out of the automobile, particularly if it has bucket seats. Vans and sports utility vehicles also create problems because of the height of the entry. Two-door vehicles fitted with bench seats offer more

TABLE 9.2   ADVANCED ACTIVITIES IN THE HOME

Activity	Procedure
Sitting on the floor	Place the prosthesis about half a step behind the sound foot, keeping the weight on the sound foot. Bend from the waist and flex at the knees and hips, reaching for the floor with both arms outstretched and pivoting to the sound side. Then, gradually lower the body to the floor. This activity is one continuous movement.
Getting up from the floor	Get on hands and knees. Place the sound leg forward, well under the trunk, with the foot flat on the floor while balancing on the hands and the prosthetic knee. Then, extend the sound knee while maintaining the weight over the sound leg. Move to an erect position by pushing strongly with the sound leg and the arms bringing the prosthesis forward when almost erect.
Kneeling	Place the sound foot ahead of the prosthetic foot, keeping the weight on the sound leg. Slowly flex the trunk, hip, and knees until the prosthetic knee can be gently placed on the floor. Clients with transfemoral prostheses can usually kneel on the prosthetic leg, but those with transtibial prostheses find that the patellar bar creates too much pressure in this position. Clients with transtibial prostheses usually kneel on the sound side. Getting up from a kneeling position is like getting up from the floor.
Falling forward	With toes against the mat, pitch forward, breaking the fall with the arms outstretched, thus absorbing the shock with slightly flexed elbows. Partial weight may then be transferred to both knees or rolled onto the unaffected hip, then shoulder.
Falling backward	Flex at the waist so that the buttocks strike the mat first, then roll backward onto the rounded back and shoulders.
Picking up an object from the floor	Place the sound foot ahead of the prosthetic foot with the body weight remaining on the sound leg. Bend forward at the waist, flexing hips and knees until the object can be reached. Care must be taken to maintain weight on the sound leg. Some individuals like to bend sideways rather than forward, while others find it easier to keep the prosthetic knee straight and bend the sound leg until the object can be picked up.

TABLE 9.3 ADVANCED ACTIVITIES OUTSIDE THE HOME

Activity	Procedure
Up and down steps	Lead with the sound foot going up, taking one or two steps at a time. To clear the edge of the step with the prosthesis, extend and slightly abduct the hip and place the prosthetic foot next to the sound foot. Although a handrail may be used for initial practice, full functional rehabilitation requires the ability to go up and down steps without a handrail. Going down, the client leads with the prosthetic foot, making sure the knee is kept locked during weight bearing. The sound leg is brought down on the same step. To go down one leg over the other, place the heel of the prosthetic foot on the edge of the step; shift the weight over the prosthesis, keeping the knee extended. When the sound leg is in position to recover on the next step, flex the prosthetic hip, allowing the knee to buckle, and let the weight go onto the sound leg. Then, extend the prosthetic knee to swing the shin forward over the next lowest step and quickly shift the body weight onto the prosthesis. Continue in a rhythmic progression.
Going up and down inclines	Lead with the sound leg going up inclines, taking a slightly longer step than usual. Hike the prosthetic hip enough to prevent the toe from catching and swing the prosthesis through; avoid abducting it. Take a somewhat shorter step with the prosthetic leg, making sure the knee is extended during weight bearing. The shorter step with the prosthesis compensates for the limited dorsiflexion of the SACH foot. Some trunk flexion may also be needed on very steep hills. Continue up the incline in the line of progression. On very steep hills or for individuals with balance problems, the diagonal method may be more effective. Ascend on the diagonal leading with the sound leg and keeping the prosthetic leg slightly behind the sound leg. On very difficult or slippery inclines, sidestepping, leading with the sound leg, may be the technique of choice. Lead with the prosthetic leg going down an incline, taking a somewhat smaller step than usual and taking particular care to keep the knee extended. Shift weight over the prosthesis and, when the sound foot is in a position to recover, voluntarily flex the prosthetic knee, catching body weight on the sound leg. Modifications include using shorter steps, using repeated single steps, and descending sideways.
Clearing obstacles	Face the obstacle with the sound foot slightly in front and the body weight on the prosthesis. Step over the obstacle with the sound leg, then transfer body weight to the sound leg. Quickly extending the prosthetic hip, forcefully flex the prosthetic hip, whipping the prosthesis forward over the obstacle. Then step forward with a normal gait pattern. An alternative method is to stand sideways to the obstacle with the sound leg closest to the obstacle. With weight on the prosthesis, swing the sound leg over the obstacle and transfer the body weight to the sound leg. Then swing the prosthesis forward, up, and over the obstacle.
Running	Step forward with the sound leg, then shift body weight to the sound leg and hop forward on the sound side. Swing prosthesis forward and shift body weight onto the prosthesis for momentary support. Immediately transfer weight to the sound leg and continue hop-skip running. Some energy-conserving or multiaxis feet allow a faster foot flat; slight dorsiflexion in foot alignment allows the amputee to take a longer stride on the sound side. Increased knee friction or a hydraulic unit helps control the swing of the shank during running.

room for entry and exit. Individuals who have a left prosthesis encounter few problems entering the driver's door but may have difficulty entering the right passenger door. On the left, they sit in the usual manner and bring the prosthesis in after them. On the right, they need to put the prosthesis in the car first. The situation is reversed for people with a prosthesis on the right. A low steering wheel may limit entrance for people with a right transfemoral prosthesis. Cars with adjustable steering wheels make entry and exit easier as do cars with electric seats. It is much more difficult to enter the back seat in a two-door car.

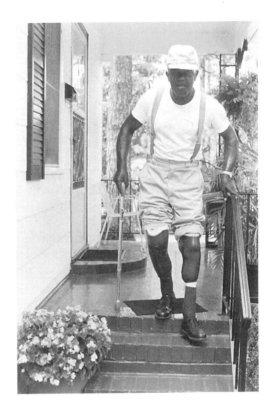

FIGURE 9.6
A client with bilateral transtibial amputations
practices going up and down steps.

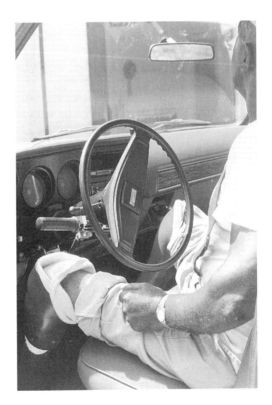

FIGURE 9.7
A client with bilateral amputations can drive with
hand controls.

Public transportation presents hazards, particularly for individuals whose agility, strength, and balance may be impaired or for those with multiple amputations. Some individuals are unable to pull themselves up the bus's high first step or cope with the stairs in and out of a subway. In some communities adapted buses are available. The so-called "kneeling" buses can lower the front end to simultaneously lower the height of the first step. Most clients have no particular problems with trains or airplanes other than the limited leg room available between seats. The individual with an amputation, particularly at the transfemoral level, may want to choose an aisle seat with the prosthesis close to the aisle. Canes or crutches may be taken by flight attendants during takeoffs and landings. Individuals who cannot ambulate independently need to make special arrangements with the airlines prior to any flight.

In some instances the home needs to be adjusted to make it possible for the person to function independently. Individuals with more than one amputation or those using a wheelchair when not wearing the prosthesis may have difficulty getting in and out of the bathroom or around a two-story house. Outside steps without a handrail pose a hazard particularly in icy weather. Early planning is necessary, and a home visit by the therapist can prevent later problems. Elderly individuals may not have the reserves for the energy demands of everyday living with a transfemoral prosthesis and may need to alter location of a bedroom or bathroom to allow the clients to function on one floor of the home. It is a good idea for the therapist to ask the family to do a home evaluation at the onset of training. There are a number of forms that can be used for the home evaluation; the client's degree of disability determines how thorough the home evaluation needs to be. Someone like Ha Lee Davis will probably not need any adaptations, whereas someone like Benny Pearl may well require special home changes. May[5] published a home evaluation form that is user friendly and adaptable to many situations.

Living with a prosthesis also means adjusting to numerous minor changes in everyday life. The person may not be able to walk as fast as in the past. He or she may need to alter type of clothing and cope with the problem of changing shoes. The prosthesis was initially aligned to one pair of shoes, and there is little adaptation to major changes in a client's other shoes' heel height. Most dynamic response feet provide some leeway (see Chap. 7), but going from athletic shoes to spike heels is not possible without totally changing feet. This problem is often not mentioned until after the client has been fitted. Many people today wear dress shoes for work, athletic shoes for leisure times, boots in the winter, and sandals in the summer. Each type of shoe has a different height heel and different configuration, yet most prosthetic feet are not adaptable to different heel heights. The prosthesis is aligned from the ground up, and heel height changes are reflected in flexion or extension moments at the knee (see Chap. 8). A felt insert in the heel of athletic shoes moderates the problem of the lower heel but does not solve the problem of higher heel shoes. Boots restrict the ankle movements of the prosthetic foot, and sandals are contraindicated for individuals with peripheral vascular disease. As discussed in Chapter 7, the human foot provides both response properties, responding to a variety of demands and providing both support and energy return, and it accommodates to various terrains and surfaces.

There are prosthetic feet that provide a high degree of response properties and others that accommodate well to varied terrains, but few seem to provide both a high degree of response and good accommodation (see Chap. 7). Different activities require different foot characteristics, but it is not practical for most people to have a different prosthesis for each activity. Prosthetic feet today come in many designs and configurations. The human foot can provide a high degree of accommodation as well as a high level of response, but it seems that prosthetic feet excel in offering one or the other characteristics but not both.[6] Selecting the prosthetic foot must include careful consideration of the individual's planned activities. High-level athletes, however, often have several prostheses including ones constructed specially for the particular sport.

Individuals with upper extremity loss likewise need to adapt to the demands of everyday life. As indicated in Chapter 10, the loss of sensation associated with upper extremity prosthetic replacement is a major loss, and many individuals find that the prosthesis does not provide enough function. Many individuals with upper extremity amputation choose not to use a prosthetic replacement. Individuals with a prosthesis must learn to integrate that prosthesis into the everyday common ADLs (Fig. 9.8).

RECREATIONAL ACTIVITIES

The importance of sport and leisure activities also needs to be considered for the client with an amputation. A full and satisfying lifestyle includes the abil-

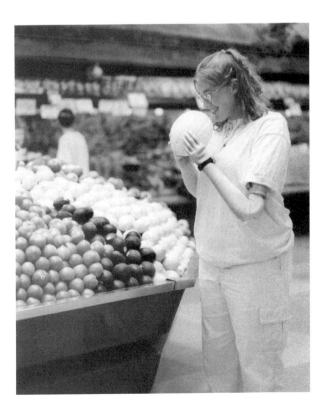

FIGURE 9.8
A woman shops for groceries.
(Courtesy of Motion Control.)
(www.utaharm.com)

ity to participate in avocational activities to improve physical fitness, sociability, self-confidence, and fun.

Many activities require little or no adaptation of the prosthesis or of movement patterns. Even those with multiple amputations and those who function primarily with a wheelchair can enjoy playing cards, gardening, or even bowling. More athletically inclined clients can engage in team or individual sports including golf, skiing, swimming, and basketball.

Kegel and associates[7] surveyed l00 individuals with unilateral lower extremity amputations to determine their involvement in sports activities. Sixty percent of the respondents were active in sports ranging from fishing to jogging. Age rather than level of amputation appeared to be the major factor influencing participation. Most returned to preamputation sports, particularly if the activity did not require running or jumping. Most found it difficult to jog or go hunting because these activities placed considerable stress on the residual limb. The majority of respondents wore their regular prosthesis for recreational activities. Seven individuals had special waterproof prostheses, eight used rotation devices in the shank of the prosthesis, and seven used assistive devices such as crutches or outriggers. Only 28 believed that the prosthetist was knowledgeable about available components for sports, and several had designed their own adaptations. Prosthetists who were also surveyed indicated that cost was a major factor in the fabrication of special prostheses for sports, particularly because most third-party payers do not fund recreational limbs.[4] Gailey[8] reported on a survey involving 1214 individuals with amputations. The sample was not totally representative, because 57 percent had lost a limb secondary to trauma. However, 60 percent of respondents stated they returned to premorbid activities within 1 year of amputation, and 76 percent indicated they participated in some recreational activities including golf, swimming, fishing, and walking. Not all individuals wore their prosthesis for all recreational activities, and about 10 percent reported not wearing the prosthesis at all. There were little differences between age groups. Although the survey questionnaires were sent to 4000 individuals across the country, Gailey suggested that more sedentary individuals who had not achieved their desired goals might not have wanted to respond.[8]

During the Vietnam Conflict (1957–1975), the U.S. Army developed a program to teach individuals who had lost limbs how to ski. Those with both unilateral and bilateral amputations learned to ski using one ski and two outriggers. The sports program expanded to include many other activities such as horseback riding, swimming, and even sky diving.[9] Most clients ski on the sound leg with one or two forearm crutches to which a short ski foresection has been attached; this is sometimes referred to as three-track skiing.[10]

Many people with one prosthesis also continue with ballroom dancing, bowling, and weight lifting. Gymnastic and fitness activities can be performed by those with two as well as one amputation with little adaptations. Individuals wearing prostheses are able to ice skate and rollerskate with little difficulty. The heel height of the prosthetic foot must accommodate the height of the skate shoe. Athletically inclined individuals should be encouraged to participate in vigorous physical activities. In too many instances, PTs and PTAs encourage younger clients to pursue exercises and active recreation but refrain from making similar recommendations to older clients who may well be in greater need of such encouragement. PTs and PTAs need to encourage all clients to participate in fitness activities and to encourage them to lead an active lifestyle.

Outdoor activities, such as camping, fishing, swimming, and water skiing are also fairly easy to perform with little adaptation. Care should be taken around water to protect the prosthesis from dampness. There are special prostheses for water activities from the Endolite Aqualimb Prostheses (Fig. 9.9A) to the Bock Swim leg. The Aqualimb is designed for showering and has a special nonskid sole (Fig. 9.9B). Some swim prostheses incorporate a hinged ankle that can be locked at 90 degrees of plantar flexion for walking or hinged to 100 degrees for swimming. The Otto Bock Co. (*www.bockus.com*) has a knee mechanism that can be used in water. Most clients including Para-

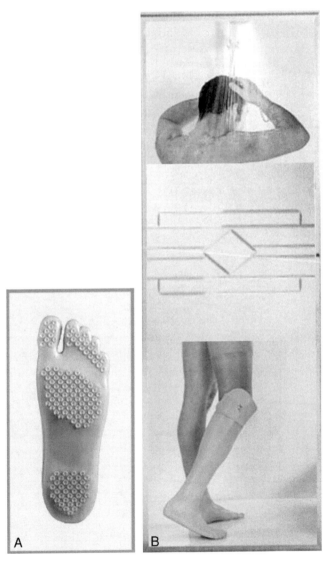

FIGURE 9.9

Endolite Aqualimb. (*A*) Sole of the prothesis designed to provide traction on wet surface. (*B*) Man showering with prosthesis. (Courtesy of Endolite USA)

lympic athletes swim without a prosthesis. Adapted swim fins are useful for individuals with bilateral lower extremity amputations. Some individuals wrap the leg in special plastic if they will be around water.

Hiking and hunting require walking over uneven ground, which is stressful on the residual limb. Some individuals use old prostheses that have larger sockets and pad the residual limb to reduce torque and rotational stress. Many of the split-keel feet provide good adaptation to uneven ground.

There are adaptations and socket designs that make participation in sports easier. The Hanger Comfort Flex socket lessens the risk of tissue trauma from constant loading and unloading through the socket design and the socket materials that contract and expand as the individual moves[10] (see Chap. 7). A torsion pylon improves shock absorption; rotational components can be installed in the shank of the transfemoral prosthesis that enable the individual to turn the body with the foot planted, as is required in golf. Some individuals, particularly those with bilateral lower limb amputations, use adapted wheelchairs.[11]

Highly motivated individuals participate in most sports. Lightweight components, specially designed knee and foot mechanisms, computer-operated limbs, new and lightweight materials, and well-suspended lightweight sockets have increased the competitive abilities of many individuals with amputa-

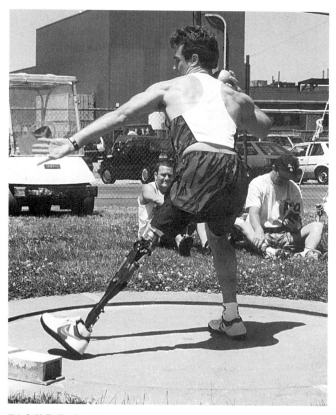

FIGURE 9.10
Mark D'Amico participates in the shotput event in the 1995 National Wheelchair and Amputee Championships.
(From Julie, Gaydos: Orthotic and Prosthetic Athlete Assistance Fund and Mark D'Amico, with permission.)

tions. There are a great number of handicapped athletic organizations for all levels of athletes. Most can be found on the Web by a search on "disabled sports" or similar. Skilled athletes have successfully participated in competitive sports events all over the world including the Paralympics that are now scheduled the month after the regular Olympics in the same city (Fig. 9.10). Prosthetic manufacturing companies sponsor a number of athletes who help test new components (Fig. 9.11). In the 2000 Paralympics, the winner of the women's 100- and 200-m dashes set new world records; each was only a few seconds slower than the winners of the regular 2000 Olympics. The winner of the men's 100-m dash was also in world record time and close to the regular Olympic time.

Enoka and associates[12] studied the running gait of 10 physically active clients with a unilateral transtibial amputation; 6 were able to run (defined as alternating periods of single support and complete nonsupport in the stride) at speeds ranging from 2.7 to 8.2 m/sec. Three others achieved periods of nonsupport from the intact limb but not from the prosthesis. Only one individual who had sustained some brain damage was unable to produce nonsupport from either extremity. Marked differences were found in the components of

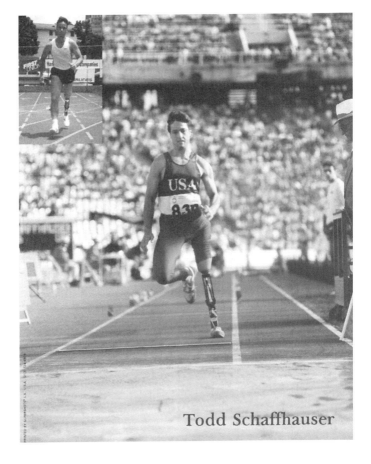

FIGURE 9.11

Todd Schaffhauser uses the Endolite high-activity limb in the 1992 Paralympics in Barcelona. (Courtesy of the Endolite Corporation.)

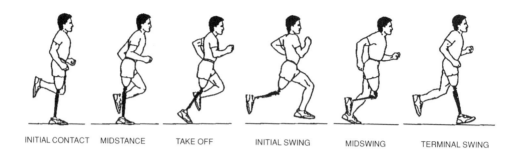

INITIAL CONTACT   MIDSTANCE   TAKE OFF   INITIAL SWING   MIDSWING   TERMINAL SWING

FIGURE 9.12

Running with a transfemoral prosthesis. (From Gailey, RS, Jr.: Physical therapy management of adult lower limb amputees. In Bowker, JH, and Michael, JW: Atlas of Limb Prosthetics: Surgical, Prosthetic ,and Rehabilitation Principles, ed 2. Mosby Year Book, St. Louis, 1992, with permission.)

the gait among clients. Over time, each achieved some skill and developed some endurance. Lightweight well-fitted prostheses with foot mobility were the most advantageous. Running can be a useful sports activity for people with one transtibial amputation, although more work is needed to develop appropriate prosthetic components.[12] Figure 9.12 depicts the running gait of an individual with a transfemoral amputation and a responsive prosthesis. Figure 9.13 depicts an individual running with the transtibial prosthesis.

Individuals with amputations also participate in team sports, although wearing the prosthesis is not always allowed. The National Federation of State High School Associations allows children with lower extremity amputations, particularly transtibial, to wear their prostheses while participating in team sports such as football. The rules specify requirements for padding and stipulate that wearing the prosthesis must not place the opponent at a disadvantage. Children with amputations play football, baseball, and volleyball, and even wrestle.[13,14,15] Individuals with amputations participate in wheelchair basketball, and many have participated in the wheelchair Olympics. The International Sports Organization for the Disabled classifies handicapped individuals for participation in various sports activities. Leisure and competitive events of all types are available to the person with an amputation.[11,14,15] Table 9.4 lists organizations that may be contacted for further information.

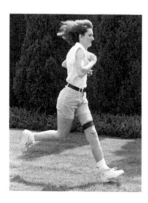

FIGURE 9.13

Running with a transtibial prosthesis.

TABLE 9.4   RECREATIONAL ASSOCIATIONS
FOR HANDICAPPED PERSONS

American Athletic Association for the Deaf
3607 Washington Blvd., #4
Ogden, UT 84403
(801) 393-8710 (voice); 7916 (TTY)

Adapted Sports Association, Inc.
Box 538
Pine Lane
Charleston, GA 30072

Aircraft Hands Control
Ed Stakleman
P.O. Box 207
Sturgis, KY 42459

American Alliance for Health, Physical Education,
    and Recreation
1900 Assoc Dr.
Reston, VA 20191

American Water Ski Association
P.O. Box 191
Winter Haven, FL 33880

American Wheelchair Pilots Association
4419 North 27th St.
Phoenix, AZ 85016

Amputees in Motion
Box 2703
Escondido, CA 92025

National Handicapped Sports
451 Hungerford Dr., Suite 100
Rockville, MD 20850
(301) 217-0960

National Wheelchair Athletic Association
3595 East Fountain Blvd., Suite L-1
Colorado Springs, CO 80910

US Association of Blind Athletes
33 North Institute St.
Colorado Springs, CO 80903
(719) 630-0422

US Les Autres Sports Association
1475 W. Gray, Suite 166
Houston, TX 77019
(713) 521-3737

US Wheelchair Racquet Sports Association
1941 Viento Verano Drive
Diamond Bar, CA 91765

Dwarf Athletic Association of America
418 Willow Way
Lewisville, TX 75067
(214) 317-8299

Adaptive Sports Program
6832 Marlette Road
Marlette, MI 48453

American Amputee Foundation
Box 55218, Hillcrest Station
Little Rock, AR 72225

American Camping Association
Bradford Woods
Martinsville, IN 46151

American Wheelchair Bowling Association
N54W15858
Menomonee Falls, WI 53051

Amputee Golfers Association
Box 5801
Coralville, IA 52241
(800) 633-NAGA

Amputee Soccer International
c/o Johnson and Higgins
1215 Fourth Ave
Seattle, WA 98161

International WC Road Racers
30 Myano Lane, Box 3
Stamford, CT 06902

Handicapped SCUBA Association
116 West El Portal, Suite 104
San Clemente, CA 92672

International Sports Organization for the Disabled
1600 James Naismith Drive
Gloucester, Ontario, K1B 5N4
Canada

US Cerebral Palsy Athletic Association
3810 W. Northwest Highway, #205
Dallas, TX 75220
(214) 351-1510

Wheelchair Sports USA
3595 E. Fountain Blvd., #L-1
Colorado Springs, CO 80910
(719) 574-1150

US Amputee Athletic Association
Box 560686
Charlotte, NC 28256

However, more up-to-date information can probably be obtained through a web search.

Living with an amputation requires physical and emotional adjustments. To a great extent, the fullness of the client's life is determined by factors that affect most of our lives—family support, financial security, and a healthy body. An amputation does not mitigate against any of these factors, and each person has to develop an individual approach to a satisfying life. The attitude of the PT and PTA can influence the client's attitude towards the amputation. Modern components and improved surgical and rehabilitation techniques can all contribute to a full and satisfying life for all individuals with amputations, regardless of age. In most instances, disability is the result of medical problems other than the amputation itself.

Summary

Rehabilitation of individuals with one or more amputations is not complete until the person returns to the most fulfilling life possible. Too often PTs and PTAs set limited ambulatory goals for the elderly individual with an amputation and rarely inform the person of the potential for participation in a full array of activities. Current reimbursement policies negatively influence the ability to help the individual develop competence in advanced activities. If full training is not possible, teaching basic and advanced activities, as well as exposure to the potential for recreational pursuits, needs to be a part of the total rehabilitation program. Long-term follow-up is also necessary to ensure the continued function of appliances and to prevent complications.

References

1. MacBride, A, et al: Psychosocial factors in the rehabilitation of elderly amputees. Psychosomatics 21:258–265, 1980.
2. Comfort, A. Sexual Consequences of Disability. George F. Stickley, Philadelphia, 1978.
3. Datta, D, et al: Analyses of prosthetic episodes in transtibial amputees. Prosthet Orthot Int 23 (1):9–12, 1999.
4. English, RD, et al: Establishment of consistent gait after fitting new components. J Rehabil R & D 32:32–35, 1995.
5. May, BJ: The home environment. In May, BJ: Home Health and Rehabilitation, ed 2. FA Davis, Philadelphia, 1999.
6. Romo, HD: Specialized prostheses for activities: An update. Clin Orthop Rel Res 361:63–70, 1999.
7. Kegel, B, et al: Recreational activities of lower extremity amputees: A survey. Arch Phys Med Rehabil 61:258–264, 1980.
8. Gailey, RS, Jr: Recreational pursuits for elders with amputation. Top Geriatr Rehabil 8(1):39–58, 1992.
9. Smith, JP: In what sports can patients with amputations and other handicaps successfully and actively participate? Phys Ther 50:121-126 1970.
10. Carroll, K, et al: Physical activity and sports: Raising expectations and improving outcomes for persons with amputations. Foot Ankle Clin N Am 4(1):159–175, 1999.
11. Kegel, B: Adaptations for sports and recreation. In Bowker, JH, and Michael, JW (eds): Atlas of Limb Prosthetics: Surgical, Prosthetic, and Rehabilitation Principles, ed 2. Mosby Year Book, St. Louis, 1992.
12. Enoka, RM, et al: Below-knee amputee running gait. Am J Phys Med 61:66–84, 1982.
13. Adams, RC, et al: Games, Sports and Exercises for the Physically Handicapped, ed 3. Lea & Febinger, Philadelphia, 1982.

14. Dodds, JW: Sports and amputees. In Karacoloff, LA, et al: Lower Extremity Amputation: A Guide to Functional Outcomes in Physical Therapy Management, ed 2. Aspen, Gaithersburg, Md., 1992.
15. Burgess, EM, and Rappoport, A: Physical fitness: A guide for individuals with lower limb loss. Department of Veterans Affairs: Veterans Health Administration, Washington DC, 1992.

CHAPTER TEN

Upper Limb Amputations

Joan Edelstein

OBJECTIVES

This chapter will enable the reader to:

1 List the etiologies for upper limb amputation.
2 Describe upper limb amputation surgery.
3 Outline a program for postsurgical management.
4 Compare the prosthetic replacements for the human hand.
5 Indicate the components of the most common transradial (below-elbow) prostheses.
6 Develop a training program for a patient fitted with a unilateral transradial prosthesis.

Upper limb amputation impacts many activities usually identified by the individual as essential to support physical, social, and psychological well-being and create a personal sense of meaningful living.[1] Because arm loss is much less frequent than lower limb loss, physical therapists (PTs), physical therapist assistants (PTAs), and other clinicians are unlikely to acquire substantial experience with such patients, unless employed by a specialized rehabilitation center. Nevertheless, it is important to recognize the basic elements of surgical and postoperative care, as well as the extent of contemporary prosthetic replacement so that one is prepared to treat the occasional patient. The purpose of this chapter is to introduce clinicians to the major considerations in management of clients with upper limb loss. Although amputation occurs at every level, from loss of a phalanx to loss of an entire limb, prosthetic use is most likely among individuals with transradial (below-elbow) amputation.[2-5] Consequently, this chapter focuses on rehabilitation of a man who ultimately will be fitted with a transradial prosthesis. Many treatment principles already described for patients with lower limb amputation apply to individuals with loss of the upper limb.

Case Study

Hector Rodriguez, 41 years old, is a machinist who sustained amputation when a faulty band saw severed his left, dominant, hand. He was referred to physical therapy 3 days after surgical revision of the wound.

■ *Case Study Activities*

1 What are the most pertinent elements of the examination?
2 What are the patient's likely psychological responses?
3 What measures should be instituted to foster optimal independence in daily activities?
4 How should he be prepared for prosthetic fitting?
5 What practice pattern(s) is the most appropriate for this type of problem?

SURGERY

By far, the most typical patient with upper limb amputation is a young man who has sustained trauma.[6] Although improvements in microsurgery occasionally enable limb reimplantation, good functional outcome is more likely in younger patients with more distal injuries.[7] Other common etiologies such as congenital limb anomaly and bone tumors affect children or young adults; consequently, healing usually is rapid. Following surgical amputation or revision of a traumatically severed limb, the arm segment is encased in a rigid plaster of Paris dressing, a semirigid Unna dressing, or simply in sterile gauze. Both the Unna dressing and the plaster cast prevent formation of edema, thus reducing postoperative pain and hastening healing.[8] The plaster cast can serve as the foundation for a prosthesis to enable the patient to grasp objects soon after surgery; such usage is associated with greater likelihood of eventual acceptance of a permanent prosthesis.[9] The limb, which has been wrapped in Unna dressing, can be placed in a temporary prosthesis. Gauze dressing is easy to remove for wound inspection but does not control edema nor permit attachment of a temporary prosthesis. Most children with congenital limb absence do not require surgical revision. Patients with tumors may be treated with a combination of surgery and radiation. The level of amputation will be determined by the site and extent of the tumor.

POSTSURGICAL MANAGEMENT

The goals of postsurgical management are to:

1. Achieve wound healing.
2. Reduce pain.
3. Maintain mobility of all proximal joints.
4. Maintain motor power at all proximal joints.
5. Enable the patient to achieve maximum independence in daily activities.
6. Address the emotional aspects of amputation.

EXAMINATION AND EARLY INTERVENTION

As with all patients, a pertinent history, systems review, and interview is conducted. The interview is used to gather information about the person's social and vocational history, determine hand dominance, and explore the individual's emotional response to the injury.

Key tests and measurements include:

1. Goniometric measurement of all remaining joints of the amputated extremity and the shoulder joint of the uninvolved limb.
2. Muscle testing of the major muscle groups of both shoulder girdles and the residual limb.
3. Observation of the condition and integrity of the skin of the residual limb.
4. Tests of sensation of the residual limb.
5. Circumferential measurement of the residual limb.
6. Measurement of remaining limb length.[1]
7. Determination of optimum electrode placement if myoelectric fitting is contemplated.

Examination for myoelectric electrode placement is an examination requiring special training. PTs are not prepared for this examination as a routine part of their education. However, PTs can take continuing education courses to learn the skills. There are also videotapes available to teach this examination technique.[10,11] Functional outcomes and the plan of care are developed from the results of the examination.

Range-of-motion measurement of all proximal joints is essential. Ample shoulder and shoulder girdle mobility is needed to operate a prosthesis using a harness and cable. Regardless of the type of prosthesis, the patient should have full range of elbow motion to facilitate grooming. Forearm motion is reduced when the interosseous membrane between the radius and ulna becomes fibrotic. Reduced mobility limits the patient's active pronation and supination. The prosthesis has a component that provides forearm motion; however, the more active the motion that is retained, the less the patient's need to rely on a mechanism. Individuals with short transradial amputations retain virtually no pronation and supination and may have limitations in elbow excursion. Although wrist disarticulation preserves the distal radioulnar joint, the patient usually has diminished forearm rotation. Lacking a hand, the person has little need to pronate and supinate. In addition, the postsurgical dressing may force the forearm bones together, fostering contracture. The most effective way of reducing contracture is by encasing the forearm in a plaster dressing that is shaped to emphasize separation of the bones.

For individuals with transhumeral amputations, the treatment plan includes exercise to maintain maximum shoulder and shoulder girdle mobility.

Most patients with arm amputation are children or relatively young adults. Consequently, motor power is usually good to normal unless the trauma that caused the amputation also injured nerves or tendons or caused excessive scar tissue. If myoelectric fitting is contemplated, a program of maintenance exercises emphasizing isometric contraction of the forearm flexors and extensors is indicated. For those who probably will have a prosthesis with cable and harness control, emphasis is on shoulder and shoulder girdle strength. Restoring functional activities is an excellent way of promoting motor power and joint mobility.

Skin inspection focuses on the condition of the surgical wound and the skin on the ipsilateral forearm and upper arm as well as the torso. Most amputation wounds heal readily, particularly if the patient has a rigid or semirigid dressing. Postoperative pain may be localized to the operative site, or it may be phantom pain, or both. Local pain often indicates infection, which may require debridement and appropriate medication. As with lower limb amputation, the patient with upper limb amputation is likely to be aware of the missing body parts. When the awareness is not painful, the phenomenon is known as phantom sensation. The patient should be reassured that this experience is normal, given the large cerebral representation of the hand. When the patient complains of burning, throbbing, electrical shocks, or other noxious sensations, the phenomenon is called phantom pain. Although no treatment eradicates phantom pain for all patients, the wide repertory of approaches should include at least one that is effective with a given patient (see Chap. 5). Some patients respond to bilateral exercise, in which the individual flexes and extends the fingers on the sound hand against resistance while imagining that the absent hand is also exercising. The PT might also use ultrasound, transcutaneous electrical nerve stimulation, massage, or functional activity. Massage is especially useful to help the patient gain tolerance to the pressure that will be applied by the prosthetic socket, as well as to prevent adhesions from occurring.[8]

Periodic girth measurements of the amputated limb will indicate when edema has subsided and, thus, when the patient is ready for fitting with a permanent prosthesis. Limb length is a critical determinant of prosthetic componentry and functional outcome. For transradial amputation, one stretches a tape measure from the medial humeral epicondyle to the ulnar styloid on the sound side. On the amputated side, the landmarks are the medial epicondyle to the end of the more distal forearm bone; if the patient has excessive soft tissue at the end of the limb, the PT or PTA should compress the tissue to obtain an accurate measurement. With the two measurements, the PT computes the percentage of limb loss. The standard measurements and nomenclature[12] for limb length are:

100 percent	Wrist disarticulation
100 to 55 percent	Long transradial
55 to 35 percent	Short transradial
35 to 0 percent	Very short transradial

For transhumeral amputation, the PT stretches a tape measure from the acromion to the lateral humeral epicondyle on the sound side. On the amputated side, the landmarks are the acromion to the end of the humerus. Transradial percentages and nomenclature are:

90 to 100 percent	Elbow disarticulation
50 to 90 percent	Standard transhumeral
30 to 50 percent	Short transhumeral
0 to 30 percent	Humeral neck
0 percent	Shoulder disarticulation

Absence of any portion of the thorax or shoulder girdle is designated as a *forequarter amputation.*

The therapist should also evaluate the patient's premorbid hand dominance. Approximately half of those with upper limb amputation lose the dominant hand. Thus, if the patient, as is true with the case study, has lost the dominant hand, an important element in early management is teaching change of dominance. The sound hand retains dexterity and sensation. Although the client may decide eventually to write with the prosthesis, other activities are generally easier with the intact hand. The patient may experience an initial period of clumsiness and frustration, but with the PT's encouragement, should retain or gain considerable independence with the sound hand in self-care activities, especially personal hygiene, dressing, feeding, writing, and similar tasks.[13,14]

Evaluation of the patient's general cognitive status and emotional response to the amputation is critical. No members of the rehabilitation team should underestimate the emotional impact of upper limb amputation. Unlike lower limb amputation, which usually follows several years of increasing disability caused by peripheral vascular disease, most arm amputations occur unexpectedly on the job or during some recreational pursuit. For most people, the hand has much more psychological importance than the foot. One holds a child's hand and strokes a loved one's brow with the hand. Loss of the hand cannot be disguised effectively. The rehabilitation team must empathize with the patient's loss, calmly accept the humanity of the individual whether or not both hands are present, and perceptively guide the patient to the realization that he or she can lead a fully satisfying work and social life even with upper limb loss. Exploring the patient's goals for rehabilitation will help clinical team members understand the degree of understanding and acceptance that the patient possesses. Psychosocial support is critical to fostering a positive rehabilitation outcome; a psychologist, social worker, or counselor can help the client cope with the emotional effects of the amputation.

PROSTHETIC REPLACEMENTS

Case Study

Mr. Rodriguez's wound has healed and he has learned to tolerate the sensation of the missing left hand. He had been an avid recreational athlete so he retained excellent motor power throughout the upper limb, as well as full range of the shoulder and elbow. Because the amputation occurred through the middle third of the forearm, pronation and supination are quite limited. He can now bathe, attend to toilet activities, and groom, dress, and feed himself independently. He still has difficulty writing rapidly with the non-dominant right hand. He is aware that several types of prostheses are available and is eager to be fitted.

■ Case Study Activities

1 Compare the passive hand, cable-controlled hand, myoelectric hand, and hook with regard to appearance, function, weight, cost, and durability. Which is most suitable for Mr. Rodriguez? Why?
2 What are the proximal components of the transradial prosthesis?

Lower limb amputation affects one's lifestyle profoundly, compelling some provision for locomotion, whether with a prosthesis or a wheelchair. In contrast, although upper limb amputation affects performance of many self-care, vocational, and recreational pursuits, numerous activities can be accomplished with one hand. Consequently, a sizeable number of individuals with unilateral upper limb amputation elect not to wear a prosthesis.[2] They find ways of accomplishing activities or foregoing those which no longer seem important, preferring to avoid problems of prosthetic discomfort, maintenance, and cost. Most individuals with transradial amputation, however, do find that a prosthesis is worthwhile, if only for selected activities or to disguise the amputation.[3–4,15]

PROSTHETIC REPLACEMENTS FOR THE HAND

Of paramount importance to the patient and the rehabilitation team is the prosthetic component that will substitute for the missing hand. No device completely replaces the appearance or function of the anatomic hand. Nevertheless, the prosthetic counterpart, called a terminal device, can contribute to the wearer's function and self-esteem. The two types of terminal devices are the hand and the hook. Either is secured to a plastic socket encasing the forearm. Table 10.1 compares terminal devices; it should be noted that manufacturers are constantly striving to make components lighter, and so weights may not be totally accurate.

Prosthetic Hands

Most patients, whether adults or the parents of children with amputation, are keenly interested in replacing the lost hand with a terminal device that resembles a hand (Fig. 10.1).[16–17] Two groups of such components are manufactured—passive hands that have no moving parts and active hands that have mechanisms permitting the patient to control finger position by appropriate action in the proximal part of the amputated limb. Both active and passive hands are made in a range of sizes to suit most children and adults, and both are covered with a flexible plastic glove that matches the patient's skin tone. Many people enhance the hand's appearance by wearing a ring or other jewelry. The glove is vulnerable to staining and tearing and should be replaced at least annually to retain optimal appearance.

As compared with an active hand, passive hands are lighter in weight, less expensive, and more durable. The fingers are made of a flexible wire covered with resilient plastic. The wearer can bend or straighten the fingers with the sound hand. Patients use the passive hand not only to restore normal appearance, but also to assist in many tasks such as holding a large package and stabilizing paper while writing with the other hand.[18] The passive hand, however, has no grasp function.

Active hands do enable grasping. Commercially available hands have a mechanism that moves the thumb, index, and middle fingers; the fourth and fifth fingers are passive. The prehension pattern is a three-jaw chuck that permits the wearer to hold many common objects securely. The hands do not open as widely as does the anatomic hand; consequently, the patient can grasp things that have a cross-section smaller than 10 cm (4 in).

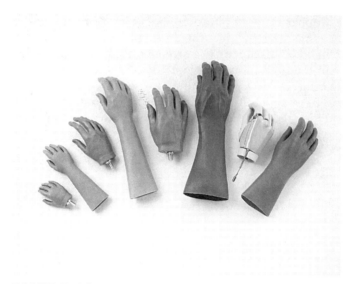

FIGURE 10.1

Prosthetic hands and gloves in child, adolescent, and adult sizes.

The most popular active hands are operated myoelectrically (Fig. 10.2).[19] The patient wears a socket that has one or more skin electrodes that contact appropriate muscle groups. When the patient contracts the muscle, the electrode transmits the microvoltage generated by the muscle to a mechanism that causes the electrical signal to operate a small motor, which, in turn, enables the hand mechanism to open or close the fingers. The motor is powered by a battery worn inside the prosthetic socket or, in the case of wrist disar-

TABLE 10.1 COMPARISON OF TERMINAL DEVICES

Component	Appearance	Function	Weight for Adult Size
Passive hand	Anthropomorphic shape. Sizes to suit 1½-year-old child to medium-sized man. Glove similar to wearer's skin color.	Can stabilize objects on a table. Wearer can adjust finger position passively.	8 oz with glove
Cable-operated hand	Same as above.	Wearer can adjust finger position by shoulder motion that causes tension in the control cable in the hand.	14 oz with glove
Myoelectric hand	Same as previous.	Wearer can adjust finger position by contracting forearm muscles that activate motor in the hand.	22 oz with glove and battery
Cable-operated hook	Shiny metal tool. Child-sized hooks available with pink or brown plastic coating.	Wearer can adjust finger position by shoulder motion that causes tension in the control cable on the hook.	3 oz

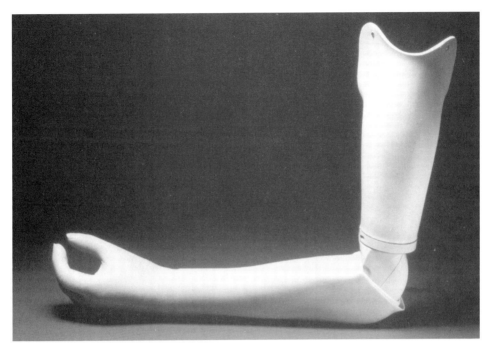

FIGURE 10.2
Utah Arm 2. (Courtesy of Motion Control) (*www.utaharm.com*).

ticulation, elsewhere on the patient's body. Manufacturers are making ever smaller and more powerful batteries and controllers to fit into very small places (Fig. 10.3). Myoelectric control can provide excellent grasp force. One version of a myoelectrically controlled hand features electronic pressure sensors in the thumb and index finger. The sensors automatically adjust grip force if the grasped object starts to slip.[20–21] Adept users control finger opening and closing easily, although patients may take many months to gain proficiency. Myoelectric hands provide proportional control, thereby allowing a small muscular contraction to translate into a greater force on the hand in a smooth manner.

The alternative type of prosthetic hand has a steel cable attached to a trunk harness. By flexing the shoulder, the patient puts tension on the cable, which pulls on the hand mechanism causing the fingers either to open (voluntary opening) or to close (voluntary closing). Relaxing tension on the cable allows the fingers to revert to the opposite position. Thus, in a voluntary-opening device, relaxation causes the fingers to close. Grasp force in the voluntary-opening device is determined by springs in the mechanism and is comparatively weak. Grasp force in the voluntary-closing device is determined by the force that the patient applies to the cable; consequently, the user can achieve substantial force. Although lighter and less expensive than myoelectric hands, cable-operated devices require that the patient wear a harness, which some patients find intrusive. The harness also tends to restrict the work space in which the patient can use the prostheses easily.[22]

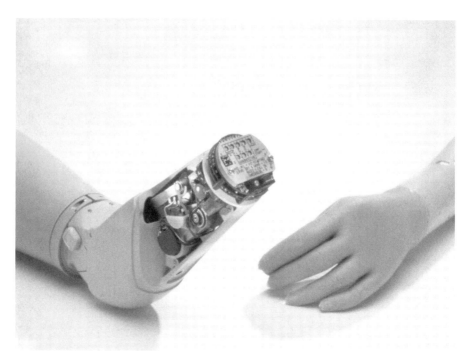

FIGURE 10.3

Myoelectric mechanism in Utah Arm 2. (Courtesy of Motion Control) (*www.utaharm.com*).

Hooks

A hook (Fig. 10.4) is the other basic type of terminal device. Made either of aluminum or steel, mass-produced hooks have two fingers that the patient can open and close. Myoelectrically controlled hooks are manufactured; however, most patients who wear hooks have cable-operated ones that are either voluntary-opening or voluntary-closing devices. The most common hook is a voluntary-opening device, in which grasp force is determined by rubber bands encircling the base of the fingers. The basic design resembles the original invention, patented in 1912.[23] Cable-operated hooks are much lighter in weight than any type of hand and are less expensive. Hooks are also more durable. Because the tips of the hook fingers are relatively small, the patient can see the object to be grasped more easily than is the case with the thicker fingers of a prosthetic hand.[24]

Terminal Device Selection

Because terminal devices are meager substitutes for a lost hand, the rehabilitation team and the patient must determine the best compromise on an individual basis. Although some patients are provided with two or more terminal devices in an attempt to increase functional restoration, most individuals find that one device serves adequately, and rarely do they use the other devices. The team and patient must weigh the relative importance of appearance, amount of grasp power needed, economy, durability, and prosthetic weight to arrive at a rational prescription (Table 10.2).[25] Vocational and social pursuits play major roles in determining the choice of terminal device. For example,

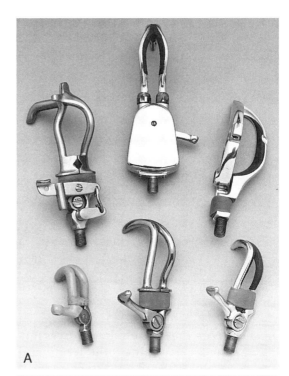

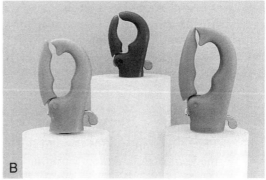

FIGURE 10.4

Hook terminal devices. (A) *Top left:* voluntary-opening hook with locking mechanism; *top middle:* voluntary-closing hook; *top right:* voluntary-closing hook; *bottom left:* infant size voluntary-opening hook; *bottom middle:* adult-sized voluntary-opening hook; *bottom right:* adolescent size voluntary-opening hook. (Courtesy of Hosmer Dorrance, Campbell, Calif.) (B) Voluntary-closing aluminum, steel, and polyurethane terminal devices; *left:* tan plastic, adolescent size; *middle:* dark brown child size; *right:* tan adult size. (Courtesy of TRS, Boulder, Colo.)

the individual whose job involves use of tools and abrasive materials will find that a hook, being more durable, is an appropriate choice. The patient with a very short transradial amputation may become fatigued after repeatedly lifting the relatively heavy myoelectric hand. Someone who has a desk job probably will find that a hand is preferable. Although a hook is conspicuously different from a hand, people who use a hook proficiently usually are able to return to the community without much embarrassment.

PROSTHETIC REPLACEMENTS FOR THE WRIST AND FOREARM

The terminal device, of whatever design, is secured to a wrist unit. In most instances, the wrist unit does not replace functions of the anatomic wrist, namely dorsiflexion and palmar flexion, and ulnar and radial deviation. In-

TABLE 10.2 COST AND DURABILITY OF TERMINAL DEVICES

Component	Cost	Durability
Passive hand	Moderately expensive.	Glove is vulnerable to stains and tears.
Cable-operated hand	Moderately expensive, more expensive than passive hand.	Glove is vulnerable to stains and tears. Mechanism may malfunction. Fingers or cable may break when moderate force is applied.
Myoelectric hand	Most expensive.	Glove is vulnerable to stains and tears. Battery requires periodic recharging and eventual replacement. Mechanism, especially its electrical components, may malfunction. Fingers may break when moderate force is applied.
Cable-operated hook	Least expensive.	Rubber lining is vulnerable to abrasion. Fingers or cable may break when extreme force is applied.

stead, the wrist unit replaces forearm motion, permitting the patient to pronate or supinate the terminal device. For individuals with high bilateral amputations, one prosthesis may be fitted with a wrist unit that allows palmar flexion as well as pronation and supination (flexion unit). The flexion unit enables the wearer to reach the midline of the body, important for eating, buttoning, and toilet activities. There are now combined myoelectric hand and wrist units that allow the patient to switch from hand to wrist positioning quickly and smoothly.

Proximal Portions of Transradial Prostheses

The wrist unit is embedded in the distal end of the socket. Sockets are custom-made of plastic and are intended to fit snugly to distribute pressure over the largest area. The proximal portion of the transradial socket terminates in the vicinity of the humeral epicondyles. A self-suspending socket supports the weight of the terminal device and wrist unit by a secure hold at the epicondyles, thus eliminating the need for harness suspension. Self-suspending sockets are often used with myoelectric hands. The same silicone and gel-suspension, shuttlelock suspension mechanism used to suspend the transtibial prosthesis (see Chap. 7) is also available to suspend the transradial prosthesis. The socket is fabricated of combination materials including carbon graphite to keep the weight minimal. Suspension is achieved through the support of the humeral condyles and the intimate fit of the sleeve locking into the forearm socket.[26]

A harness is necessary to suspend the socket, which is not supported by the epicondyles or a shuttlelock system, or to transmit shoulder motions to a cable, or for both functions. The harness is made of Dacron webbing (Fig. 10.5). The customary design, a figure-of-eight, has a loop around each shoulder that connect in back. One strap from the loop on the amputated side is buckled to the cable that controls the terminal device. The other strap from the loop on the amputated side is buckled to an inverted "Y" strap that lies on

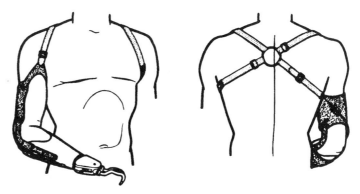

FIGURE 10.5
Figure-of-eight harness for a transradial prosthesis with tricep pad and hook.

the anterior surface of the upper arm and suspends the prosthesis. The loop on the sound side is known as the *axillary loop.*

Proximal Parts of the Transhumeral Prosthesis

The prosthesis for the individual whose amputation is at the elbow disarticulation level or higher includes a terminal device, a wrist unit, a forearm shell to replace the length of the absent forearm, an elbow unit, a socket, and a suspension mechanism (Fig. 10.6). All elbow units have a hinge for elbow flexion and a locking mechanism to enable the wearer to retain the desired flexion angle. For the patient whose amputation is at the standard transhumeral level or higher, the elbow unit also incorporates a turntable that allows the individual to rotate the forearm shell medially and laterally. The elbow unit connects the forearm shell with the socket. A harness, typically a transhumeral figure-of-eight, suspends the prosthesis and transmits shoulder and shoulder girdle motions to the cable system. Ordinarily, one cable operates the terminal device and the elbow hinge, and a second cable operates the elbow lock.

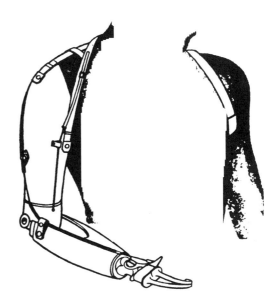

FIGURE 10.6
Transhumeral prosthesis with figure-of-eight harness.

PROSTHETIC TRAINING

The elements of upper limb prosthetic training are donning and doffing, control training, functional use training, and vocational training or retraining. Careful evaluation of prosthetic fit and function of all components should precede training.[27] Prosthetic training is frequently done by the occupational therapist (OT), but is sometimes performed by the PT.

Donning and Doffing

Regardless of prosthetic componentry, it is essential that the patient be able to don the prosthesis independently. Otherwise, the individual is almost certain to abandon wearing the prosthesis after discharge from the rehabilitation center. Donning a prosthesis that has a figure-of-eight harness involves (1) applying a sock or liner, (2) inserting the amputation limb in the socket, and (3) inserting the sound limb through the axillary loop. To doff the prosthesis, the client reverses the steps—removes the axillary loop, withdraws the amputation limb from the socket, and removes the sock.

To don a myoelectrically controlled transradial prosthesis, the patient (1) dons a cotton stockinet tube, taking care that the proximal margin of the stockinet is above the antecubital fossa; (2) applies the socket; and (3) pulls the distal end of the stockinet through a hole in the socket, thereby drawing the superficial tissue of the forearm snugly into the socket. The patient thus does not wear a sock. Ordinarily, the prosthesis has no harness. Doffing requires gently tugging on the distal part of the prosthesis until it is off the forearm.

Controls Training

Controls training encompasses teaching the patient to operate every element of the prosthesis correctly. Early structured training is a key determinant of long-term prosthetic acceptance.[28] The transradial prosthesis has only two components that the patient must control, namely the terminal device and the wrist unit. Although the transhumeral prosthesis is more complex, the basic principles of controls training for a transradial prosthesis are pertinent.

Terminal Device Training: Myoelectric

Before the prosthesis is made, the patient undergoes preliminary training to determine the best site for electrode placement.[29] The PT or OT uses a surface electrode and a voltmeter to explore the forearm for sites where the patient can produce the greatest electrical response. Although the therapist usually starts exploration at the motor point on the muscle belly, the final electrode placement is determined empirically. Most myoelectric systems have an electrode on the flexors and another on the extensors. Thus, preliminary training is devoted to locating optimum sites and to guiding the patient to contract one muscle group isometrically while maintaining relaxation of the antagonists. When the sites have been identified, the patient practices with a test socket that has electrodes. The test socket facilitates alteration in electrode positioning. Once final electrode positions are determined, the prosthetist fabricates the permanent socket that incorporates electrodes. With the permanent socket, the patient practices contraction of the flexors to cause the hand to close and extensor contraction to open the hand. The goal is accurate hand function without unwanted finger motion. The patient concentrates on the movement of the hand by watching the way the fingers move; eventually the person develops proprioceptive appreciation of the amount of muscular activity necessary to produce the desired amount of finger motion.

Terminal Device Training: Cable-Operated Units

The PT or OT instructs the patient to flex the shoulder to operate the terminal device, whether voluntary-opening or voluntary-closing. Initially, the patient's elbow should be flexed 90 degrees so that the individual can see the terminal device easily and cable alignment is optimal. Sometimes it is necessary to resist shoulder flexion so that the patient can put enough tension on the cable to affect the terminal device. Once the patient realizes the relation of shoulder flexion to terminal device operation, training is devoted to refining control motions. The patient should keep the contralateral, sound arm relaxed. Training will help the patient recognize that the same body motion is effective whatever the position of the elbow and shoulder. The therapist then places the terminal device close to the patient's chest and asks the person to operate the device. Scapular abduction is necessary because shoulder flexion would cause the terminal device to move away from the chest.

With a voluntary-opening terminal device, the patient should practice maintaining slight tension on the control cable to prevent the hand or hook fingers from closing completely; this skill is used when handling fragile objects (Fig. 10.7). With a voluntary-closing terminal device, the patient should practice applying gentle tension on the control cable, which will be necessary when dealing with objects which might crush (Fig. 10.8).

Wrist Unit

Most wrist units are passive, that is, the patient changes the position of the unit by turning the terminal device with the sound hand, or nudges the terminal device against the edge of a table, the chest, thigh, or contralateral forearm. If the wrist unit has a locking mechanism, the therapist teaches the patient how to lock and unlock it by means of a lever or rotating rings on the unit. If the wrist unit is controlled by a cable or by myoelectric mechanism, the therapist teaches the patient the correct sequence of motions to effect change in terminal device position.

Once the patient understands how to control the wrist unit, the PT introduces a formboard to help the individual integrate terminal device and wrist unit operation. The formboard consists of objects of various sizes, shapes, textures, and weights. The purpose of formboard training is to increase skillful use of the prosthesis. The patient does not use the sound hand. Of course, one acknowledges the artificiality of formboard training; in a real-life situation, the patient would grasp an object with the sound hand. Because the purpose of a unilateral prosthesis is to assist the sound hand in complex maneuvers, the individual must be able to control the prosthesis independently (Fig. 10.9).

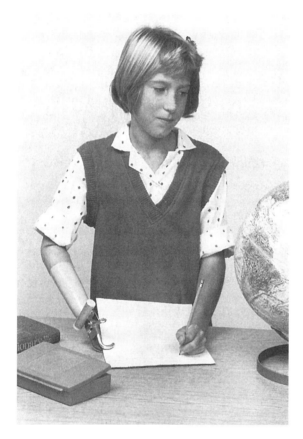

FIGURE 10.7

Child using a transradial prosthesis with electrically controlled voluntary-opening hook. (Courtesy of Hosmer Dorrance, Campbell, Calif.)

It is relatively easy to grasp a hard rubber cube; the patient pronates the terminal device, opens it so that the fingertips are slightly farther apart than the width of the cube, then closes (or allows the fingers to close). More difficult is managing a thin metal disk. The patient will find that placing the terminal device in midposition between pronation and supination affords the best approach to grasping the disk.

An object that is easy to deform, such as a paper cup or a foam rubber ball, requires the patient to maintain tension on the control cable with a voluntary-opening terminal device, to apply minimum tension on the control cable with a voluntary-closing device, or to contract forearm flexors gently with a myo-electrically controlled device.

Functional Use Training

Functional use training is the next step in rehabilitation. The patient is guided to use the prosthesis to assist the sound hand in the performance of bi-manual activities. Because most daily tasks can be accomplished with a single hand, the therapist must be creative in selecting those that are easier to execute bimanually. The basic principle is that the prosthesis performs the more static part of the task. For example, when cutting meat with a knife and

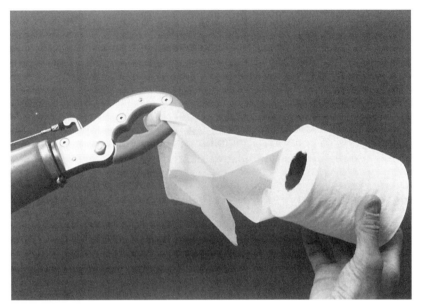

FIGURE 10.8
Grasping toilet tissue with voluntary-closing terminal device. (Courtesy of TRS, Boulder, Colo.)

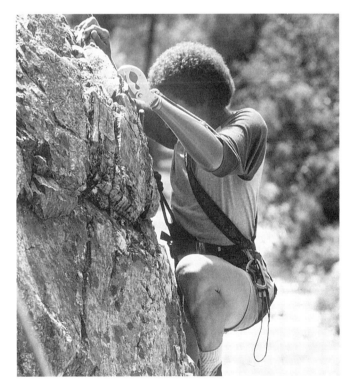

FIGURE 10.9
Adult using a transradial prosthesis with voluntary-closing terminal device to aid in mountain climbing. (Courtesy of TRS, Boulder, Colo.)

fork, the patient stabilizes the meat with the fork held in the prosthesis and uses the knife with the sound hand. Other bimanual activities are opening and applying an adhesive bandage, hammering nails, pulling on socks, folding a letter and inserting it into an envelope, and wrapping a package. Some tasks, such as tying shoelaces, can be done either one-handed[30] or with a prosthesis.

Prior to discharge, the patient should be assessed regarding the practicality and ease of use of the prosthesis, the individual's ability to don and remove it, and care for the prosthesis and the skin. The client's positive expressions of comfort, acceptable appearance, and effectiveness of the prosthesis are the ultimate indicators of rehabilitation success.[1]

Vocational Training

Because most people who sustain upper limb amputation are men of working age, it is important to explore vocations that can be pursued with or without a prosthesis. Preparing to return to work is highly motivating for many individuals. Very few jobs are beyond the capability of people with upper limb amputation. Although the rehabilitation program generally is not designed to include specific job training, the clinical team should conduct prevocational exploration or vocational assessment, or refer the patient to a job training center.

Functional Outcomes

The ultimate goal of rehabilitation is to return the patient to the lifestyle that most closely reflects the his or her physical, cognitive, and emotional abilities and interests. In this light, surveys of functional outcomes may reflect successful rehabilitation even though many individuals opt to limit or eliminate prosthetic use because they can accomplish meaningful tasks unimanually. Full-time prosthetic use appears to be unusual,[2] particularly among those with traumatic amputation,[31] although early prosthetic fitting and training are more likely to result in long-term usage.[32] Adults with wrist disarticulation and transhumeral amputation are least likely to continue prosthetic wear, as are those with limitation of shoulder motion or brachial plexus injury. In contrast, individuals with bilateral amputation are most apt to persist with prosthetic use.[5] Among children with congenital amputation, rejection of a prosthesis most often occurs when fitting is delayed until the youngster is older than 2 years; adolescence is the other peak period for prosthetic rejection.[33]

Summary

Upper limb amputation is a relatively unusual occurrence. The most common etiology is trauma, particularly affecting young men. Surgical management may include use of a rigid or a semirigid postoperative dressing. Postsurgically, the therapist is concerned with wound healing, pain reduction, maintaining joint mobility and motor power, and enabling the patient to resume independence in daily activities. The team also addresses the emotional impact of amputation. The transradial prosthesis consists of a terminal device, either a hand or a hook; a wrist unit; and a socket; if the terminal device is cable-operated, then the prosthesis also has a harness. The steps in training are donning, controls training, functional use training, and vocational training. Relatively few patients wear unilateral prostheses on a full-time basis, presumably because they are able to accomplish most tasks with one hand.

PTs who find themselves working regularly with individuals with upper extremity amputation need to take a continuing education course to learn current interventions. Prosthetic componentry changes so fast that therapists are advised to consult the Web pages of manufacturers. Initial access can be obtained through *www.oandp.com.*

Glossary

Cable	The metal cord that connects the harness to the terminal device and transmits the power to the terminal device from shoulder motion.
Hook	A type of terminal device that has two metal figures.
Myoelectric	Type of control using muscle contraction to provide an electrical current to a terminal device.
Terminal device	Part of the prosthesis that replaces the hand. The terminal device may be an artificial hand or hook.
Test socket	A preliminary socket constructed to ensure proper fit and power attachments.
Voluntary closing	A terminal device that closes with muscle movement and opens with relaxation.
Voluntary opening	A terminal device that opens with muscle movement and closes with relaxation.

References

1. APTA: *Guide to Physical Therapist Practice.* Alexandria, Va.: American Physical Therapy Association, 1997.
2. Jones, LE, and Davidson, JH: The long-term outcome of upper limb amputees treated at a rehabilitation centre in Sydney, Australia. Disabil Rehabil 17:437–42, 1995.
3. Millstein, SG, et al: Prosthetic use in adult upper limb amputees: A comparison of the body powered and electrically powered prostheses. Prosthet Orthot Int 10:27–34, 1986.
4. Sturup, J, et al: Traumatic amputation of the upper limb: The use of body-powered prostheses and employment consequences. Prosthet Orthot Int 12:50–52, 1988.
5. Wright, TW, et al: Prosthetic usage in major upper extremity amputations. J Hand Surg 20:619–22, 1995.
6. Ouellette, EA: Wrist disarticulation and transradial amputation: Surgical principles. In Bowker, JH, and Michael, JW (eds): Atlas of Limb Prosthetics: Surgical, Prosthetic, and Rehabilitation Principles, ed 2. Mosby Year Book, St. Louis, 1992.
7. Graham, B, et al: Major replantation versus revision amputation and prosthetic fitting in the upper extremity: A late functional outcomes study. J Hand Surg 23:783–91, 1998.
8. Malone, JM, et al: Immediate, early, and late postsurgical management of upper-limb amputation. J Rehabil Res Dev 21:33–41, 1984.
9. Brenner, CD: Wrist disarticulation and transradial amputation: prosthetic principles. In Bowker, JH, and Michael, JW (eds): Atlas of Limb Prosthetics: Surgical, Prosthetic, and Rehabilitation Principles, ed 2. Mosby Year Book, St. Louis, 1992.
10. Sears, HH: Approaches to prescription of body-powered and myoelectric prostheses. Phys Med Rehabil Clin N Am 2(2):1047–51, 1991.

11. Training the Client with an Electric Arm Prosthesis. Videotape available from Motion Control, 2401 S 1070 W. Suite B. Salt Lake City, UT 84119.
12. Geraghty, TJ, and Jones, LE. Painful neuromata following upper limb amputation. Prosthet Orthot Int 20:176–81, 1996.
13. Muilenberg, AL, and LeBlanc, MA: Body-powered upper-limb components. In Atkins, DJ, and Meier, RH (eds): Comprehensive Management of the Upper-Limb Amputee. Springer, New York, 1989.
14. Atkins, DJ: Postoperative and preprosthetic therapy programs. In Atkins, DJ, and Meier, RH (eds): Comprehensive Management of the Upper-Limb Amputee. Springer, New York, 1989.
15. Burger, H, and Marincek, C: Upper limb prosthetic use in Slovenia. Prosthet Orthot Int 18:25–33, 1994.
16. Billock, JN: Upper limb prosthetic terminal devices: Hands versus hooks. Clin Prosthet Orthot 10:57–65, 1986.
17. Datta, D, and Ibbotson, V: Powered prosthetic hands in very young children. Prosthet Orthot Int 22:150–54, 1998.
18. Fraser, CM: An evaluation of the use made of cosmetic and functional prostheses by unilateral upper limb amputees. Prosthet Orthot Int 22:216–23, 1999.
19. Edelstein, JE, and Berger, N: Performance comparison among children fitted with myoelectric and body-powered hands. Arch Phys Med Rehabil 74:376–80, 1993.
20. Otto Bock develops SensorHand™and ErgoArm. O&P Business News, December 1, 1999, pp 32–34.
21. Tura, A, et al: Experimental development of a sensory control system for an upper limb myoelectric prosthesis with cosmetic covering. J Rehabil Res Dev 35:14–26, 1998.
22. Stein, RB, and Walley, M: Functional comparison of upper extremity amputees using myoelectric and conventional prostheses. Arch Phys Med Rehabil 64:243–48, 1983.
23. Craig, B: Dorrance design: The split hook unchanged after 88 years. O&P Business News, April 1, 2000, pp 66–68.
24. Murphy, EF: In support of the hook. Clin Prosthet Orthot 10:78–81, 1986.
25. Radocy, B, and Beiswenger, WD: A high-performance, variable suspension, transradial (below-elbow) prosthesis. J Prosthet Orthot7(2):65–67, 1995.
26. Upper-limb electronic technology moves forward. O&P Business News, December, 1999, pp 20–23.
27. Atkins, DJ: Adult upper-limb prosthetic training. In Atkins, DJ, and Meier, RH (eds): Comprehensive Management of the Upper-Limb Amputee. Springer, New York, 1989.
28. Lake, C: Effects of prosthetic training on upper-extremity prosthesis use. J Prosthet Orthot 9:3–9, 1997.
29. Spiegel, SR: Adult myoelectric upper-limb prosthetic training. In Atkins, DJ, and Meier, RH (eds): Comprehensive Management of the Upper-Limb Amputee. Springer, New York, 1989.
30. Edelstein, JE: Special considerations—rehabilitation without prostheses: Functional skills training. In Bowker, JH, and Michael, JW (eds): Atlas of Limb Prosthetics: Surgical, Prosthetic, and Rehabilitation Principles, ed 2. Mosby Year Book, St. Louis, 1992.
31. Gaine, WJ, et al: Upper limb traumatic amputees: Review of prosthetic use. J Hand Surg 22:73–6, 1997.
32. Pinzur, MS, et al: Functional outcome following traumatic upper limb amputation and prosthetic limb fitting. J Hand Surg 19:836–39, 1994.
33. Postema, K, et al: Prosthesis rejection in children with a unilateral arm defect. Clin Rehabil 13:243–49, 1999.

CHAPTER ELEVEN

The Child with an Amputation

OBJECTIVES

At the end of this chapter, all students are expected to:

1 Classify congenital amputations according to standard terminology.
2 Differentiate between congenital and acquired amputations.
3 Develop an assessment program for a child with a unilateral amputation.
4 Develop a treatment program for a child with a unilateral amputation.
5 Discuss the role of the family in working with children with amputations.

Case Studies

Michael Donnagin is a 6-month-old boy brought to the clinic by his mother. Michael was born with only half a humerus on the right side and only the medial two toes on the right foot. The rest of the extremities are normal. He is an only child. His father is a loan officer in a bank, and his mother is on leave from her job as a legal secretary.

Jenny Smith, 6 years old, had a left transfemoral femoral amputation secondary to a farm accident 4 weeks ago. An attempt was made to reattach the limb, but it failed. She was discharged from the hospital about 4 days after the amputation and has been at home with visiting physical therapy and nursing services. She is referred to an amputee clinic for evaluation and treatment. She lives with her parents and four older siblings on a moderate-size dairy farm about 60 miles from the city.

Mario Jonas is a 3-year-old boy with a left longitudinal deficiency femur, partial **proximal focal femoral deficiency (PFFD),** Category D, who is referred to the amputee clinic for prosthetic fitting. He lives in a small town in Mexico with his mother and five older siblings. He has been walking on crutches. He has been referred to the U.S. clinic through an international aid organization. He has never been treated for his disability. He does not speak English.

■ *Case Study Activities*

1 Classify Michael's amputations using appropriate terminology.
2 Compare and contrast acquired versus congenital amputations.
3 Determine the appropriate practice pattern(s) for each child.
4 Using the practice pattern as a guide, develop an appropriate examination plan for each child.
   a What critical data do you need that can best be obtained through interview?
   b What critical historical data do you need?
   c What tests and measurements would you perform today? Why?
   d What might be the parents' concerns at this time?
   e What information would you like to have from the parents?
5 Would you fit each of these children?
   a If yes, briefly describe the components you would use.
   b If no, justify your decision and determine your alternative plan of action.
6 Compare and contrast the prosthetic rehabilitation program for each of these children and an adult with a similar disability.

The habilitation of children with single or multiple limb loss is a complex, long-term process involving specialists from many disciplines with training in pediatric care. This chapter provides a brief overview of this topic offering general guidelines for the physical therapist (PT) who may occasionally work with a child who has lost one limb. Most PTs and physical therapist assistants (PTAs), knowledgeable in the prosthetic care of adults, can provide effective therapy to a child with one limb loss. The care of the child with multiple limb deficiencies requires considerable expertise, and such children should be referred to special centers for optimum care.

PTs and PTAs need to be cognizant that the child is not a miniature adult. Children have special problems related to developmental tasks, parental adjustment, and adjustment and acceptance of the artificial limb themselves. The rehabilitation program involves the whole family, and the attitudes of the parents, other siblings, and family members have considerable influence on the adjustment of the child. Children who are born without a limb or a part of a limb usually adjust to limb replacement on the basis of comfort and utility. Their major goal is to emulate their peers and participate in the activities of other children. Children who are born without one or more limbs are very adaptable; if missing their hands, they will learn to use their feet. Prosthetic replacements must fit a functional need to be used.[1]

Children with acquired amputations, unless very young, will have a sense of loss. Their acceptance of a prosthesis will usually be influenced by function and attitude of parents and siblings. In general, children with lower limb amputations adjust to the prosthesis better than those with upper limb loss. The higher the level of upper limb loss, the more complicated the prosthesis, and the more difficult the adjustment.[1] Function and cosmesis are important considerations in acceptance of upper limb prostheses; they are basically tools and must provide greater function than the residual limb and be cosmetically satisfactory to be acceptable.[2,3]

CLASSIFICATION

Juvenile amputations are classified into two broad categories, acquired and congenital. Acquired amputations occur after birth and result from trauma, tumor, infection, or disease. There are approximately twice as many acquired amputations from trauma than from disease; there are more acquired than congenital amputations, although exact current figures are not available. Most traumatic amputations are the results of accidents with power tools, lawnmowers, or farm implements. The major disease causing amputations is malignancies, but this number is dwindling as limb-sparing surgery has become more common.[4]

Congenital amputations are the result of a prenatal or birth defect. Many congenital amputations require subsequent surgical amputation for conversion of the anomaly to enable better prosthetic fitting. A different nomenclature is used for congenital amputations than for acquired juvenile amputations. The International Standards Organization (ISO) has developed a classification scheme for limb deficiencies present at birth based on skeletal elements (Table 11.1).

Limb deficiencies are classified as transverse or longitudinal. Transverse deficiencies are described by the level at which the limb terminates. The limb is normal proximally to the level named; distally, there is no skeletal component. A child missing the skeletal component below the elbow has a transverse total forearm loss. If part of the bone is present, such as the loss of the component below the middle of the femur, it is classified as transverse middle femoral loss.

Longitudinal deficiencies refer to those with a reduction or absence of skeletal components with normal components present below the affected part. Identification of longitudinal anomalies includes:

1. The names of the affected bones in a proximal to distal order.
2. Indication of whether each bone is partially or totally absent.
3. Indication of the amount of absent bone.
4. Digits, metacarpals, metatarsals, or phalanges that are present.

TABLE 11.1   LONGITUDINAL CONGENITAL LIMB DEFICIENCIES

Limb Segment	Bone Segment (UE) May Be Partial or Complete	Bone Segment (LE) May Be Partial or Complete
Proximal	Humeral (Hu)	Femoral (Fe)
Distal	Radial (Ra)	Tibial (Ti)
Distal	Central (Ce)	Central (Ce)
	Carpal (Ca): if partial, indicate row left. Metacarpal (MC): if partial, indicate ray left. Phalangeal (Ph): if partial, indicate phalanx left.	Tarsal (Ta): if partial, indicate row left. Metatarsal (MT): if partial, indicate ray left. Phalangeal (Ph): if partial, indicate phalanx left.
Combined	Indicate bone segments that remain. Indicate if partial or complete. Indicate specific carpal, ray, or phalanx left.	Indicate bone segments that remain. Indicate if partial or complete. Indicate specific carpal, ray, or phalanx left.

For example, an individual with a normal tibia attached directly to the pelvis, no fibula and the first two rays of the foot is described as having a longitudinal femoral-fibular deficiency with two partial rays.[5]

Congenital anomalies vary. A **vestigial** component may be attached to a proximal part, digits may not be separated, and individuals may sustain multiple limb deficiencies or anomalies. An innovative and creative approach to surgical interventions and fitting is used by members of the child limb deficient clinics.

Proximal Femoral Focal Deficiencies

One special problem that is seen with some regularity is the longitudinal deficiency femur with PFFD. PFFD is classified in relation to the position of the foot, the condition of the hip joint, and the length of the femoral and tibial segments. A very short femoral segment that is held in flexion, abduction, and external rotation characterizes this deficiency of the proximal end of the femur. The quadriceps muscle is frequently **hypoplastic** with a correspondingly small or vestigial patella. Often, there is associated ipsilateral paraxial fibular **hemimelia.** The total limb length of the affected side is about the level of the knee joint on the unaffected side. The condition may be bilateral or unilateral. There are a number of variations of PFFD that can be differentiated radiographically after the child is 9 to 12 months old.[6]

Representative anomalies will be discussed briefly in this chapter.

SURGICAL INTERVENTIONS

Lower Extremity

The aim of amputation surgery, if performed, is to produce a limb that is adequate for a prosthesis and that will remain adequate through the remaining growth period and through adulthood. Lower limb surgery should allow pain-free weight bearing, stability, an adequately sensate limb, near-normal gait, maximum bone growth, and satisfactory cosmetic appearance. Amputation for cosmetic reasons alone should not be done until the child is old enough to share in the decision.

The child who has a traumatic or surgically elected amputation should be placed on a carefully planned postoperative program that includes exercises and activities to prevent contractures and to maintain the function of the residual limb. Parents should be informed of the effect contractures have on the usefulness of the prosthesis. Parents also need instruction in a home program that may include assisting the child to use the **anomalous** limb to perform functional activities in an atypical manner.

Upper Extremity

Reconstructive surgery is frequently used to improve congenital deformities. Function first and cosmesis second are the primary concerns. The surgeon must consider bone loss and incompletely developed muscles and ligaments that may affect joint function. In the upper extremity, reconstructive surgery plays a major role in the management of **syndactyly** and **polydactyly** as well as radial and ulnar deficiencies that lead to poorly positioned hands. Surgery, designed to provide the child with as functional a hand as possible, should be performed early. Amputation of a functionless part is performed if it will enhance function. Procedures are designed to improve both function and appearance rather than to enhance prosthetic fitting. Prostheses are designed to adapt to the limb.[7]

Lower Extremity

In the lower extremity, reconstructive surgery is often delayed to allow for the greatest amount of bone growth possible. Maintenance of long bone growth plates allows for the greatest development of limb length.[8] Individuals with short proximal skeletal pieces may eventually develop a usable residual limb. Severe deformities that interfere with early fitting or with function require early surgical intervention. The surgeon considers overall function and related muscular development. It is important to prevent progressive deformities that may occur as a result of muscle and nerve imbalances.

Hemimelias

Hemimelias are longitudinal deficiencies in which part or all of one long bone is missing. In the lower extremity there may be tibial, fibular, or femoral hemimelias. Fibular hemimelia results in leg length discrepancy and bowing of the tibia. Surgical leg lengthening has met with minimal success. Surgical arrest of the growth plate of the other limb is also used. More recently the Ilizarov technique has been used with some success. The Ilizarov technique involves progressive fracturing of the tibia with callus distraction and limb protection. The limb is maintained in a rigid external apparatus during this process that can be quite protracted.[9] The child is fitted with a shoe lift to equalize leg length until old enough for the lengthening procedure. Leg lengthening cannot be used if the expected discrepancy is likely to be more than 7.5 cm. In such cases, Syme amputation is usually performed.[8] If the foot is removed at a young age because of unfittable deformity, then the Syme amputation will become a transtibial as the child grows (Fig. 11.1*A* & *B*).

Tibial hemimelias are usually treated with knee disarticulation amputation.[8] If part of the tibia remains, it is sometimes possible to attach the fibula to the remnant of the tibia, and then perform an ankle disarticulation.

Amelias

An **amelia,** the total absence of a limb, may be unilateral or bilateral. They are usually treated like a disarticulation. Remaining digits may be kept if they can be useful to provide sensory input or perform self-care activities.

Proximal Femoral Focal Deficiencies

Treatment of PFFD is long term and may involve surgical reconstruction as well as prosthetic fitting. As the child grows, total leg length becomes progressively shorter than the other extremity. One method of management involves fitting the child with an adapted prosthesis until maximal bone growth has occurred and reconstructive surgery can be performed (Fig. 11.2). Once the child has reached the teen years, the knee may be fused and a Syme ampu-

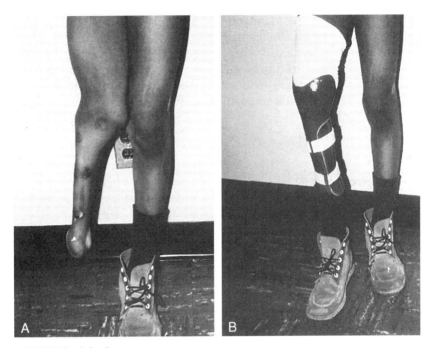

FIGURE 11.1

(A) Syme amputation in infancy will become a transtibial level amputation as the child grows. (B) A Syme prosthesis is still needed because of the larger distal end.

tation performed to provide a functional transfemoral residual limb. On some occasions, a Van Ness 180-degree rotational osteotomy of the tibia is performed that allows the ankle to be used as a knee joint and the child to be fitted with a transtibial prosthesis.[10,11] In a recent study of the gait characteristics of 9 individuals who had had Syme amputations compared to 10 individuals who had had Van Ness rotational osteotomy, the authors reported that those with Van Ness rotational osteotomies had a more functional gait and less nonprosthetic limb compensatory mechanisms than those with Syme amputations.[12] In cases of bilateral PFFD associated with upper extremity deficiencies, the feet may not be removed because the child may learn to use the feet for prehension.[8] Some clinics advocate early ablation of the foot.

The prior discussion may lead the reader to believe that most congenital anomalies are single bone problems. This is rarely the case. There may be associated deformities of the lower segments of the involved limb or involvement of other extremities and related loss of muscles and ligaments. Surgical intervention is individualized, and prosthetic fitting is adapted to the residuum and the total needs of the child. Surgery may be performed early or late, depending on the state of bone growth and the potential for a functional outcome.

Acquired Amputations

The surgical procedures used in acquired amputations are much like those with adults. Special considerations in relation to amputation surgery in children relate to bone growth. Many acquired amputations in the pediatric popu-

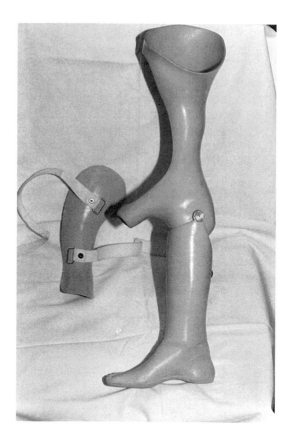

FIGURE 11.2
Prosthesis for proximal focal femoral deficiency.

lation are performed because of cancer. In recent years, the number of amputations has decreased as tumor resection and bone reconstruction techniques
have become more sophisticated and effective. Follow-up studies have yielded
similar percentages of recurrence and longevity among individuals treated
by amputation and those treated by tumor resection and limb reconstruction.[13,14,15] In another study, the authors compared the functional results of individuals undergoing amputation versus those undergoing tumor resection
and reconstruction. Several standardized tests were used to evaluate functional results including the SF-36. Results indicated somewhat more disability for individuals undergoing amputation, although the differences were not
as great as anticipated.[16] There are a great many factors that go into the decision to perform an amputation or attempt resection and reconstruction. In
some instances, when high amputation has been indicated, bone grafts have
been used to increase the length of the residual limb and eventual prosthetic
function.[17] Improvements in surgical reconstruction and in adjuvant therapy
provide the surgeon with many alternatives in the treatment of children with
malignancies.

Although surgical procedures for adults and children are similar, there are
concerns with children not present in adults. The surgeon tries to preserve
length and bone growth plate, particularly in younger children. Function,
cosmesis, and expectations for future development are all considerations. In
addition, there are some problems that can occur with children following amputation surgery.

Terminal Overgrowth

Bone overgrowth occurs most often in the femur, fibula, tibia, and humerus, especially if the amputation is through the growth areas. This is one reason that disarticulation amputations are recommended. Radiologically, the overgrowth appears as a sharp **spicule** of poorly trabeculated bone that extends from the end of the cut bone. Irritation of the soft tissue sometimes produces a bursa. Bone overgrowth occurs more often following acquired amputations or amputations to convert anomalies. Multiple surgical revisions may be required before bone maturity if overgrowth does occur and capping is unsuccessful. Full-thickness skin coverage is desirable at the end of growing bones for comfortable prosthetic fit. This problem occurs in 8 to 12 percent of cases.[4,8]

Bone Spurs

Bone spurs are small bony spicules that may develop at the edge of the bone end. Spurs rarely cause problems in children and must be differentiated from overgrowth.

Adventitious Bursae

Adventitious bursae may develop in the soft tissue over an area of terminal overgrowth. They may be treated by steroid injection, socket modification, or aspiration, but permanent relief usually necessitates surgical excision of the **adventitious bursae** and underlying bone.

Scarring

Frequent surgical reconstructive surgery may lead to scarring of the residual limb. These rarely cause problems in the prosthetic fitting of children.

PROSTHETIC FITTING

The prosthesis for a congenital amputation is generally fitted as early as possible, consistent with motor development, to enable the child to meet the motor milestones. An upper extremity prosthesis is indicated when the child begins bilateral activities (between 3 and 5 months), and a lower extremity prosthesis is indicated when the child demonstrates the desire to stand (usually when the child is between 6 to 9 months). For an acquired amputation, the prosthesis is fitted as soon as the residual limb heals. The early prosthesis may be a simple brace-like device. The goal should be to provide a prosthesis that is functional and acceptable to touch and sight.

Upper Extremity

Many children with a congenital upper extremity amputation are fitted with a passive mitten that is soft and well padded to avoid injury to self and others. The early prosthesis is not powered and is suspended by a simple chest harness. As the child develops motor control, a padded hook may substitute for the mitten and eventually be attached to a cable for power. Early prostheses need to be simple, but as children grow, they need to try different terminal devices to determine which is most functional. **Myoelectric** prostheses become an option for children 18 months and older; the myoelectric hand has voluntary control of both opening and closing and stronger pinch force than the cable-controlled hook. It operates independently of elbow position. However, it is heavier, cannot be placed in water, and the cosmetic glove requires regular replacement. Young children adapt to myoelectric prostheses fairly readily, depending on motor development. The child's size and degree of development also affects the selection of components because not all components are made in all sizes.

Children with unilateral upper extremity loss become dominant on the unamputated side. Some become adept at using the residual limb for bilateral activities and may reject the prosthesis. Early fitting for both congenital and acquired amputations helps the child integrate the prosthesis into daily life.

It is important to consider appearance as well as function when selecting components for children with upper extremity loss. Children need to fit in with their peers both in activity and in looks; the more cosmetic the prosthesis, the better the chances of acceptance. Children grow fast and prostheses require new parts, sockets, and components on a regular basis. Using multi-layered sockets and heavy socks expands the life of prosthetic sockets.[18] Finally, components need to be durable to support an active lifestyle. Upper extremity prosthetic components are discussed in greater detail in Chap. 10.

Lower Extremity

Lower extremity prostheses must also support developmental activities. As in the upper extremity, simplicity and durability are the keys to selecting components. Cosmesis becomes important in the preteen years for both boys and girls. Generally, the child with a unilateral lower extremity amputation is fitted when ready to pull to stand. There is little point in fitting earlier, because rolling and crawling can usually be done more easily without a prosthesis, and suspension is very difficult to attain. The major considerations in fitting an infant are to select a socket that will allow for linear and circumferential growth and to provide suspension without interfering with activity. Complex prosthetic feet and knee joints are not necessary for children who are just beginning to walk. Some very young children with transtibial amputations may slip out of a patellar-tendon bearing (PTB) prosthesis and require a corset for suspension. The infant with a transfemoral amputation is fitted without a knee joint, and the child with a hip disarticulation is fitted with a hip joint to allow sitting but not with a knee joint. When the child begins to gain control, a manual lock knee may be used as a transition to a fully articulated limb. Feet in children's sizes are available for 6-month-old infants, and knee units are manufactured for 2 year olds. Hydraulic knee mechanisms and suction sockets are usually not used until a child is about 10 years or older.

Children with limb anomalies and partial limb remnants require adaptation of standard sockets. Roentgenograms are taken prior to prosthetic fitting to determine the bony structure of the incomplete extremity. Subsequent roentgenograms allow assessment of development for required prosthetic modifications as the child grows. The child must be followed closely to avoid skin problems and socket discomfort due to growth. Bone growth in the congenitally deficient limb will likely be diminished at least in part because of abnormal, asymmetric, or reduced muscle pull and weight bearing. Children with PFFD are fitted with adapted ischial weight-bearing prostheses. If the foot remains, it is placed in plantar flexion to fit more cosmetically while allowing some weight bearing on the bottom of the foot.[19] Alignment techniques for the child's prosthesis are similar to those for the adult's prosthesis.

In cases of bilateral involvement, when both limbs terminate at or above the knee, stubbies may be used in the transitional stage. Stubbies consist of sockets with foot pieces that usually have a rocker bottom that is slightly elongated posteriorly. A Silesian bandage is usually sufficient for suspension unless the residual limbs are short, in which case a pelvic band with hip joints is used. Shoulder straps may be used prior to 5 years of age because bilateral pelvic bands limit hip motion. The socket is flexed a few degrees to prevent an excessive lumbar lordosis. Stubbies are indicated as an initial prescription when the child is too young for a secure balance on longer articulated prostheses as a primary fitting.

Multiple Limb Loss

Children with multiple limb loss or limb anomalies require adapted sockets and components and are usually treated through juvenile amputee programs. The number of children born with congenital limb deficiencies increased exponentially in the 1950s and 1960s as a result of the drug thalidomide.[20,21] New surgical techniques and new prosthetic and mobility aids were developed to help these children achieve as much function as possible. Special juvenile amputee clinics throughout the country are important resources especially for children with multiple congenital deformities.[22]

Sports Prostheses

Sports and other vigorous activities are an important part of a child's development. Prostheses need to be durable enough to withstand the stress of strenuous activities as well as to protect both the child and any opponents from injury. Many recreational programs are available for children with limb deficiencies, and many adaptations can be constructed to aid in sports activities. Adapted skis are common for children and adults. Old prostheses can be made usable in water for fishing or rafting. Special rotators allow translatory movements in both upper and lower extremities.[23] Many sports activities require no special prosthesis. PTs and PTAs who may work with children need to be aware of the potential for participation in sports.

TRAINING

Working with children with limb loss really means working with parents. The parents have the primary responsibility for helping the child adjust to the prosthesis, learn to incorporate it into daily life, and accept themselves as a person who has a limb loss. As the child grows, peer acceptance becomes important. Children with congenital or acquired amputations may be at risk for long-term psychological and social maladjustment. The long-term stress of coping with a handicap that limits function sets the person apart and makes daily life difficult. Varni and associates[24] studied a group of children with congenital and acquired limb loss and suggested that children with low levels of support from peers, family, and teachers were at greater risk for depressive symptoms and low self-esteem. Early referral of parents and children for evaluation and social services is recommended. Some prosthetists and therapists have used amputee dolls to help children understand prosthetic replacements. Svoboda[25] created a series of dolls with various limbs missing as well as miniature prostheses. Children are encouraged to play with these dolls to act out their feelings and gain a better understanding of prosthetic replacements.

Upper extremity prosthetic training is usually performed by occupational therapists. Children learn fairly easily as long as the training is at an appropriate level for their development and the activities are interesting. Most children require minimal training in the use of lower extremity prosthetic devices. The parents should be given systematic instruction in the therapy program with regular review because they will continue with it at home. Play is the primary motivation for desired movements and activity. Therapists must be careful not to expect more from the child than from his or her peers with normal extremity function. The normal child does not establish heel-to-toe gait until about 2 years of age. At about 20 months, the normal child can stand on one foot with help; at 3 years, on one foot momentarily; at 4 years, on one foot for several seconds; and at 5 years, on one foot for longer periods.

The knee of the transfemoral prosthesis is nonarticulated or locked until the child is secure in stiff-legged walking. Prosthetic heel-strike to toe-off gait is not usually attained until the child is about 5 years old or can demonstrate sustained one-legged standing. Efforts to develop a smooth alternating progression should follow. The major causes of gait deviations are growth or wear of prosthetic parts.

Children grow longitudinally and circumferentially. A new prosthesis is indicated when the old prosthesis is more than 1 cm (0.4 inch) short. A delay in the replacement of a short prosthesis may result in the development of scoliosis. A new prosthesis or socket is required about every 1 to 2 years for circumferential growth. Follow-up is usually necessary every 3 to 6 months but may need to be more frequent during adolescent growth spurts. Parents must be instructed in and responsible for the care of the residual limb and prosthesis for the young child.

Case Studies

Michael Donnagin's evaluation involves mostly play as you determine his developmental level. He may already be using the residual limb for bilateral activities. A great deal of information regarding the parents' attitude toward the disability and the potential support for therapeutic activities can be gathered through informal interview. It would be expected that Michael would be developing normally and should be ready for initial fitting with a nonarticulated arm and a soft passive hand. The loss of toes will not limit his standing and walking when he is ready and may not be a problem throughout his life. It will probably be helpful to the parents to talk to other parents attending the clinic. They may have a tendency to be overprotective, and it would be helpful for them to learn early that Michael is a boy first and a handicapped child second.

Jenny Smith's evaluation will be similar to that of an adult with a transfemoral amputation. You will need information on the residual limb and hip range of motion and strength. It will be important to determine when the limb will be ready for fitting because it is desirable to fit a child as soon as possible. Residual limb wrapping may not be an issue unless there is considerable edema. It would be anticipated that Jenny would have learned to walk on crutches while still in the hospital. The attitudes of both the parents and the child are critical, particularly if the parents blame themselves for the accident. Trauma is associated with failed replantation. Jenny and her parents may have many questions that will need to be answered fully. When the residual limb is fully healed and free of edema, Jenny can be fitted with a lightweight transfemoral prosthesis, probably with a constant friction knee and SACH foot. She will need some gait training and would be expected to do well with the prosthesis.

Mario Jonas's needs for prosthetic care and replacement are dictated to some degree by where he lives and how often he will be able to return to the clinic. Depending on the extent of leg length differences and whether the foot is usable, he may be fitted with an adapted PFFD prosthesis with the foot encased and used for partial weight. It is too early to consider amputation of the foot. The family will need to learn how to care for the prosthesis and what to do as the child grows. Again, the parents are the pivotal partners in the care of the child and need to be as fully informed as possible.

Summary

Care of the child with an amputation is a specialized type of practice that usually can be best carried out by a pediatric amputee clinic team, particularly with a child with multiple limb deficiencies. Many resources, such as the Association of Children's Prosthetic-Orthotic Clinics, exist for the PT or PTA who only occasionally encounters a child. It is important to consider the child's developmental needs and utilize prosthetic replacements and management to enhance normal development as much as possible. Many children will use nonstandard prostheses. Creativity is needed in defining one or more functional limbs. The parents are integral members of the rehabilitation team and need to be involved in all aspects of care.

Glossary

Adventitious bursa	A fluid-filled sac, usually around a joint, that develops in response to friction or pressure.
Amelia	Congenital absence of one or more limbs.
Anomalous	A deviation from normal.
Hemimelia	Longitudinal deficiencies in which part or all of one long bone is missing.
Hypoplastic	Defective development of tissues.
Myoelectric	Muscle movement that is stimulated by electricity.
PFFD	Proximal focal femoral deficiency.
Polydactyly	Multiple congenital abnormalities of the hand and wrist.

Spicule	A thin sliver of bone.
Syndactyly	The congenital joining together of digits.
Vestigial	A small, incompletely developed structure.

References

1. Fisk, JR: Introduction to the child amputee. In Bowker, JH, and Michael, JW (eds): Atlas of Limb Prosthetics: Surgical, Prosthetic, and Rehabilitation Principles. Mosby Year Book, St. Louis, 1992.
2. Patterson, DB: Acceptance rate of myoelectric prosthesis. J Assoc Child Prosthet Orthot Clin 25:73–76, 1990.
3. Weaver, SA: Comparison of myoelectric and conventional prostheses for adolescent amputees. Am J Occup Ther 42:78–91, 1988.
4. Tooms, RE: Acquired amputation in children. In Bowker, JH, and Michael, JW (eds): Atlas of Limb Prosthetics: Surgical, Prosthetic, and Rehabilitation Principles. Mosby Year Book, St. Louis, 1992.
5. Day, HJB: The ISO/ISPO classification of congenital limb deficiency. In Bowker, JH, and Michael, JW (eds): Atlas of Limb Prosthetics: Surgical, Prosthetic, and Rehabilitation Principles. Mosby Year Book, St. Louis, 1992.
6. Aitken, GT: Proximal femoral focal deficiency: Definition, classification, and management. In Proximal Femoral Focal Deficiency: A congenital anomaly. National Academy of Science. Publication No. 1734, Washington, DC, 1969.
7. Light, T: Upper-limb deficiencies: Surgical management. In Bowker, JH, and Michael, JW (eds): Atlas of Limb Prosthetics: Surgical, Prosthetic, and Rehabilitation Principles. Mosby Year Book, St. Louis, 1992.
8. Kruger, LM: Lower-limb deficiencies: Surgical management. In Bowker, JH, and Michael, JW (eds): Atlas of Limb Prosthetics: Surgical, Prosthetic, and Rehabilitation Principles. Mosby Year Book, St. Louis, 1992.
9. Frankel, VH, and Lloyd-Roberts, GC: The Ilizarov technique. Bull Hosp J Dis Orthop Inst 48:17–27, 1988.
10. Cummings, DR, and Kapp, SL: Lower-limb pediatric prosthetics: General considerations and philosophy. JPO 4(4):196–206, 1992.
11. Aitken, GT: The child with an acquired amputation. Int Clin Info Bull 7:1–15, 1968.
12. Fowler, EG, et al: Contrasts in gait mechanics of individuals with proximal femoral focal deficiency: Symes amputation versus Van Nes rotational osteotomy. J Pediatr Orthop 19(6):720–31, 1999.
13. Whooley, BP, et al: Primary extremity sarcoma: What is the appropriate follow-up? Ann Surg Oncol 7(1):9–14, 2000.
14. Weis, LD: The success of limb-salvage surgery in the adolescent patient with osteogenic sarcoma. Adolesc Med 10(3):451–58, 1999.
15. Rytting, M, et al: Osteosarcoma in preadolescent patients. Clin Orthop Res (373):39–50, 2000.
16. Davis, AM, et al: Functional outcome in amputation versus limb sparing of patients with lower extremity sarcoma: A matched case-control study. Arch Phys Med Rehabil 80(6):615–18, 1999.
17. Mohler, DG, et al: Augmented amputations of the lower extremity. Clin Orthop Res 371:183–97, 2000.
18. Supan, T: Upper limb deficiencies: prosthetic and orthotic management. In Bowker, JH, and Michael, JW (eds): Atlas of Limb Prosthetics: Surgical, Prosthetic, and Rehabilitation Principles. Mosby Year Book, St. Louis, 1992.
19. Oglesby, DG, Jr, and Tablada, C: Lower limb deficiencies: prosthetic and orthotic management. In Bowker, JH, and Michael, JW (eds): Atlas of Limb Prosthetics: Surgical, Prosthetic, and Rehabilitation Principles. Mosby Year Book, St. Louis, 1992.
20. Marquardt, E: The management of infants with malformation of the extremities. In Limb Development and Deformity: Problems of Evaluation and Rehabilitation. Charles C. Thomas, Springfield, Ill., 1969.
21. McBride, WG: Thalidomide and congenital abnormalities. Lancet 2:1358, 1961.

22. Marquardt, E: The multiple-limb-deficient child. In Bowker, JH, and Michael, JW (eds): Atlas of Limb Prosthetics: Surgical, Prosthetic, and Rehabilitation Principles. Mosby Year Book, St. Louis, 1992.
23. Page, CJ, and Messner, DG: Juvenile amputees: Sports and recreation program development. In Bowker, JH, and Michael, JW (eds): Atlas of Limb Prosthetics: Surgical, Prosthetic, and Rehabilitation Principles. Mosby Year Book, St. Louis, 1992.
24. Varni, JW, et al: Effects of stress, social support and self esteem on depression in children with limb deficiencies. Arch Phys Med Rehabil 72:1053–58, 1991.
25. Svoboda, J: Psychosocial considerations in pediatrics: Use of amputee dolls. JPO 4:207–12, 1992.

Index

Page numbers followed by an "f" indicate figures; page numbers followed by a "t" indicate tables.